Hormones and
Your Health

Also by Winnifred B. Cutler

Love Cycles: The Science of Intimacy

Hysterectomy: Before and After

The Medical Management of Menopause and Premenopause: Their Endocrinologic Basis (with Celso Ramon Garcia, MD)

Menopause: A Guide for Women and the Men Who Love Them (with Celso Ramon Garcia, MD and David A. Edwards, PhD)

Menopause: A Guide for Women and Those Who Love Them, Second Edition (with Celso Ramon Garcia, MD)

Searching for Courtship: The Smart Woman's Guide to Finding a Good Husband

Wellness in Women after 40 Years of Age: The Role of Sex Hormones and Pheromones (with Elizabeth Genovese, MD)

Hormones and Your Health

The Smart Woman's Guide
to Hormonal and Alternative Therapies
for Menopause

Winnifred B. Cutler, PhD

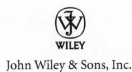

John Wiley & Sons, Inc.

Published by John Wiley & Sons, Inc., Hoboken, New Jersey
Published simultaneously in Canada

Illustrations copyright © 1986 by Athena Institute for Women's Wellness, Inc. Tom Quay
General Counsel

The information contained in this book is not intended to serve as a replacement for professional medical advice. Any use of the information in this book is at the reader's discre-
tion. The author and the publisher specifically disclaim any and all liability arising directly
or indirectly from the use or application of any information contained in this book. A
health care professional should be consulted regarding your specific situation.

For general information about our other products and services, please contact our Cus-
tomer Care Department within the United States at (800) 762-2974, outside the United
States at (317) 572-3993 or fax (317) 572-4002.

Wiley also publishes its books in a variety of electronic formats. Some content that appears
in print may not be available in electronic books. For more information about Wiley products, visit our web site at www.wiley.com.

Library of Congress Cataloging-in-Publication Data:
Cutler, Winnifred Berg.
    Hormones and your health : the smart woman's guide to hormonal and alternative
therapies for menopause / Winnifred Cutler.
        p. cm.
    Includes bibliographical references and index.
    ISBN 978-0-470-28902-0 (cloth)
    ISBN 978-1-68442-899-1 (paperback)
    1. Menopause—Hormone therapy—Popular works.   2. Menopause—Alternative
treatment—Popular works.   3. Women—Health risk assessment—Popular works.
    I. Title.
    RG186.C9268   2009
    618.1'75061—dc22

                                                                    2008055869

Printed in the United States of America

10 9 8 7 6 5 4 3 2 1

*To the research scientists who left a trail the author followed,
and to the smart women and physicians who join
this expedition.*

Contents

Acknowledgments

Grateful acknowledgment is due to many friends and colleagues who have contributed to this book, and to the hundreds of cited scholars whose published studies and commentaries shaped my conclusions.

To Loretta Barrett, my literary agent, for her vision in helping me define the scope of the book and in guiding its early editorial focus, and for her extraordinary professionalism in producing this work for women and their physicians who can benefit from it.

To Stephanie Young, whose editing work on the entire text and journalist's expertise have dramatically enhanced its readability.

To the Athena Institute for Women's Wellness management team: Tom Quay, Esq., for his legal erudition about the FDA, Big Pharma, due process, and withstanding scrutiny, and his editorial contributions to every aspect of the book. To Glynis Gould for helping to edit for clarity and good English usage every chapter several times. To Jodie Cohen for creating the computer data management system used in tracking the 900 references and her "lighter" editing from a reader's perspective.

To the professional experts in medicine and scientific research whose detailed critiques increased both clarity and accuracy and helped lead me to my independent conclusions occasionally at variance with theirs, especially two fellows of the American College of Obstetricians and Gynecologists: Drs. Millicent Zacher in the United States and Regula Burki in Switzerland. To Dr. Elizabeth Genovese, who kept feeding scientific papers to me and sharing her expertise in quality assurance and internal and occupational medicine. I thank Dr. Janet Daling of the Fred Hutchinson Cancer Center for her substantial critique of the breast chapter. Her epidemiological studies of HRT and breast cancer have spawned a significant group of trained scientists and an important body of knowledge. Dr. T. Maruo in Japan for his correspondence on uterine myoma and for sending the research papers of his extraordinary team of scientists. To Mary Lou Ballweg, one of the founders of the Endometriosis Association, who encourages important research in this difficult field.

To the wonderful Athena Institute college student interns who worked as manuscript assistants during the six years the research was under way: Maggie Parlapiano, Suzanne Smith, Leigh Bausinger, Rachel Nagourney, Lauren Fell, Amy Midgley, Kara Gillam, and Kendra Johnson.

To the participating Athena Institute staff: Cathy Peluso, Alice Sarajiandenty, Julia Liebhardt, Maria Kenny, Laura Gergel, Cindy Wilson, and Cynthia Allen.

Thanks to those women who reviewed chapter drafts, offering critiques aimed at improving intelligibility for end users, especially Lynne Avram, Melanie Wilson, Susan Kersch, and Anna Mae Charrington.

And, finally, to the excellent team of editors at John Wiley & Sons for their faith and guidance in bringing this book to press: Tom Miller, Christel Winkler, Lisa Burstiner, and Patricia Waldygo.

Introduction

YOU CAN DROP OFF YOUR CAR for routine maintenance and repair, but you shouldn't leave the diagnosis, the cure, and the routine maintenance of your body to impersonal "experts." Only at your peril do you give up control of the magnificent body in which you live and move and experience life.

I wrote this book in an attempt to combine good sense and good science. In it, I summarize current research so that women and their physicians can work together to improve the quality of health care for women. This is the mission that drives my work.

It also fulfills a promise I made thirty years ago to my late mentor and graduate-study adviser, Celso Ramon Garcia, MD, of the University of Pennsylvania. He was a renowned surgeon, a brilliant intellect, and one of the fathers of the oral contraceptive "the Pill." In 1979, with a biology PhD in hand, I left the University of Pennsylvania for Stanford as a postdoctoral fellow in physiology to cofound the Stanford Menopause Study. Eventually we reported that, contrary to then current gynecological texts, the sex lives of menopausal women were not defunct. In 1983, Dr. Garcia and I wrote *Menopause: A Guide for Women and the Men Who Love Them* with Professor David Edwards at Emory University. This led to a medical publisher's invitation to coauthor a textbook for physicians, *The Medical Management of Menopause and Premenopause: Their Endocrinologic Basis.* Four other books followed. Unfortunately, a few years later, one large study sent us back into the Middle Ages, because its data were misunderstood, misinterpreted, and misreported.

In 2002, panicky headlines announced that the Women's Health Initiative (WHI) Study, a massive federally funded trial, was being abruptly halted because women who were taking hormones were suffering more strokes and breast cancer than those on a placebo. But the Food and Drug Administration (FDA), certain medical societies, and many physicians misunderstood the atypical population that was studied and incorrectly jumped to the conclusion that the WHI results applied to *all* women and *all* hormone therapy regimens. Doctors told their patients to stop taking hormone-replacement therapy. What a shame that was! Panic trumped good science.

In this book I have explained what good scientific analysis teaches relevant to your unique needs to help you recognize the various agendas behind the advice from media, clinicians, big drug manufacturers, disease associations, and promoters of alternative medicine. As you will see, I believe that some hormone regimens are fabulous for women but that other products (and services) serve the purveyor's best interest rather than yours. You need to know that I have *never* received any research funding, tips, trips, or consulting or speaker's fees for products or services that I pan or praise. I have no hidden agenda.

Hormones and Your Health is for both you *and* your doctor. It represents thirty years of careful study of published scientific research and tries to answer the big question: What's a woman to *do* to improve her health, increase her longevity, avoid preventable conditions, and live life to its fullest? If you are willing to commit to learning the material in this book, you will be able to navigate this minefield to achieve your optimal health. The task is worth the effort!

1

Take Ownership of Your Health

YOU ARE IN CHARGE OF YOUR HEALTH. No one else should do it for you. No one else can feel what you feel when your energy is soaring, your sense of joy is boundless, your bones and muscles are vibrant as you stand erect and move gracefully through your days, and your immune system is strong enough to fight off the never-ending bombardment of pathogens. Don't accept less than what is best for you. As a functioning, intelligent adult, you have many decisions to make that will affect both the quality and quantity of your remaining years. Let's start with the first decision you make: your choice of physicians.

Your Choice of Physician

You need and deserve a relationship with a compassionate physician who respects your intelligence, your dignity, and your time. If a doctor keeps you sitting in the waiting room for an hour past your appointment, without explanation or apology, that treatment is disrespectful. Find a doctor who respects you.

Most doctors simply do not have time to read all of the scientific papers I explain in this book. As a scientist, I have studied more than three thousand peer-reviewed, published papers, and I cite nearly nine hundred here as references.[173] Your physician will appreciate the rigorous research that this book clarifies for both of you.

Your Doctor's Economic Dilemma

Contrary to a widely held view, your doctor may not be rolling in money. Medical school is hugely expensive: $200,000 for tuition and related costs is not uncommon. Malpractice insurance for gynecologists who perform even minor surgery can easily exceed $100,000 per year. Medical insurance companies and HMOs systematically reduce payments to doctors. To cover costs, more patients must be seen, with less "face time" being spent with each one.

Divergent Agendas and Interests

Your physician must rely on pharmaceutical sales representatives and Big Pharma–sponsored continuing medical education courses to stay up-to-date on essential information about drugs and medical devices. The reps and the speakers *do* present truthful, FDA-approved data, but they have no incentive to discuss their competitors' products. And funded speakers, as well as medical societies, are usually reluctant to pan the products of a drug company that has provided trips and money. Conflicts of interest are very serious, and they are endemic. On February 28, 2007, the *Philadelphia Inquirer* reported, "Ex-FDA Chief Must Pay $90,000 in the Stock-Disclosure Case"[864]—stock in drug companies that he was regulating, which he forgot to disclose. This news is not reassuring. Similar disclosures have been in the news about journal presentations as well. Editors and medical society leaders who control which research gets presented to physicians and scientists should disclose, not hide, their own, as well as their protégés', funding sources.

Fearing malpractice attorneys, your doctor may practice "defensive medicine" by ordering redundant, expensive tests for you. Or sometimes doctors may stick to defensively postured practice guidelines that serve their, rather than your, best interests, in order to minimize their liability. You need to take charge of your own health and well-being; consult with the best medical people you can find and decide which recommendations to accept.[754] And you need to identify the economic interests behind the recommendations that are offered to you.

Media Need Catchy Sound Bites

Have you seen articles titled "Estrogen Replacement Therapy Triples Risk of Breast Cancer"? This statement is more false than true and is definitely misleading. The "triple" actually meant an increase from 1 woman in 10,000 to 3 women! And the statistic applied only to a group of women taking a regimen of synthetic progestin every day with a horse-derived oral estrogen, a regimen I believe you should avoid. Don't be misled by catchy headlines that are designed in part to sell newspapers.

Alternative natural therapies abound. The FDA, however, does not evaluate herbal or other alternative remedies. Do not trust advertisements for such products and services that claim to "cure" serious diseases "with no side effects."

Generic Drugs Flourish

The FDA *does* regulate generic drugs and assures us that they are as reliable as brand-name drugs. But some recent published studies cast doubt on whether their quality is equal.[434, 719] If you can afford brand-name drugs, you might be better off buying them.

Your Power as a Health Consumer

As a patient, did you know that competition for your business is real? Consider the inherent conflicts when you get medical advice. Your doctor can help you only within his skill set. Will he or she refer you to another physician who can offer you a less-invasive or less-costly treatment?[543] No law says that a doctor must do this.[698]

From Age Forty Onward: The General Order of Things

The chapter topics in this book follow the order of health issues that women will encounter beginning in their early forties—or sooner, if they undergo a hysterectomy before then.

1. The perimenopausal changes that women experience from age forty to forty-eight (hot flashes, night sweats, and unexpected bleeding) signal the loss or decline of progesterone, followed by erratic changes (plummets and peaks) in estrogen. These early body signals are storm warnings that your sex hormone production is winding down for its eventual sharp decline.

2. There are two kinds of remedies to consider: hormones and alternative treatments. You will learn which hormones are being marketed and which ones you should know to request or avoid, and why.

3. The following pelvic problems and their prevention and correction are addressed because they occur in the majority of women.

   • Bleeding abnormalities that 80 percent of women experience in their forties drive them to doctors, who often incorrectly prescribe a hysterectomy. This actually exacerbates the hormonal problems and shortens the woman's lifespan.

   • A weakening of the pelvic floor and the consequent urinary incontinence (experienced by 30 percent of thirty-five-year-olds and 65 percent of sixty-year-olds) can often be prevented by taking appropriate hormones, beginning an exercise program, and cultivating other healthful habits.

   • Prolapse problems (65 percent of women will have them by age sixty) also lead doctors to suggest surgery, whereas exercise is more often a better remedy (it's cheaper, safer, and usually more effective than surgery).

   • Fibroid tumors (80 percent of women develop them) are related to the hormonal changes that begin in the forties, but fibroids are seldom life threatening. Many doctors will prescribe a hysterectomy, but it should be avoided, if possible, because more effective treatments are now available.

4. Waiting in the wings are the following dramatic but hidden changes that occur as a woman ages:

   • Bone loss begins around age forty for most women, just as their progesterone production is declining. This degenerative, crippling disease is preventable if you take action by age fifty.

Otherwise, osteoporosis can affect 80 percent of women. The widely marketed bone drugs are not nearly as effective or risk free as proper hormone-replacement therapy, exercise, healthy eating, and practicing good balancing exercises to avoid slips and falls that crush fragile bones.

- Blood vessel changes begin with the transition into menopause or are caused by certain types of widely prescribed hormone therapy, as well as by a sedentary lifestyle and unhealthful eating habits. These blood vessel changes can lead to irreversible atherosclerosis. There is a lot you can do to promote healthy vessels and a vibrant circulatory system.

- The terror that women feel about breast cancer is driven by the marketplace. The actual incidence of this disease is one-eighth that of blood vessel deterioration and maybe one-fourth as serious as bone loss, but the "breast" people are top-notch marketers, and they prey on your fear. I hope to dissipate this media-driven fear of femininity and female hormones. Fear itself promotes hormonal changes that are bad for your health!

5. Once you make intelligent decisions regarding your hormones, your bones, your blood vessels, and living a healthy lifestyle, you'll find it easy to follow the advice on sexual function and cognitive capacity in this book's final chapters.

The motto we have adopted at Athena Institute for Women's Wellness is one that you might appreciate:

> When a woman refuses to be treated with disrespect and condescension, she becomes empowered to evaluate options and make intelligent choices. By doing the work of learning about her body and improving her health habits, she is in a position to assert her power. Power begets dignity. Dignity is essential to well-being.

2

Taking Hormones for Good Health: Why You Will Benefit from Hormonal-Replacement Therapy (HRT)

A CAREFULLY SELECTED PRESCRIPTION for sex hormone–replacement therapy (HRT) can be a powerful asset for your well-being if you make informed, judicious choices about what's right for you. Your own hormones inevitably change as your fertility begins to wane in your early forties, or even earlier after pelvic surgery. Hormonal therapies (HT) become an option worth considering. But hormone prescriptions vary. They are not interchangeable. And be aware that inappropriate regimens, incorrect doses, and poor timing can create serious risks in a minority of users. HRT and HT are used interchangeably by some experts. Others confine HRT to reflect formulations that are replacing natural human hormones with chemically bioidentical substances.

Timing Matters

The inevitable decline in the ovarian secretion of estrogen and progesterone causes severe symptoms in about 25 percent of women as they age.[555] Women vary. Progesterone imbalance is usually the first hidden change. Its consequence can be excessive bleeding. Estrogen changes usually occur next. For some women, an abruptly plummeting estrogen level occurs in the mid-forties, five to seven years before the average age of menopause. For others, the decline is gradual, or there may be huge spurts and troughs.[174] These are signals. They tell you about your life and your hormone status.

If you have a regular sex partner, you are less likely to experience abrupt roller-coaster-like changes in estrogen. But if you suddenly end a sexual relationship, your estrogen levels are likely to suddenly drop.[169] If you begin a judicious prescription of hormones when the deficiency signals first start, you can eliminate symptoms within days. Starting early makes a big difference in preserving the health of your blood vessels, too.[145]

Symptoms of Declining Estrogen and Progesterone Levels

- Hot flashes
- Sweating/night sweats
- Mood swings
- Insomnia
- Vaginal dryness or atrophy
- Painful or uncomfortable intercourse
- "Abnormal" bleeding

The Innate Wisdom of Your Body

These symptoms of hot flashes, vaginal dryness, and sleep disturbances provide valuable signals. Uncomfortable intercourse due to vaginal dryness isn't a wonderful experience, but it's telling you to *do* something. Like an early warning signal of an impending hurricane, these symptoms are calling you to take notice so that you can avoid the storm. Listen to the signals your body sends, and you can take preventive actions that will enrich the second half of your life.

Of course, you can grit your teeth, be uncomfortable, and accept the inevitability of growing older and eventually disabled. But keep in mind that the majority of postmenopausal women who do *not* use hormonal-replacement therapy will not merely experience unpleasant symptoms; they will risk diseases brought about by loss of bone, loss of blood vessel elasticity, and decreased protection from cardiovascular disease.[121, 555] You may not need hormones. You may have a body that produces all you need. Or you may not be a good candidate due to your family history. Ask your clinician to discuss options related to your own personal health history. But read this book first!

Hormone Therapies Are Just Better— for Some Deficiencies

Hormone-replacement therapies are obviously not the only route to good health. There are alternative paths to maximize your health that I describe throughout the book, such as exercise, weight loss, and quitting smoking. But for hot flashes, bone loss, atherosclerotic change, and sleep disturbances, correct hormone therapies appear to offer the most efficient, effective remedies. They have consistently outperformed alternative remedies, including placebos, tranquilizers, sedatives, herbal remedies, and other drugs.[168, 171, 175, 759] Unlike other prescriptions from your doctor, they can be used to *prevent* disease. (Of course, exercise and other healthy habits are still important, with or without hormone therapy.)

Long-term hormone therapy is associated with lower death rates in older women.[582] I believe that a powerful argument can be made *against* the current recommendation that hormones are all right but in "as low a dose as possible for as short a time as possible."[582] The data published by hundreds of outstanding biomedical scholars convince me that carefully chosen long-term therapy may extend the length and the quality of your life leading up to menopause and for many years thereafter.

Your Longevity Clock Ticks On to Menopause

"Menopausal" describes the part of your life that follows your last menstrual cycle—not only the cessation of menses, but also the change in ovarian secretion of hormones that drive the menstrul cycle: estrogen and progesterone most notably. Worldwide, this occurs at the average age of fifty. The later the onset of menopause, the longer a woman is likely to live.[579] Unfortunately, ten years into the course of untreated menopause, atrophy (degeneration) of the urogenital tissues affects up to 47 percent of women.[731] Later effects of postmenopausal hormonal deficiencies include declining strength in the bones and the cardiovascular system.

Postmenopausal hormonal deficiencies can lead to:

- Decline in bone quality
- Diminished cardiovascular health
- Urogenital atrophy
- Wrinkled skin
- Blood vessel thickening and atherosclerosis
- Cognitive decline
- Increase in fat, decrease in muscle

Having a hysterectomy speeds up your aging clock. The surgical removal of the uterus accelerates your entry into menopause.[579] Having an ovariectomy speeds up the aging process even more,[593] because your estrogen-progesterone factories, your ovaries, have been removed.

After a hysterectomy, women have an even higher risk of developing hormone-related deficits than intact aging women have.[216] It's best to keep all of your healthy internal organs as you age.[593] If the uterus was removed but the ovaries were retained, the normal menopause-related decline in the ovarian production of estrogen and progesterone hormones is likely to occur much earlier than the intact woman experiences. Unfortunately, this leads to serious consequences: even lower bone density, increased cardiovascular disease (CVD) risk, and more severe estrogen-deficiency symptoms.[216, 236] How severe? It depends on how early in life the surgery was performed.

For women who were hysterectomized at age 42, menopause seemed to follow within 2 years, instead of in 8 (at age 50). For those hysterectomized at age 44, ovarian failure occurred with in one year. And for 45-year-olds, it was immediate,[705] a 5-year acceleration of their aging.

This is not trivial. If you have had a hysterectomy and/or an ovariectomy, you can take effective action—the earlier, the better.

By 2005, a large and well-done analysis had proved that at no age was it ever beneficial to remove healthy ovaries during a hysterectomy. Avoiding castration (ovariectomy) until age 65 clearly benefits the long-term survival of women who undergo a hysterectomy for a benign disease. The incidence of developing ovarian cancer after a hysterectomy is 40 percent lower than in the general population,[593] so there is no logical reason to remove healthy ovaries. But the most sensitive risk was coronary heart disease; having an ovariectomy increases the risk of cardiovascular disease, the main cause of death for women.[593] The younger a woman is when she has an ovariectomy, the greater the chances for harm.

Unfortunately, despite the facts, in 2005, data from the Centers for Disease Control (CDC) showed that 78 percent of women in the United States who underwent a hysterectomy between the ages of 45 and 64 were also castrated. A survey of Taiwan gynecologists found that the same practice was common there.[128] What this means to me is that women need to recognize their right to refuse suggested surgery.[396, 428] You should refuse to accept castration unless cancer is looming.[170, 592]

By 1989, medical societies routinely showed their member physicians the many benefits of HRT. Hundreds of studies had been published to prove that women could be spared osteoporosis, vaginal atrophy, and many other age-related diseases that were apparently the result of declining levels of sex hormones. But it took some time for the medical establishment to get on board.

Finding the Right Way to Prescribe Hormones

From the get-go, medical science didn't get it quite right. First, estrogen, unbalanced (or unnopposed) by progesterone, was widely prescribed.[167, 171] Only after researchers discovered that women risked developing endometrial hyperplasia when they took unopposed estrogen (which increased the rate of uterine cancer) did it become apparent that Mother Nature had it right in generating the sequential pattern of secretion of ovarian sex hormones in fertile women. Women needed progesterone, ten to fourteen days a month when they took estrogen every day. Some brilliant work on optimizing prescriptions for hormonal balancing for uterine health by gynecologist Dr. R. Don Gambrell has spanned more than thirty years. Until his death in 2007, he continued to publish his studies calling for other physicians to recognize which regimens women need to optimize their hormonal therapy.[257, 258] I call it nature's design.

Dr. Gambrell showed that the closer a prescriber came to providing the progesterone the way Mother Nature designed in a woman's fertile years, the better off the woman's uterus was.[174, 258] She needed progesterone for about half of the month, when she took estrogen every day. As you will see in later chapters, these sequential regimens also lower the risk of breast cancer and build better bones, better mental function, and a healthier cardiovascular system.

Why aren't women routinely offered this choice? Unfortunately, two large randomized, controlled trials (RCTs) tested a regimen that did *not* mimic nature, and the outcomes were not so good. I believe that the incorrect interpretation and the publicized results triggered a very serious health setback for women.

How Hormones Got a Bad Name

Two very large studies were conducted with the aim of finding out how hormones would benefit women. It is worth noting that these studies used a specific regimen, but their results were generalized to give *all* hormones a bad name.

What: The first study, called HERS (the Heart and Estrogen/ Progestin Replacement Study), was a randomized, blind, placebo-controlled trial of the effect of Prempro (a pill combining a horse-derived estrogen and a synthetic progestin) on coronary heart disease (CHD) risk.

Who: 2,763 postmenopausal women with documented CHD.

Result: The regimen did not improve things.[286] Overall, Prempro did not help lessen future CHD problems in women who already had them.

What: The second study of this same regimen was called the Women's Health Initiative (WHI).

Who: 161,809 healthy postmenopausal women.[656]

Result: It, too, did not produce positive results in the early analyses of the extensive data.[856] The WHI results, to the shock of many, led to a worldwide HRT panic. Here is how it started.

The Enormous WHI Study Unfolds

Between 1993 and 1998, the WHI enrolled 161,809 postmenopausal women between 50 and 79 years old at 40 clinical centers in the United

States in a set of clinical trials of postmenopausal hormone use. This was a government-sponsored study, in which Wyeth agreed to supply its HRT drugs, Premarin and Prempro. The FDA approved Prempro in 1993. The goal as stated was a noble one: to assess the major health benefits and risks of the most commonly used combined hormone preparation in the United States.[656] The phrase "most commonly used" was misleading because Prempro was *not* in use, according to three medical scholars who investigated this.[402] Although initial results were widely misinterpreted, I want to emphasize how valuable are the data collected in the HERS and WHI studies for later analysis by researchers. The study still goes on, as the women continue to be followed. The WHI began with three "arms."

The First Arm

What: The Women's Health Initiative Observational Study (WHIOS).

Who: A large proportion, 75,343 of the 102,692 women who were reported on, either refused to be told what hormone (or placebo) to take or were ineligible.[611]

What they did: These women said that they were willing to be studied so that investigators could accumulate data covering the experiences of women who made their own decisions. Of these women, 75,343 did not agree to blindly take a drug for the next five years that *might* be a placebo or *might* be a sex hormone. The plan in the WHIOS was to study ongoing health history (up to a woman's first heart attack or death from cardiovascular disease). This trial was observational, which means that the scientists studied outcomes of what women chose to do, not what they were told to do.

Result: The health outcomes of the women who made their own decisions about hormonal therapy were largely positive. When women listened to their bodies, they seemed to do well on hormones and make good choices. (See chapters 9, 11, and 12.)

RCT: The Two WHI Randomized Control Trials of Postmenopausal Women

Overview: The Second and Third Arms

In these two groups, the women each agreed to take a pill daily. Neither they nor the researchers knew whether they were taking active hormones or placebo (inactive) pills. Controlled trials are beneficial because they offer a placebo comparison, but they are limited to the drug chosen—and the age group studied—without individualization of dose. The two arms had one key difference.

The Second Arm: Women without a Uterus—Placebo or Premarin?

Who: Enrolled in the study were a total of 10,739 women who previously had undergone hysterectomies.[741] About half of them were assigned to test the placebo; the other half, an "estrogen-only" pill, Premarin. The thinking—at the time—was that a woman without a uterus did not need any progesterone. Since the prevailing medical opinion had been that progesterone's (only) function was "opposing estrogen to protect the uterus," a hysterectomy was believed to obviate the need for progesterone. (*I do not agree with that view.*)

The point: Hysterectomized women could be studied to learn whether an estrogen was more helpful than a placebo taken every day for many years.

The Third Arm: Women with a Uterus—Placebo or Prempro?

Who: In the study, 16,610 intact postmenopausal women were randomized to receive either a placebo or the hormone. The hormone chosen for 8,508 was a combination of two separate FDA-approved hormonal preparations.[402] Called Prempro, the pill combined Premarin with Provera. Provera is the trade name for one of the synthetic progestins: medroxyprogesterone acetate (MPA). It was used for the WHI at a daily dose of 2.5 mg. Premarin is the trade name of the most widely used conjugated *equine* estrogen at that time, made by Wyeth. The name Premarin reflects its manufacturing derivation: *pregnant mare urine.* In other words, Premarin is a natural estrogen—*for a pregnant horse.*

The point: Intact women could be studied to learn whether an estrogen-progestin combined in one pill was more helpful than a placebo taken every day for many years.

The problem: The intact women who qualified to enroll were long past their transition and early menopause years: on average, they were 17 years into menopause. Since they had no obvious symptoms, such as hot flashes, they could not tell whether they were taking hormones. That's good for the purposes of the study (providing the results are not misinterpreted to apply to other ages or drug products).

Why the Panic Button Was Pushed

On May 31, 2002, the safety monitoring board recommended stopping the third arm, the Prempro trial of the intact (nonhysterectomized) women in the study. There was evidence that compared to a placebo, the Prempro caused 8 extra cases per year of breast cancer per 10,000 women.[391] Basically, the risk of taking Prempro had exceeded its benefits. Stopping such a study is a dramatic, headline-producing event, and the media grabbed hold of it.

Keep in mind that the WHI results cannot be extrapolated to sequential regimens with human-type estrogen and progesterone (which, I conclude, scientific studies prove are the best regimens for most women).

The Rush to React

Based on these very preliminary trends from the WHI, the FDA decided that hormone therapies must carry a warning: hormone-replacement therapy causes an increased risk of breast cancer. All hormones, no exceptions. A blind panic erupted. Newspaper headlines trumpeted that hormones cause breast cancer. Medical societies told their members to take their patients off hormones. Many women also stopped their hormones cold turkey without consulting their doctors. Given the defensive-medicine posture that physicians have been forced to assume in recent years, it really is not surprising that the FDA's decision and the resultant reaction by physicians had significant effects on women.

Here are some examples of these widespread effects: Within the first six months in five different cities in the United States, 37 percent of women, ages 40 to 80 years old, stopped using hormonal therapy.[102]A year later, according to one Minnesota health pharmacy database, 63 percent of the according Prempro users had discontinued it.[650] In Spain, a significant change in physician and patient attitudes toward HRT was reported.[121] In Switzerland, 1 in 3 intact women had stopped using HT.[529] In Germany,[336] the discontinuation rate was half as severe; in Chile, it was one-eighth as severe.[336]

Some Voices of Reason

The quieter, more rational voices could not be immediately heard against the alarmist media sound bites. Their story was perhaps too tame for the media. But by 2005, this situation had begun to change.

- **One result cannot be applied to all**, said Dr. Fred Naftolin, an eminent biomedical scholar at Yale University. He commented that the WHI had been inappropriately used to create guidelines (for physicians) that are incorrect for any group other than the overweight, average-seventeen-years-postmenopausal population on which the particular regimen was tested.[549] I agree!

- **The study participants weren't particularly "healthy."** WHI participants ranged in weight from simply overweight to frankly obese, with an unusually high incidence of arterial hypertension at entry and high drug use to control these pathologies.[75] Nearly 50 percent of the study population had several serious cardiovascular risk factors.[656]

- **The WHI was not a preventive study.** Dr. Martin Birkhaeuser, in an editorial for the International Menopause Society's journal, pointed out that the WHI, contrary to its claims, was not designed to study the primary prevention of CVD since the disease was clearly already there, given high proportions of hypertension, obesity, and statin and aspirin use.[75] Contrary to its "well-women claim," the WHI was a "secondary prevention trial" in women who already were past the stage of life where they could prevent atherosclerosis.[402] (*Secondary prevention trial* means the study was testing whether disease could be prevented from occurring after evidence of its presence reveals that the test subject is already at high risk of recurrence or occurrence.)

- **Not all progestins are alike**, and furthermore, that erroneous logic in the United States attributing a "class effect" to all progestins is not supported among scholars outside the United States.[75]

Sadly, women were caught in the crossfire. Many thriving hormone users gave up their HRT and suffered as their bodies began to pay the toll with a cascade of expected physiological changes that reflected their abrupt state of estrogen deficiency.

The Panic Subsides

The International Menopause Society forged a leadership role. First, it fought the too-quick conclusions of the World Health Organization International Agency for Research and Cancer, which, in June 2005, issued its classification for combination hormone contraception and menopausal therapy as carcinogenic in humans.[682]

And by 2006, the American medical journals were beginning to recover from the panic that the misinterpretation of the WHI data incorrectly caused. Authorities now pointed out that risk-benefit ratios were significantly influenced by the time when hormone therapy is initiated[18](and by the woman's state of health) and by the type, the regimen, and the route of hormone therapy. Dr. Joanne Manson, one of the co-investigators of the WHI, noted that *natural progesterone* appears to be more favorable than *synthetic progestin* preparations such as MPA (medroxyprogesterone acetate) on lipids and that transdermal estrogen appears to be more favorable than oral estrogens to reduce the risk of venous thromboembolism (stroke).[493](MPA has accounted for most prescriptions in America for the progestin component of HRT.) Complex analysis, instead of simplistic thinking and eye-catching headlines, began to make its way into editorials and medical meetings. One well-respected expert in progesterone research noted, "Following the WHI publications, the role of progestins on HT have unfortunately been directed toward progestins as a class which is a grave error because of the striking differences that exist among different progestins."[714] (The phrase "grave error" certainly stings.)

More Experts Weigh In, More Studies Begin

Other careful analysts concluded that, in retrospect, the 2002 release of the preliminary data generated a global turmoil that was not justified in view of the more detailed information that was subsequently published.[603] And that many clinicians and consumers made decisions about HT based on poor-quality, biased, sensational sound bites that were inaccurate.

Just contrast the data with these statistics: The facts about taking prophylactic aspirin for primary cardiovascular disease protection do not generate panic, despite the increased risk of hemorrhagic stroke by 40 percent (up to 4 additional cases per 10,000 people per year of use) and for major GI bleeding by 70 percent (up to 8 extra cases per 10,000 people per year of use). But similar risks of hormone therapy (26 percent increased risk of breast cancer detection, 8 extra breast cancers detected per 10,000 women per year) generated a global turmoil that obscured reality. Clearly, breast cancer scares more women than stroke does. Dr. Amos Pines, the president of the International Menopause Society, concluded correctly, "Knowledge and wisdom were lacking in the WHI scares."[603]

By 2006, in the United States and in Australia, two new randomized, controlled trials were underway; they were designed to test whether other regimens and earlier ages at inception would yield more positive results.[483, 493] Meanwhile, an enormous body of observational studies has consistently found that women who *choose* hormones seem to do very well. Dr. Manson noted that although it is probable that the observational studies have overestimated the benefits of HT, it is also possible that the life phase of the volunteers was a key factor. The randomized, controlled trials (HERS and WHI) were all timed to a late menopause era, but observational studies generally followed women who began HT when symptoms began in early menopause but before aging effects had occurred. By 2007, Dr. John Studd, an eminent British researcher and a gynecological surgeon, said that the misapplication of WHI's research resulted in "devastating effects on the health of tens of thousands of women, now afraid to take the therapy that they require."[752]

What was the conclusion by expert researchers? In addition to healthy changes in lifestyle and dietary management, hormone replacement therapy remains a principal tool in preventing illness and maintaining quality of life.[549] This is my conclusion, too, and I intend to show you which hormones make the most sense—and I'll provide the citations that support my claims.

The Unambiguous Benefits of Hormonal Therapies

The last twenty-five years have produced a solid body of research. Much of that science demonstrates the profound benefits of hormone replacement therapy. Hormones impact an astonishing array of body parts, systems, and senses, including the skin, the vagina, the nose, the voice, the teeth, the eyes, sleep, the cells, and intestinal function. Let's examine the details.

1. *Estrogens and skin.* Much of the wrinkling and the aging appearance of older skin is due to the loss of underlying subcutaneous

tissue and bony architecture.[218] (See chapter 8.) Most women know that attractiveness is often central to one's sense of power. And power can be economic; holding one's own in the workplace is easier when you look good. Being concerned about one's image is not groundless. Perceptions exist that a woman who can take care of herself can likely take care of business.

Compassionate physicians recognize that it is not trivial to consider the quality-of-life issues, that is, the social and emotional needs of the patient.[772] Timing appears to be very important in hormonal therapy.[60] *Early* action can preserve the stores of collagen and hyaluronic acid in the body, as well as the amount of elastic tissue.

Long-term benefits of hormonal therapies on skin rigidity and wrinkles were reported in a study of 65 postmenopausal women (who were an average of 7 years postmenopausal) at Yale-New Haven Hospital. The result: hormone users had fewer wrinkles and less loss of elasticity.[849] This was a nice result.

When researchers looked for estrogen receptors in skin, they found them.[96] Estrogen receptors are tiny cellular structures that combine—like a lock and a key—with estrogen and then turn on the DNA machinery of cells. Our faces are at their best when our estrogen level is higher. Postmenopausal women who use estrogen have better skin. Estrogen users fared significantly better on measurements of skin youthfulness: thickness, water-holding capacity, fewer wrinkles, greater blood flow, and faster wound healing.[96, 849]

Topical preparations of two different naturally produced human estrogens, estradiol at .01 percent and estriol at .03 percent, were tested. When about 1 gram of cream was applied each day, there was no change in the blood levels of hormones, whether the women were using estriol or estradiol cream. The hormone supplied locally was too small to make any difference within the overall blood supply. But there was a significant improvement in all local measures of skin wrinkling, elasticity, pore size, and moisture after 6 months of daily use.[677] "Crow's feet" wrinkles had significantly decreased by 6 months.

Both preparations (estriol and estradiol) were equally effective. Estrogens are good for your skin, whether you apply them directly on the skin (topically) or take them into your body first (e.g., by swallowing) in a sufficient dosage to raise the concentration in blood.

2. *Estrogen and urinary and genital tissues.* About 50 percent of post-menopausal women experience estrogen deficiency symptoms in their urogenital functions: vaginal dryness, intense genital itchiness (pruritus), painful intercourse (dyspareunia), painful urination (dysuria), urinary urgency, urinary frequency and nighttime need to use the bathroom (nocturia), increased vulnerability to urinary tract infections (due to the thinning of the epithelium), increased rigidity of tissues, and decreased closure pressure in the urethra.

Hormonal therapies that are supplied early in menopause (before age 60) unambiguously provide relief.[205, 587, 744, 810, 831] But timing counts. Unfortunately, for postmenopausal women over age 60, the HERS and WHI studies reported an adverse effect of Prempro: it increased the incidence of urinary incontinence.[744]

3. *Estrogen and the vagina.* Normally, healthy vaginal tissue of premenopausal women is able to produce the acidity that is necessary to prevent infections. Once the tissue of postmenopausal women had been deprived of estrogen for more than 3 months, it was unable to fully respond during one full year of estradiol-17β therapy.[281] It may, however, require a higher dose to restore the tissue than was given in that experiment.

Other aspects of healthy vaginal physiology, besides acidity, are more responsive to estrogen therapy, even after a period of postmenopausal deficiency. A reversal of atrophied cells occurred in women up to age 67 who were studied and who started treatment on ultra-low doses of unopposed estrogen applied as a skin patch.[381]

Topical estrogen (Premarin cream) also helped restore atrophic tissue within two months at higher doses in women up to age 70 who were studied.[636] And posthysterectomized women (with an average age of 54 and more than 5 years postsurgery) who had the expected sexual complaints of vaginal dryness, dyspareunia (painful intercourse), and anorgasmia (absence or loss of orgasmic experience) tested either the oral pill Premarin or the cream applied vaginally. Both routes helped solve the vaginal dryness and the dyspareunia but not the anorgasmia.[468] (See chapter 12.)

4. *Estrogen and hot flashes and night sweats.* More than fifty years of research and hundreds of published studies have clearly established that hot flashes result from the dramatic sudden plummeting in

estrogen. Not surprisingly, those flashes are cured with estrogen therapy. When hormone levels are changing in a roller-coaster fashion, a woman is pretty likely to experience these annoying discomforts. Once the blood levels of estrogen even out, the healthy body seems to adjust and hot flashes tend to stop. But for many women who use no hormonal therapy, this can take seven or more years of embarrassing, distressing, and uncomfortable flashes of heat and sweat that occur unpredictably.

Here's how hot flashes happen: Core body temperature starts to increase approximately seventeen minutes before each flash and continues to rise until the time of the hot flash. Increases in energy expenditure and panting have been recorded with each hot flash when women were studied in a laboratory.[116] The body becomes inflamed—in a sudden fever—with rapid breathing; then the flashing heat occurs in the face and the chest as the woman breaks out in a sweat and the heat is rapidly dissipated. This is not pleasant!

Each of the sex hormones—estrogen, progesterone, and testosterone—can alleviate these flashes.[616] In recent years, big pharmaceutical corporations concluded that a low-dose, or ultra-low-dose, hormone regimen would be marketable, so low-dose formulations have been tested. They do help, but not as much as higher doses.[703, 792] Every regimen that has been studied seems to work, provided that it is able to even out the estrogen level in blood. You want to find a regimen that doesn't just work a little but works a lot. No more hot flashes.

5. *Estrogen and progesterone and your nose.* Anatomical and physiological changes in nasal tissue coincide with declining levels of estrogen. These include a reduction in water content, a sensation of nasal stuffiness, and less mucus production.[552] Since your nose is the first line of defense against airborne infections, such changes reduce your ability to fight colds and viruses, including those that cause the flu. Probably, a susceptibility to pollen also occurs. Hormonal therapies can help.

In a study of fifty-five postmenopausal women, *sequential hormone therapy* (progesterone about half the month, estrogen every day) was significantly better than continuous-combined regimens for restoring the lining of the nose, the upper respiratory regions, and the vaginal walls.[118] Sequential regimens also produced positive results via an intranasal spray that delivered the hormones directly to the nasal mucosa.[551]

6. *Estrogen and your voice.* The larynx, the box-shaped part of the respiratory tract between the base of the tongue and the top of the windpipe, "the voice box," is an estrogen-receptive organ in the same way that the vaginal mucosa is. Under a microscope, swabs from the cells from either surface look exactly alike.[119]

An observational study of healthy, surgically postmenopausal women from 46 to 60 years old found that of the 48 who had been using estrogen therapy, compared to the 49 who had not, the estrogen users had significantly fewer voice complaints.[119] For example, only 16 percent of estrogen users but 62 percent of those using no hormones reported a problem with hoarseness. Similar benefits for estrogen users were found for a deepening of the voice (11 percent versus 31 percent) and for a change in the timbre (0 versus 37 percent). The author concluded that estrogen may prevent and possibly treat pathophysiology such as vocal cord dystrophy, which can occur in postmenopausal women.

7. *Estrogen and your teeth.* Estrogen can keep you smiling longer. In a study of 330 postmenopausal Japanese women, those with a longer duration of estrogen use had more total and more posterior teeth remaining.[763] That is not really surprising, considering the relationship between the underlying bone and the maintenance of the teeth. Chapter 8 reviews the enormous body of research on how estrogen and progesterone protect your bones.

8. *Estrogen and progesterone and your eyes.* Certain diseases of the eye are more common as women age. Overall, it seems that hormone users enjoy better vision and fewer age-related pathologies.

The Beaver Dam Eye Study was a total community sample. It found that the postmenopausal use of estrogen was associated with a reduced risk of more severe macular sclerosis of the eye.[403] A longer period of sex hormone secretion, that is, an earlier age at first menstruation and an older age at menopause, reduced the risk of the cortical opacities. The authors concluded that estrogens offer some protection in the lenses of women.

Other benefits of hormonal therapy on visual system physiology have also been reported. In 1948, the Framingham Eye Study enrolled men and women as part of the Framingham Heart Study. Fifty years later, the survivors provided a subgroup that could be studied for their use of hormones and visual losses. Women who took estrogen for more than 10 years had a 60 percent lower incidence of opacities of the lenses of their eyes, compared to the women who did not take estrogen. Surgical menopause (removal of the uterus and the ovaries) significantly increased the risks; up to 30 percent of the postsurgical group, unfortunately, showed these impairments of their vision.[851] The authors concluded that postmenopausal estrogen users have fewer visual impairments. Since progesterone was not commonly prescribed until after 1980, the researchers were unable to analyze its effects.

Visual acuity was also shown to be *much improved* after one year of an HRT regimen but *unchanged* at one year in a placebo group; Italian women ages 52 to 70 tested a conjugated equine estrogen combined with the Big Pharma progesterone, dydrogesterone at 5 mg. Both tests revealed the power of HRT to improve the visual system: women could see more clearly and their eyes were more responsive in tearing to an irritant one year after having been on HRT.[299] Those who tested a placebo got worse. Another study reported that sequential hormonal therapy improved tear production in aging eyes, which are otherwise prone to dryness.[6]

But one large observational report found that "never-users" of hormones had the lowest incidence of dry-eye syndrome (5.9 percent), while up to 9 percent of those who used oral estrogen therapies reported dry eyes.[675] Progesterone use along with estrogen worked best.

One study of 102 women who were 60 to 82 years old searched for but could not find any benefit *or* risk of hormones on age-related maculopathy because ischemic heart disease obscured the effect of hormones.[3] So although the studies show some variation in design and outcome, it seems that our eyes tend to benefit from sex hormones.

9. *Estrogen and progesterone and sleep quality.* Postmenopausal women more frequently reported difficulty sleeping than did premenopausal women.[673] HRT helps to promote better sleep.

The WHI showed that HT users had a superior quality of sleep compared to placebo users. HRT produced a better quality of sleep and a significantly better quality of life among 2,428 menopausal women in Italy as well: "Never users" more frequently reported sleeping badly.[673] And a study from Finland concluded that it was progesterone that contributed to the sex hormone improvement in breathing during sleep, which improved its quality.[607]

10. *Estrogen as an antioxidant.* Estrogen has been shown to act as an antioxidant that buffers (that is, "sops up" or puts a stop to) the damaging power of oxygen "free radicals." These free radicals generate a cascade of damaging effects by attacking the cell membranes that line the blood vessels. Collectively, the damage inflicted by oxygen free radicals is termed "oxidative stress."[393] Free radicals are formed during various physical stresses such as exercise and from psychological stress as well. More than twenty-five years ago, animal experiments at Stanford University by Dr. George Feigen revealed that vitamin C and estrogen were synergistic in buffering free-radical damage. Each substance helped the other more effectively buffer free radicals.[168]

11. *Estrogen and gut/intestinal function.* Estrogen can help the absorption of certain key minerals and can maintain overall healthy functioning of the gut. Both bones and the central nervous system require adequate calcium. But digestion and the absorption of nutrients decline with age. Elderly women who were given estrogen showed an immediate increase in the capacity of their intestines to absorb the calcium they ingested.[805]

In postmenopausal women after hysterectomy, estrogen (Premarin) was shown to increase blood levels of "substance P." This hormone is widely found in the gastrointestinal tract, the spinal cord, the vagus nerve, and many other peripheral nerves. It regulates blood flow, pain signal transmission, gut immune response stimulatory action, and smooth muscle activity. But some products don't work; Prempro did *not* increase this substance; neither did raloxifene, a drug that is used for bones instead of HRT.[426]

12. *Estrogen, blood sugar, and type II diabetes.* As women age, they are significantly more prone to age-related aberrations in insulin levels if they do not use hormone therapy.[762]

After meals that contain sugar or any form of carbohydrate, insulin levels rise at a rate that is affected by the type of food we choose.[762] Insulin and glucagon are the two "sugar-regulating" hormones, and both are secreted from the pancreas gland whenever sugar in the blood is too high or too low. This tight regulation of the blood levels of sugar is essential for life. Too little or too much results in coma and death. It's that serious. Insulin is the choreographer, directing the molecular events that remove sugar from the blood, then moving it into muscles, nerves, and other tissues where it is consumed for energy. Or, if there is more than is needed to stoke the engine, the excess sugar is placed into storage as fat. (Glucagon, the other choreographer, rises when blood sugar is too low, and it signals the storage centers to melt down the fat, convert it to sugar, and return some to the blood.)

Fasting levels of insulin are not changed by hormonal therapy. But with the typical age-related declines in sex hormones, things can get a bit out of whack. For example, too much insulin could be produced after a meal that is not "moved" out fast enough. A high level of lingering insulin that fails to return to normal in time is a potential precursor of type 2 diabetes. Fortunately, elevated insulin levels are less likely when postmenopausal women take hormone therapy.[762]

These menopausal aberrations do not produce any immediate negative effects of glucose or insulin levels in plasma, but experts state that "it is well known" that they increase the risk of impaired glucose tolerance and type 2 diabetes mellitus.[163] (Glucose tolerance tests measure the insulin response to a test dose of glucose.) HRT improves eating-related insulin function pretty fast. Within twelve weeks of transdermal estrogen, followed by twelve weeks of estrogen-progestin combined therapy, women who had a previously exaggerated insulin response to swallowing a high-sugar drink showed a 30 percent reduction in insulin to this same test.[163] That's good: it restored the system to normal.

The prevalence of type 2 diabetes is increasing worldwide.[689] Factors that increase the risk include:

- Obesity
- Hypertension

- Hyperlipidemia (excess fats in the blood)
- Hyperglycemia (excess sugar in the blood)
- Lack of exercise
- Cardiovascular disease

Metabolic syndrome describes a *combination* of these risk factors.

Hormone therapy appears to help reduce the likelihood of developing metabolic syndrome and type 2 diabetes.

The HERS study of women with coronary heart disease had 2,029 women without diabetes when the study began. The Prempro group experienced a significantly lower incidence of developing type 2 diabetes: 6.2 percent versus 9.5 percent of the placebo group.[384] Comparisons among different regimens in another study showed that the sequential regimens appeared to be most helpful.[689]

Estrogen and body fat. Too much fat can damage your health, from a cellular to a structural level. Like the ovary, adipose (fat) tissue is a manufacturing site for estrogen. While the ovarian production of estrogen decreases after menopause, the fat cells' manufacturing activities seem to increase with age. Adipose secretion of hormones is not affected by taking estrogen therapy. Rather, your local fat cells' production of estrogen (which can be twenty times higher than circulating levels; see chapter 10) can be very bad for your health. It may "play a pivotal role in the increase in estrogen-dependent malignancies in the postmenopausal years."[525]

Hormonal therapies may be bad for women who are seriously overweight because of the combined dangers that they may add to an already local overabundance of estrogen.

Hormone Therapies Are Not All the Same

Some HTs increase, while others decrease, the risks of your developing cardiovascular disease, osteoporosis, cognitive dysfunction, and sexual debilities, and some improve your general well-being, whereas others don't. It is vital for you to learn which hormone therapies represent your personal best choice.

Aren't FDA-Approved Drugs Safer?

It is true that hormone therapies from Big Pharma undergo extensive trials before finally achieving FDA approval.

The FDA-approved labeling is extensive, listing all of the side effects that have been reported. But it will also tell you that hormones cause breast cancer or stroke, for example, without advising you that some regimens won't.

The investment behind an approved drug (testing trials, advertising, and marketing costs) is so huge that once Big Pharma gets FDA approval, it has no incentive to offer a regimen that is economical or marginally better. Therefore, Big Pharma is "stuck" with pitching its patented drug and listing the class-adverse reactions of *all* sex hormones. It is up to us, objective scholars and consumers, to investigate elsewhere to learn of potentially better options for individual care.

Does My Doctor Know Best?

There's no easy answer to this question. The scientific literature on women's hormonal health provides massive amounts of sometimes fragmented, often contradictory, information. During the last thirty years, I have tried to study it without bias.

For me, the literature reveals that some hormonal regimens offer a much better choice for you than others do. Why don't doctors have this information at their fingertips? I have observed that physicians who attend medical meetings to learn this information are not offered it by the leaders of the continuing medical education courses. Why not? The medical meetings are almost always led by lecturers who have received money from the pharmaceutical industry. The same goes for the officers and the program directors of the medical societies. Because I have never taken any fees from any pharmaceutical company and do not work at an institution whose critical funding depends on the goodwill of the drug industry, I am liberated to tell you what I conclude through research without bias.

It's not only what you take, it's how you take it. Dr. Gambrell tried to teach that *sequentially* taken progesterone is a beneficial adjunct to any estrogen regimen.[258] I think he got it right!

The biological design of an intact, healthy fertile female endocrine system can offer clues about the importance of sequential progesterone when we study how fourteen days a month are what it takes to do its optimal job on the bones, the breasts, the brain, and the pelvis. Women are not like men, who have unvarying levels of hormones and behavior across the month. Taking progestin all thirty days a month might have been rational for drug-development profits, but it never was for women's biology. So, come along with me on a journey and see whether you agree that progesterone is important for every woman, about half of every month, whether or not she still has her uterus. Because she still has her brains, heart, bones, breasts, and her sexual interests, and these are designed to function in a feminine way, with symphonic ebb and flow.

3

Prescription Hormones: How to Choose Them, How to Take Them

IF YOU DECIDE TO EXPLORE the possibility of taking hormonal therapy, recognize two essential truths. First, hormones are powerful and should never be used without prescriptions from a physician who knows you, has examined you, and is monitoring your health. (And, of course, your doctor will tell you whether your medical history disqualifies you from using them.) Second, don't buy a "natural hormone product" in a health food store. A clerk in this store is not licensed to advise you in such matters or to practice medicine. To take any hormone on your own is folly. It is dangerous. Don't do it. Learning about your options will help you work effectively with your doctor to find an individualized regimen that is right for you.

The Essential Estrogens

Before you see your doctor for a prescription, take the time to read about what you're trying to replace. Here's what you should know.

Not All Estrogens Are Alike

Three major forms of estrogen circulate in your blood: estradiol, estriol, and estrone. Of the three, estradiol is the most active hormone, the one that researchers test in women. It's also the choice for experiments on biological tissues. Estradiol produces measurable effects on every physiological system and body part on which it has been tested: bone, skin, brain, and sexual response. It is considered a *strong* estrogen because of that kind of wide-ranging power. (Estradiol in the body is found in two variants, like left- and right-handed, called 17α and 17β.) But estriol, considered the weak estrogen, also has some powerful effects: it reduces wrinkles on the face and can restore aging (technically, atrophic) vaginal skin (see pages 19–20). Think of the third estrogen, estrone, as the storage "reservoir tank" that can be measured from a sample of your blood. Experts who measure the biochemical conversions report that estrone and estradiol seem to continually convert back and forth, from one biochemical form into the other.[167] Perhaps they convert from estrone storage into the active form of estradiol, as needed by the body. You might call it a bit of shape-shifting magic by Mother Nature.

The top two rows of data within table 3.1, "How Do You Measure Up?" on page 33 show average *existing* blood levels of estrone and estradiol that are typically found in pre- and postmenopausal women who are *not* using hormonal therapy. The next rows show the average *resulting* blood levels found in postmenopausal women *after* they use different doses of three widely prescribed estrogen products. These numbers provide you with a good reference point for comparison, but remember that each woman is different so these are just averages. When your blood levels are high, like those of young women, your bones are strong, your blood vessels tend to be healthy, and your vagina is well lubricated. If you get your own blood levels tested, you can compare your estrone and estradiol to these averages to recognize how high or low your own levels are and whether you want to make changes. Then you can discuss with your doctor the significance of the readings.

Different Delivery Routes, Different Effects of Estrogen Products

The differences among prescribed estrogen products in potency and their varying effects on your physiology depend on their chemical structure and how they are delivered into your bloodstream. Delivery routes include injection, swallowing a capsule or a tablet, applying a skin patch, smoothing gel or cream onto your skin, or inserting a vaginal pill. You can also place a hormone tablet under your tongue or between your gum and your cheek, where it melts and is absorbed into the tiny blood capillaries nearby. Eventually, every route brings the hormone into your bloodstream for distribution throughout the entire body.[714] These variations affect the way estrogens influence breast tissue, sexual and mental function, and lipid changes (such as potentially elevating harmful triglyceride levels—but only if you take an oral swallowed form).

Differences in Your Unique Biology Affect Hormone Levels

Some days your body will absorb—and use up—more estrogen, other days less. And your body will send signals that provide important clues to what is happening. Table 3.1 shows how you can get a clear picture of your estrogen status from a small blood sample.[86] For example, (looking at the first line) blood samples from a woman who is premenopausal will reveal an estrone level between 40 and 170 and an estradiol level between 50 and 250 picograms, per milliliter of blood depending on which day of her cycle the blood is drawn. Around ovulation she will show the higher levels; around her menstrual period she will be at her lowest levels.[169] The next line shows that a postmenopausal woman's blood test results do not vary across the month (since she does not cycle) and the estrogens' levels are much lower if she does not use HRT.

Listen to your body: if you take any form of estrogen and your breasts feel painfully full, the estrogen levels may be too high. Skipping a day or reducing the dose should quickly resolve this problem. Likewise, episodes of vaginal dryness or hot flashes can signal that the body is estrogen-starved and would thrive with a higher dose of estrogen or with some extra estrogen applied topically directly where it is needed, at the vagina. (Vaginal estrogen is very effective but not advisable before intercourse, or you will be giving your partner some estrogen to absorb through the skin of the penis.) But you need to recognize the safe limits for day-to-day adjustments, along with your clinician. In the early years when HRT first became available, women felt (and looked) great on the very high doses of estrogen their doctors had prescribed. They had fewer facial wrinkles, and they slept better.

Table 3.1 How Do You Measure Up?

	Blood Levels of Estrone (pg/ml)	Blood Levels of Estradiol (pg/ml)
No HRT: premenopausal women	40–170	50–250*
No HRT: postmenopausal women with ovaries intact	35	14
HRT users: postmenopausal women		
Type of Estrogen Used		
Premarin Swallow Tablets (conjugated equine estrogen)		
Dosage strength: 0.3000 mg	76	19
Dosage strength: 0.6250 mg	153	40
Dosage strength: 1.250 mg	200	60
Estrace Swallow Tablets (micronized estradiol)		
Dosage strength: 1.0 mg	150	40
Dosage strength: 2.0 mg	250	60
Estradiol Skin Patch (transdermal estradiol)		
Dosage strength: 50 mcg	51	72
Dosage strength: 100 mcg	57	120

*Because the estrogen levels of a fertile woman change throughout the month, the range shown (50 to 250 pg/ml) reflects the lowest and highest levels that typically circulate within a month.

But the doses were too high and were inadequately balanced with progesterone. This imbalance caused excessive tissue growth in the uterine lining, called endometrial hyperplasia, which led to uterine cancer in 3 to 7 percent of cases (see chapter 5).[167a] Increasing the duration (to more days per month) and sometimes also *the dose* of progesterone solved this problem, restoring tissue to normal.

A closer look at delivery methods, their pros and cons, can also help your decision-making process.

Pills

When you swallow a pill, the drug (in this case, estrogen) goes into your stomach. There it's broken down, then moved into the intestines en route to the liver. The liver gets these particles, still highly concentrated, before they are subsequently channeled into the bloodstream and diluted by the five liters or so of blood that your body circulates. Think of a bouillon cube that you add to a recipe. If you first dissolve the cube in a tiny bit of fluid, this highly concentrated syrup may be too strong to taste good. But when you further dilute it, the cube adds good flavor to the soup.

The Cons

The strong concentration in the liver—from the oral route—causes certain significant reactions that lead to an elevation in blood triglycerides and other dangerous substances. That could be bad news for your blood vessels. It may also increase your risk of developing metabolic syndrome.

The Pros

Pills are neat and easy to take. And pills may not put you at any risk, depending on your personal cardiovascular health profile. Among the oral options, there are further decisions to be made. Ask your physician and even your pharmacist, who is a professional with expertise on the types of pharmaceutical dosages.

Your Options

More than 80 percent of the market share for oral estrogens in the United States has been for one version, Premarin. This sales dominance is largely due to the enormous research and marketing investment made by its Big Pharma manufacturer. Although this is the one oral product most likely to be prescribed by your doctor, it does not mean this is the best hormone for you. You can and have the right to request a different prescription that you believe would better fit your needs. The key is to find a doctor who is willing to work with you. It is your body. You do not have to buy a product that you conclude better serves the purveyor than it does the purchaser.

Premarin, oral conjugated equine estrogen pills, actually contains many different ingredients.[791] Table 3.2, "What Are You Swallowing?" shows the eight most common ones.[86] Many of the horse components

Table 3.2 What Are You Swallowing? The Most Common Components in Premarin

Composition of conjugated equine estrogen USP[86]

Sodium estrone sulfate

Sodium equilin sulfate

dihydroequilen-17α

Estradiol-17α

Equillenin

Dihydroequilen-17β

Delta-dehydroestrone

Estradiol-17β

---

are naturally found in the pregnant horse but are not found in women. Note that the words *equine* and *equilin* mean "derived from the horse." And many of these components build up in the blood of the women who take them, since they are not metabolized by human bodies. [167] Although these accumulating equine products have not been shown to produce any damaging effects, I do not see how they serve the woman's best interest. I would not recommend them unless there were no alternatives—but there are.

Another Option

Other FDA-approved estrogens are less frequently prescribed (and have less substantial research behind them than Premarin), but they are just as good, maybe better. Estrace is a pill of estradiol in a micronized form that enables rapid absorption. It's a chemical copy of an estrogen that your body manufactures naturally. Taking this form of estrogen does not cause an accumulation of components that are foreign to the human body. This Big Pharma product and its generic versions can be easily obtained at drugstores with your doctor's prescription. They contain *no horse components*. Having researched hundreds of relevant studies, I conclude that natural estradiol, such as Estrace or other estradiol-17β products, is better for you, even though it is less widely marketed to doctors. You should consider it.

Yet Another Option

A new form of oral estrogen, estradiol acetate, is rapidly converted to estradiol once it is absorbed. It, too, is identical to naturally occurring hormones produced by the ovaries. FDA approval is anticipated, due to the results from recent experimental trials.[731]

Other Delivery Routes for Estrogen

Non-oral modes of delivery include patches and gels, vaginally inserted estrogen pills, a slow-release ring that is placed in the vagina, tablets you place under the tongue, or lozenges you place between your gum and cheek. These other routes all avoid the "first pass" in the liver, something like diluting the bouillon cube fully before it gets into the soup pot. These nonswallowed routes more closely mimic what happens in the fertile woman's body as her ovaries secrete hormones into the bloodstream, in tiny, repeating pulses all day long. (I think nature's design is the most rational. When in doubt, copy Mother Nature.)

Estrogen can also be provided by your doctor in fixed dosages, which relieves you from day-to-day decision making but also of control. These routes include surgical implants, an intrauterine device, or monthly injections. If you get your hormones this way, you are not able to take an active role in listening to the signals your body sends and you cannot beneficially titrate (adjust) the dose in response to these signals. You cannot skip a day occasionally or add more hormones. You do gain the advantage of not having to remember to do anything, but isn't this abdication?

Medicinal Lozenges

Estrogen can be placed under the tongue (sublingual) or between the cheek and the gum (transbuccal) in a lozenge form. Within a few minutes, it is absorbed directly across the highly porous epithelial cells that line the area under your tongue. With this route, the hormone enters directly into the bloodstream and is rapidly diluted, instead of going to the liver.

One investigator in Australia tested the bioavailability of hormones, including estrogens and progesterone, when a hormone lozenge was placed in the mouth between the cheek and the gums.[852] He used a medicinal lozenge that was compounded by a local pharmacist, and the results were good. His studies of 6 women, ages 45 to 60, consistently revealed a rapid absorption, allowing this route to readily duplicate physiological patterns of all natural hormones that were delivered by lozenge. If you choose this route, your physician would need to write such a prescription for your pharmacy to compound. Women's Health America is one of the excellent compounding pharmacy (nationally accessible) organizations (www.womenshealthamerica .com). Another good compounding pharmacy is College Pharmacy (www.collegepharmacy.com).

Estradiol showed this good pattern of rapid absorption—at two standard test doses (0.5 mg and 2.0 mgs).[852] Other researchers have confirmed that the lining of the cheek works as a route for sex hormone therapy.[717]

More than twenty-five years ago, estradiol pills that were designed for swallowing, such as Estrace (a Big Pharma estradiol), were considered equally able to be absorbed under the tongue (sublingual). But there has been little pharmaceutical interest in promoting this route, so your physician may be unfamiliar with it. Big Pharma's estradiol, Estrace, taken along with a progesterone tablet compounded by a pharmacist, can be conveniently absorbed sublingually.[167, 168] But doctors rarely have the time to read this research and won't hear it covered at continuing medical education courses because no Big Pharma product is being marketed this way. Ask your doctor to prescribe your estrogen this way, and you will find that it is an excellent way to take it. Or ask your pharmacist for information, too.

Patches

Patches have been well studied because a number of pharmaceutical companies manufacture and promote these products to doctors and, via ads, to women. For estrogen, they serve as pretty good delivery routes. But they do not work for everyone because of extreme inconsistencies from one woman to the next in how well the estrogen in them is absorbed.

The Cons

Patches, like bandages, can irritate your skin if you are sensitive to them. Women also vary tremendously in the blood level of hormone they achieve when they wear a skin patch. The patch is typically applied to the arm, the buttocks, or the belly. In one study of thirty women using the Alora estrogen patch, a 2-inch square patch placed on the skin produced a huge difference (after six days) between the woman with the lowest absorption and the one with the highest. The lowest showed less than 1 picogram (pg) per ml of estrogen. The highest absorption added 98 pg/ml.[419] You can't be sure with the patch how much hormone you're absorbing. If you refer to table 3.1 on page 33, you can see that the 98 pg/ml level reflects a premenopausal level. But for a woman who added only 1 pg/ml of estrogen to an already low postmenopausal hormone level, the patch would be useless. So you can imagine that some women with inadequate estrogen would still have hot flashes or vaginal dryness, and others would find these symptoms cured if enough estrogen was absorbed.

The same research also showed that contrary to the instructions that tell women to change their patches every three days, most women could replace them every six days to get the same benefit. If a woman used her own body's signals to tell her when she had stopped absorbing estrogen from her patch (for example, she experienced a return of hot flashes), she would not have to buy as many patches. For most of the women tested, this would mean half the cost. The authors suggested, therefore, that it would save women money to titrate the dose to the symptoms they experienced.[419] Because women vary, a simple written prescription rigidly adhered to by every woman would be irrational. One size does *not* fit all.

Results like these support the idea of working with your doctor to find a range of usage that adjusts your dose based on your body's feedback signals. This is not a license to double and triple the dose. Rather, it respects the intelligence of the woman who occasionally will skip a day of estrogen or tweak the dose to a preset higher level when her signals call for more. Your intelligence and your body should be respected.

Gels
Introduced in 2005, these products require spreading a measured amount of gel over the arms or the legs each day. Estrogel is one such FDA-approved product that is manufactured by Big Pharma (Solvay).

The Cons
The daily use of the gel costs twice as much as the patch—about $97 compared to $49 per month—at the wholesale price in 2006.[555] The

gel may feel cold when it's spread across the arms or the legs because of the alcohol base, and it takes about five minutes to dry. It must not be washed off before it is all absorbed, which may take more than an hour. But these may be trivial inconveniences for you.

The Pros
If you opt for the gel, you will get the hormone absorbed transdermally without having to wear a bandage in one place for days at a time.

Vaginally Inserted Forms
Vaginally inserted forms have shown good absorption into the bloodstream. Estrogen cream can be delivered via a plunger or by a tablet that dissolves. There is also a narrow rubberlike tubing "ring" that is left in the upper vagina, where it releases a measured amount of hormone every twenty-four hours. At low doses, the vaginally placed estrogen acts only locally and is effective in restoring degenerating genital tissue.[636, 728, 831] At higher doses, the blood levels of estrogen rise, achieving bodywide circulation that is equivalent to other routes. At these higher levels, vaginally delivered estrogen can be as effective as other routes.[308]

The Cons
Women may not stick with it if they find it uncomfortable, intrusive, or messy.

The Pros
Absorption is pretty dependable and is not affected by digestive disturbances that can disrupt absorption if you swallow a pill. Neither is absorption affected by fat deposits in the skin, which can disrupt absorption with patches or gels. Also, with vaginal delivery, fluctuating levels are avoided and that can lessen side effects.[17] Finally, the overload on the liver is avoided.

Experiments comparing one ring, the ESTring, to an inserted vaginal tablet, Vagifem, provide a rare comparison study. Results showed that both were equally effective for local tissue atrophy after forty-eight weeks of test use.[831] But the dropout rate was much lower among the women testing the tablet than for the ring: 1.9 percent versus 21 percent. Dropouts were mainly in the first three months, due to slippage of the ring or discomfort in the lower back or the abdomen. And dropouts mean no compliance, which means no hormone benefits.

If you want to try a vaginal route for some or all of the estrogen therapy your doctor prescribes, tell your doctor your preference. The FEMring provides doses that will raise your blood levels of estrogen, unlike the low-dose ESTring. You might find that a liquefying tablet is less intrusive than an inserted rubbery device. So might your sex partner.

What You Should Know about All Delivery Routes

The delivery route that you will keep using is your best choice. And you can test each one before you choose. You can exert control over the delivery system you use. You insert, apply, or swallow. Most estrogen regimens are used every single day, all through the month.

Side effects are generally trivial and usually disappear after women adjust to—or modify—their regimens. But if you take a hormone that continues to cause nausea or pain, listen to this signal. Breast pain usually resolves by lowering the dose of estrogen or skipping a day. But other types of pain or discomfort should signal you to ask your doctor for a different regimen. Never take a regimen that makes you feel ill! Hormones should help you feel good.

The Powerful Progesterone

Progesterone is the other main female sex hormone. Unlike estrogen, which a fertile human ovary manufactures and secretes into the bloodstream every day of the month, progesterone is produced and then secreted into the bloodstream only during the second half of the month—from the day before ovulation and every day thereafter until menstruation occurs. For this reason, progesterone can be measured from a blood sample drawn from the arm of a fertile woman only if the blood is drawn during the second half of her monthly cycle. The quantity of progesterone a woman is circulating in her blood can best be measured by a blood test. So the salivary testing of hormones that is promoted by some laboratories and compounding pharmacies may not be a good use of your money. The amount of hormone in saliva does not accurately reflect the amount circulating in the bloodstream.[289, 483]

Many different synthesized progesterone products are for sale by prescription and are collectively termed "progestins" or "progestagens." They were named *progestagens* because pregnant women (women who were "gestating") secrete high levels of the hormone. Literally, the word means "for gestation." The first scientists who coined the term saw this; however, medical schools started to teach doctors that the only function of the hormone was "progestational." This is incorrect! Mother Nature never made a hormone with only one role.

Progesterone's crucial health role in the female body balances against estrogen—much like the yin and the yang of all creative forces. The sequential rising and falling each month of progesterone, balanced against estrogen, generates the command signals to remodel your bones and keep your breasts healthy, your mind sharp, and your sleep sound. Regular sexual contact, as a steady drumbeat, sets the rhythm for this hormonal symphony, which plays out within the monthly cycle of the moon.[169]

Here are the main points you should know.

Not all progesterone is alike. "Progestin" is the shorthand that is widely adopted for any progestational drug. At least eighteen different progestational products are currently manufactured by Big Pharma, including one that is bioidentical to human progesterone. All of the other progestins are not bioidentical to women. So I will use the correct term, *progesterone,* to refer to the hormone that your body naturally makes or to mean a man-made copy that is identical in its chemical makeup and that the drug industry makes. The nonbioidentical products I call "synthetic progestins."

Why are there so many synthetic progestins? Unfortunately, Big Pharma's early efforts to synthesize (to manufacture) an oral bioidentical progesterone pill were not successful. The oral formulation that was first used was so rapidly metabolized (within a few minutes), it just vanished too fast—so fast that not enough progesterone reached the uterus to do its job of balancing the estrogen therapy. For this reason, synthetic progestins derived from testosterone and from other molecules were invented, such as the widely prescribed Provera, which is the "pro" in Prempro. Its chemical name is MPA (medroxyprogesterone acetate), and it is a very strong drug with many adverse effects, such as an increased risk of developing cardiovascular disease. (See chapter 9.) Natural progesterone does not have these adverse effects.

The human form of progesterone was subsequently micronized, then added to peanut oil and formulated into a capsule for swallowing. This led to an FDA-approved Big Pharma product, a natural human-type, bioidentical progesterone called Prometrium. Progesterone can also be made by compounding pharmacies with your doctor's prescription for under-the-tongue or across-the-cheek delivery in a tablet or a lozenge. The brain metabolizes progesterone (but not necessarily all synthetic progestins) into active nerve hormones (which are technically called "neurosteroids"). And while progesterone synergizes with estrogen to protect nerve firings and cognitive function,[266] MPA does not—and might even oppose the same action. (See chapter 11 for details.) (*Neuroprotective* means that it exerts protective effects on the central nervous system, as shown in measurements of nerve firing patterns, and cognitive function. See chapter 11.)

The bottom line: avoid MPA unless you need it for a pelvic problem. (See chapters 5, 6, and 7 for details.)

Most women are well served by progesterone. Study after study shows the profoundly valuable benefits that progesterone can offer you. Progesterone can improve nasal and visual integrity, as described in chapter 2. In addition, progesterone plays a key role, when balanced with estrogen, in the physiology of the bones,[613] of healthy breasts (see chapter 10), and in mental alertness (see chapter 11). The limited view of progesterone's role (on the uterus) that is held by many medical "authorities" has proved to be shortsighted and wrong!

For all HT-using women, and especially after a woman undergoes a hysterectomy, progesterone can cause maximum benefits with minimal side effects if prescribed correctly.[258] This means that the progesterone is sequentially used, for the last 10 to 14 days of each month, along with using estrogen every day of the 29-day monthly cycle.

Natural is better than synthetic. According to one highly respected progesterone expert, Dr. Regine Sitruk-Ware, the synthetic progestins used in hormone therapy have various pharmacological properties, and one cannot simply consider them all as one "class" of

Table 3.3 The Wide World of Synthetic Progestins (grouped by their hormonal tendencies to exert biological action)

Progesterone Derivatives	Testosterone Derivatives
"Pure" progestational	**Partly masculinizing**
(19 norprogesterones)	Norethisterone
Nestorone	Norgestrel
Nomegestrol acetate	Desogestrel
Promegestone R5020	Gestodene
Demegestone	Norgestimate
Trimegestone	**Antiandrogenic**
Minimizes masculinization	Dienogest
Cyproterone acetate	
Chlormadinone acetate	
Drospirenone	
Nomegestrol acetate	
Trimegestone	
Partly glucocorticoid	
Medroxyprogesterone acetate	
Antimineralocorticoid	
Drospirenone	

Adapted from Sitruk-Ware (2003),[716] Rudolph (2004),[658] and Kuhl (2007).[425]

drug. For example, some synthetic progestins *reduce* insulin levels, and others dramatically *increase* them.[715] Some increase the risk of stroke, but natural progesterone does not.[112]

Read labels. Know what you're putting into your body. These commercially available forms of progestins have significant effects, such as masculinization (translation: growing a mustache!). Table 3.3, "The Wide World of Synthetic Progestins" above, lists eighteen different *synthetic* progestin products sold worldwide by Big Pharma. Although the names are difficult to pronounce, their various effects matter to your health. You need the products' names to know which ones you will say, "No, thank you" to, if offered. The information on this list should also help you discuss choices with your doctor. I think that you and she will be convinced that chemically identical human progesterone, rather than any of the listed synthetic progestins in table 3.3, might best serve your needs unless you have a pelvic problem.

Natural Progesterone Options

Progesterone can be formulated into a capsule in oil, a tablet you place under your tongue or between the gums and the cheek, a cream, or a gel. The absorption pattern of progesterone is not the same as for estrogen. Here are your options.

Pills

Micronized oral progesterone capsules in oil (Prometrium) absorb well when swallowed. Prometrium is not listed in table 3.3 because it is not a synthetic progestin. This is a Big Pharma product, and it is a bioidentical human progesterone.

Lozenges

Progesterone in a tablet or a lozenge also absorbs well when placed either under the tongue or between the cheek and the gum. Natural progesterone, once absorbed, gets used up quickly. Therefore, you will probably need to take half of the dose each time, twelve hours apart, rather than the full dose at one time, due to its rapid metabolism. You need to refuel.

The published studies convince me that swallowing a Prometrium capsule or using bioidentical progesterone tablets, either under your tongue or as a lozenge absorbed inside the cheek, provides a better form of progesterone. Any form of adequately dosed synthetic progestin or progesterone, however, will protect the endometrial lining of the uterus from the overgrowth of tissue (endometrial hyperplasia) that taking only estrogen would risk. These sublingual tablets or capsules can be prescribed by your doctor for a compounding pharmacy to make in standard 100-milligram doses.

Patches

Although transdermal skin patches of estradiol have been established as a reasonable option, neither progesterone nor synthetic progestin works well when delivered by patch.[257]

Creams

Creams that are spread on the arms or the legs also seem like a poor choice. One investigator tested a 4 percent progesterone cream that was transdermally applied and did report good results but conceded that further testing was needed.[445] The gold standard of scientific research—randomized controlled trials—have not yet been conducted and their results published to confirm these claims. Unlike the well-tested forms of progesterone, the creams do not change the signals of bone metabolic activity that would suggest adequate absorption.[852] For this reason, it is premature and unsafe to use progesterone or synthetic progestin via topical creams.

Gels

The absorption rate of progesterone is likely to be better with an alcohol-based gel than with cream formulations.[86, 289, 737] If you choose this route, query your doctor and maybe your pharmacist on what is currently available. Then ask them whether studies of the products have been published in peer-reviewed scientific journals. Otherwise, your body might fail to absorb what you need.

Beware of These Side Effects (from Synthetic Progestins)

Synthetic progestin steroids may cause undesirable side effects that natural progesterone does not cause. Bloating, weight gain, androgenization (male-pattern hair growth and deepening of the voice), and metabolic disturbances are all implicated with synthetic progestins.[854] The chapters on protecting your breasts (10), your brain (11), and your cardiovascular health (9) also provide extensive research suggesting that progesterone is consistently a more benign choice. European experts have been very vocal about the failure of WHI researchers to recognize the negative effects of MPA.[437, 647] I think that the side effects listed here and the data in the detailed chapters to follow provide sufficient reasons for you to avoid continuous MPA (Provera) and some of the other synthetic progestins.

R. Don Gambrell, MD, amassed and in 2006 published long-term data of 1,200 patients: 400 with surgical menopause (removal of the uterus and the ovaries) and 692 with natural menopause.[258] He prescribed a variety of estrogen and progestin regimens to individualize the dose in accordance with each patient's signals. (That's called "titration"; think of it as "proportioned individually"—the farthest distance from "One size fits all.") He used 18 different synthetic progestins and 16 different estrogens. And he reported that synthetic progestins *can* be given to postsurgical menopausal women with minimal side effects if it is done correctly. Rejecting the general trend of telling a woman with no uterus that she did not need progesterone, Dr. Gambrell believed that the progestin hormone was so important that he intentionally treated 73 percent of the surgically menopausal women with it. The dosage strength and frequency were determined from his patients' *responses* and were not based on blood levels of estradiol or testosterone. Convinced that women must feel good or they will not continue therapy, Dr. Gambrell listened to his patients. (A doctor-scholar who listens—that is someone you hope to find.) Although I prefer natural progesterone because of its whole-body benefit, for the purpose of endometrial protection, any progestin works if it is correctly dosed.

Dr. Gambrell believed that taking progesterone daily (which does not mimic nature's design) had the unfortunate physiological effect of rendering the progesterone "invisible" to the body's receptors, thus blocking the beneficial progesterone effects. Dr. Gambrell pointed out that women who used the WHI Prempro (continuous-combined synthetic progestin Provera with Premarin) regrettably did not experience the protection from uterus lining (endometrial) cancer that appropriately prescribed progesterone should offer. There were more than 100 cases of endometrial cancer reported on those regimens. That rate could have been lowered with a sequential regimen of progesterone.[258] Dr. Gambrell's research stands out as a beacon to show the way. Sequential progesterone makes sense to me. Not every day of the month but, as nature designed it, fourteen days per month at the most. The sequencing of progesterone—for half of each month, while estrogen is prescribed daily—is termed a "sequential regimen" of HT. It is better for you than a "continuous-combined regimen" that adds progesterone every day of the month.

What You Should Know about Sequential Hormone Therapy

Sequential HT regimens are likely to cause a monthly menstrual-type flow, if you still have your uterus. Such bleeding can occur regularly, each month, or irregularly.

Remember that estrogen taken unopposed by any progesterone or synthetic progestin causes endometrial tissue to proliferate (grow), and, after two weeks of unopposed estrogen, progesterone causes the tissue cells of the endometrium to stop multiplying. Then the tissue sloughs off, as in menses. This painless, menstrual-like bleeding may occur monthly for as long as the uterus retains enough youthful capacity to respond to the estrogen and then to the progesterone. Unfortunately, there are no published data to define how long the aging uterus will act young.

Investigators in Italy have compared various hormonal regimens to evaluate withdrawal bleeding. (*Withdrawal bleeding* was so named to denote the withdrawal of hormonal support that had stabilized the nestlike endometrial lining in preparation for a fertile egg. The nest washed away, until the next cycle.) They concluded that natural progesterone might be superior to synthetic progestins from a metabolic point of view. They also noted that human bioidentical forms of progesterone produced more irregular bleeding than did any of the synthetic progestins tested, using the dosage regimens they chose.[211] Because the human bioidentical form of progesterone is more rapidly metabolized by the human body, it makes most sense to split the prescribed dosage to half in the morning and half in the evening to regularize the withdrawal bleeding. The Italian researchers suggested that higher doses of the human bioidentical form of progesterone would likely be the best option for human bodies. I think that half the dose in the morning and half in the evening might do as well. It is normal for bleeding patterns to become irregular as a perimenopausal uterus approaches its last years of menstruation. This reflects the changing balance and levels of estrogen and progesterone secretion that an aging ovary manufactures. Eventually, the withdrawal bleeding becomes scanty and finally stops.

But bleeding can occur for other reasons, not only from the hormonal supply being withdrawn from the endometrial lining. Your relationship with your gynecologist must include keeping her fully up to date to assure that your bleeding is normal, that is, not a sign of disease. See chapter 5. (A detailed description of this "normal" menseslike blood flow, experienced by users of sequential regimens, can also be reviewed on pages 60 to 62 of *Hysterectomy: Before and After*.[168])

In 2004, investigators compared three synthetic progestins to the human bioidentical form of progesterone in experiments in vitro (in laboratory test dishes outside the body). They were searching for which hormone product formulation would best inhibit the dangerous unchecked growth of the endometrial cells that can (rarely) lead to cancer. The natural progesterone was most effective.[523] Finding the right dose is always a key issue.

Women can learn how to use the signals their bodies send to work with their physicians and ultimately come up with a healthy prescription that is right for them. This is not so difficult when one understands the underlying process. Does your typical pattern of bleeding start too soon? If you did not get a chance to take at least ten days of the progesterone, then the uterus needed more progesterone to balance the estrogen.[173] Usually, half of the standard dose of progesterone taken in the morning and half in the evening better controls the timing of bleeding than does the total dose taken once a day, because of the rapid metabolism of progesterone.

Defining One Cycle for Sequential HRT

Whenever a menstrual-like bleeding begins, this is the first day of a new cycle. It restarts the clock. Day 1 of the new cycle begins. A good sequential regimen would be done this way: Take estrogen unopposed for the first 14 days of the new cycle. Then take progesterone along with estrogen from days 15 to 29 or until the bleeding starts.

Progesterone: A Wrap-up

Progesterone is important to all women who take estrogen. The relevant scientific literature makes it clear that the chemical form should be identical to the human form to minimize adverse effects. The optimal routes appear to be either a capsule taken orally, a tablet under the tongue, or a lozenge between the cheek and the gum. It seems rational to me that the best sequential regimens mimic nature's design: take about ten to fourteen days of progesterone per month if you use estrogen every day.

Traces of Testosterone

The so-called androgen hormones, which include testosterone, DHEA, and androstenedione, were once considered to be exclusively male sex hormones. Thanks to improved detection methods, it is now well recognized that women also circulate these androgen hormones, which lend power, force, and sexuality to both mind and body. Their risks and benefits in postmenopausal hormone prescriptions have been less thoroughly investigated than those of the estrogens and the progestins. But they clearly serve an essential role in sexual satisfaction and genital sensation. Overdosing on these can be disastrous to a woman's cardiovascular health. When taken as needed, however, they can provide some extraordinary benefits in a carefully monitored hormonal regimen prescribed under the care of a knowledgeable physician. For information on testosterone, a hormone that your doctor can prescribe, see chapter 12.

The research on DHEA is in its infancy and is still investigational.[173] It has not been systematically studied because DHEA is not considered a drug but a food supplement. For that reason, its use in HRT is not described in this book.

Labeling: Synthetic versus Bioidentical

Synthesize means "to make or manufacture"; *natural* means "found in nature" and *can* refer to a synthesized, chemically exact copy of what is found in nature, such as Estrace or Prometrium. *Synthetic* refers to a chemical variation that renders the end result different from what is found in nature, such as the MPA Provera.

Bioidentical means "biologically identical." A pharmacist can synthesize a natural or a synthetic hormone. So can Big Pharma.

Unfortunately for women who try to find their way through this maze, the term *bioidentical* is politically charged. Here's why: Big Pharma opposes its competitors, the compounding pharmacies. In legal battles, the state pharmacy boards that control the practice of pharmacy, including compounding, have prevailed in lawsuits that the FDA brought to assert federal control over the states. Neither Big Pharma nor the FDA was permitted to block pharmacists from issuing hormones that physicians prescribe.

This legal battle for consumer dollars was ended in 2002 by the Supreme Court. So your access to a compounding pharmacy has not been blocked, despite Big Pharma's efforts to use the FDA for this purpose. You can work with your doctor to obtain a hormone prescription for bioidentical hormones that match your human female chemistry. Or you can use drugstores for your physician's prescription of a Big Pharma or generic copy. It's your choice and it's backed up by the Supreme Court of the United States. The law states that the federal government (in this case, the FDA) does not control either the practice of medicine or the practice of pharmacy. The individual states do.

We Are Not Horses

The original intention of the word *bioidentical* was to describe a substance that was biologically identical (bioequivalent) to what the body manufactured. So, used this way, a conjugated equine estrogen, such as Premarin or Prempro, contains a bioidentical or natural estrogen *for pregnant horses*, since the hormone is extracted from the urine of confined pregnant mares. (The *prem* in Prempro stands for Premarin; the *pro* stands for Provera, which is MPA.) But it is not bioidentical to a human's hormones. So you could be prescribed a "bioidentical" hormone that is compatible with a horse but might not be as compatible for a human. Check it out. The estrogen sold under the trade name Estrace—which the label states is a synthesized 17 beta estradiol, sold by Big Pharma—is bioidentical to the human hormone, not to the pregnant horse hormone. Likewise, Prometrium, a Big Pharma formulation of progesterone, is bioidentical to the human hormone. And both Estrace and Prometrium are high-quality Big Pharma products. There are many other hormone products, some of which are bioidentical, that have been scientifically studied.

What You Should Know: Bioidentical Is Not Benign

The term *bioidentical* is used differently by various professionals, so you want to be sure when you hear it that you can discern the meaning intended by the user. The published studies continue to reveal various risks from different products. Because this is so, I have taken care to list the type of drug tested and discuss these variations in tables for your reference throughout this book. For example, in early 2007, an excellent study of 271 stroke victims in France, compared to 610 other women, revealed clear differences in users of oral versus transdermal 17 beta estradiol. This is a human bioidentical estrogen manufactured by Big Pharma. The "swallow" forms increased the risk of stroke; the transdermal (skin) forms did not. In other words, taking the same human bioidentical form of estrogen but via different routes of entry into the bloodstream results in different outcomes on risk of stroke.[112]

The 2007 French study also showed that for progesterone and progestin the issue is not the route. It is the form of synthetic progestin being taken. The "swallow" routes for either natural micronized progesterone or some forms of synthetic, nonbioidentical progestins did not increase the risk of stroke; whereas oral (swallowed) forms of other synthetic progestins increased the incidence of stroke fourfold! Thus, using the same route (oral) of delivery but taking different synthetic progestins produces different outcomes. Unfortunately, the French study did *not* link specific results with specific synthetic progestins. Instead, the study grouped together "Progesterone derivatives" as a class. Therefore, I cannot confirm that any specific synthetic progestin was safe for risk of stroke. The study listed only the progestins confirmed as dangerous. And MPA is not usually prescribed in France (see chapter 10) so it cannot be scored. While the authors concluded that "Progesterone derivatives" were not harmful for stroke, only the currently prescribed forms should have been scored. Therefore, the study's design prevents me from agreeing with that overly broad conclusion.

With hormones presenting a real possibility for you to achieve your best health, I hope you will think carefully about which products make sense for you as you read the chapters on protecting your bones, your cardiovascular system, your cognitive abilities, your breasts, and your sexual and overall well-being.

4

Complementary and Alternative Practices: Some Good, Some Bad

W HAT WOMAN DOESN'T WANT TO FEEL great every day? Who wants the discomfort of hot flashes, sleep disturbances, joint pains, and headaches? Those are just some of the symptoms most healthy women begin to experience after age 40. About half of women ages 42 to 55 who do *not* use hormonal therapy acknowledge these symptoms.[44, 180, 572, 761] These physical disturbances follow the dramatic loss of progesterone and the volatile patterns of estrogen secretion that mark the seven-year transition from fertility to menopause. These "external" symptoms also signal changes within: declining bone mass, increasing risk factors for heart disease, and changing blood-sugar tolerance that can lead to diabetes and obesity.

Understandably, many women are driven to seek remedies. And many remedies are either in addition to, or instead of, help from their medical doctors.[264] According to a recent study in partnership with the Centers for Disease Control, such complementary and alternative medical therapies were used by almost half of the women surveyed.[394] Women who have also undergone a prior hysterectomy reported the highest number of symptoms (whether or not they also had their ovaries removed) and the highest use of these complementary practices.[394, 572, 761]

What Remedies Are Women Using?

Complementary practices, or alternative medicine, may involve healing rituals,[387, 835] eating or exercise regimens, lifestyle changes, or herbal remedies. Some are dangerous, some safe. Some—such as healing rituals—do work.[835] They utilize a powerful "placebo effect" that engages the psyche to solve the distress. Consider a woman who is experiencing debilitating hot flashes. Cynics may think it foolish for her to assume a yoga position, chant, take a sugar pill, or drink a special herbal tea. But about half the time, such actions actually reduce hot flashes. Hormone therapy (HT), by comparison, will work about 95 percent of the time if the dose is adjusted to provide adequate relief. And HT will always show a significantly greater benefit than will a placebo, exercise,[7] health food store phytoestrogens, and all of the other alternative remedies that have been tested in comparison to HT.

The Key Dangers of Complementary Practices

You need to assess your choice of remedy for its effectiveness and safety. Do your own research and don't rely on an untrained salesperson as your adviser. (Reading this chapter counts as part of your research.) Many of the untested treatments that are available in health food or vitamin stores may have effects that render them just plain unsafe to use.[20, 149, 575] Often, it's the consumers' perceptions about these products that can get you into trouble. Do you make any (or all) of the following assumptions?

- "If it's herbal, it's harmless." Not so. Many of these plant-based remedies have measurable biological actions in the body. They can affect the function of your body, as any drug can.
- "It's been sold for years, so it must be safe." Consider kava and comfrey: they were sold for years but have been withdrawn from the market because they can cause liver failure. One manufacturer of herbal weight-loss products that contained ephedra concealed thirteen thousand complaints of adverse effects, including heart palpitations and death.
- "If it's herbal or plant-based, it's more pure than pharmaceuticals." Many traditional herbal medicines contain toxic amounts

of lead and other metals. Others have even been adulterated with prescription drugs. Is the herbal product from China? The Chinese government executed the head of its food and drug oversight organization for fraud, so it may be a while before that nation has enough new laws in place to regulate safety.

If you find such information alarming, you are right: be alarmed. Any FDA-approved drug your doctor can prescribe is backed by at least two well-controlled studies that prove its effectiveness compared to a placebo and also monitor thousands of test subjects for each drug's toxicity on the bone marrow, the kidneys, and the liver. No herbal remedy has ever been exposed to such scrutiny. Recent news about contamination, heavy metals (which oxidize and generate damaging free radicals), and the erroneous labeling of products is alarming and worth your serious consideration.

So, be cautioned that even when good scientific results are reported from a particular substance, you may be unable to buy an unadulterated, accurate portion of this substance. And yet some people incorrectly assume that these herbal pills and potions are safe to swallow every day "or else they wouldn't be allowed on the market." In July 2007, *three* ex–surgeons general testified that "politics can trump science" sometimes. But fraud does not ordinarily trump the science of the FDA and the NIH (National Institutes of Health).

Physicians are legally liable and can lose their medical licenses, as well as their financial security, if they recommend a product that is untested and that might even be dangerous.[94]

Trust the science, not a salesperson. No license is needed to be a salesperson in a vitamin or health food store. Consult your physician, who knows your health practices, before you take herbal remedies.

Herbal Supplements Specifically Touted for Menopausal Women

The many women who turn to botanical and dietary supplements for menopausal changes should recognize that these are not regulated by the FDA. No law requires proof of their safety and effectiveness before they are marketed.[674]

In the United States, botanicals fall under the Dietary Supplement Health Education Act, which classifies them as dietary supplements, not drugs, and which are not intended for the diagnosis, prevention, or treatment of disease and therefore are not subject to strict regulation by the FDA.[264]

Consumers should be aware that the brand, the dose, and the contents are not uniform, and what you read on the bottle's label might not be the entire contents or even an accurate representation of what it contains. Let's consider the scientific proof for—and, mostly, against—these natural remedies.

"Natural" Estrogens

Phytoestrogens are plant-based estrogens (such as isoflavones and genistein). These naturally occurring compounds have a structure similar to that of human estrogens. They are found in a variety of plants, ranging from legumes (especially soybeans) to cereal grains. Phytoestrogens can also be purchased as supplements; the range of quality and safety of these can vary.[738]

A number of published experiments have tested whether phytoestrogens can be used effectively to provide relief for menopausal symptoms. The results are not consistent. Many experiments have produced occasional positive but very modest findings on plasma lipids.[150, 161, 162, 209] What are the red warning flags I see from the studies?

There's No Known Effective Dose

One reviewer of eleven studies suggested that at least 15 milligrams per day of specific phytoestrogens (genistein) will significantly reduce menopausal symptoms such as hot flashes.[844] But other experiments testing these same "adequate" and much higher doses reported the opposite. Isoflavones (which are relatively "weak" estrogen compounds made from plant extracts, or genistein) or soy protein produced effects no better than a placebo, even at much higher doses, on hot flashes, night sweats, loss of libido, vaginal dryness, and urinary frequency.[254, 411, 420, 560, 734]

They Don't Even Touch the Effectiveness of HT

In 2004, a daily high dose of 54 milligrams per day of genistein as a supplement was compared to a placebo and to HT in a randomized, controlled trial of 99 healthy women who experienced distressing hot flashes. The results showed that the number of hot flashes per day declined in all three groups: the best results were obtained for low-dose estrogen (1 mg estradiol; see table 3.1, in chapter 3) in a combined HT (54 percent reduction in hot flashes compared to a placebo); the results were half as good for genistein (24 percent compared to a placebo).[161] A 24 percent reduction means that instead of ten hot flashes a day, a woman endures eight per day. These are not very good results!

They Don't Hold Up to Food-Based Supplements

In 1998, a randomized controlled trial of women suffering from hot flashes (45 to 65 years old) compared a bread supplemented with 45 grams per day of soy grits, providing 53 milligrams/isoflavones, versus linseed versus wheat to test their effects on hot flashes after 12 weeks. (These kinds of doses can be purchased at many health food stores, but this may not always be wise.) The isoflavones were not helpful. Here's how the results stacked up:

- Hot flashes were significantly reduced by 60 percent on the wheat diet.
- Hot flashes declined by 45 percent on the linseed diet.
- Hot flashes were *not* significantly reduced on the soy-based diet.

None of the tested regimens corrected the vaginal dryness, painful intercourse, and deterioration of tissue.[179]

So, depending on which physiological problem was measured, the various sources of phytoestrogens at these doses helped but not substantially.

In 2005, a randomized controlled trial of 124 women who experienced more than 5 hot flashes per day tested a "cocktail" of soy isoflavones, supplements, and vitamins against a placebo of olive oil. Results: the "cocktail" was no better than olive oil after 6 or 12 weeks, although menopausal symptoms improved with both.[802]

In another trial, which tested lower doses, there was no benefit to using isoflavonoids over a placebo. The phytoestrogens in this trial were tested at 114 milligrams per day of total isoflavonoids, of which about 8 milligrams were the touted genistein.[560]

- Another study of 62 women tested 60 milligrams of *genistein* and *daidzen* versus a placebo and after 6 months found no benefit on hot flashes or blood flow through the arteries.[601]

- *Black cohosh* (the plant name is *Cimicifuga*) and red clover do have some research behind them, but the results do not support taking them.[463] Despite the widespread use of black cohosh for menopausal symptoms there are five published studies, each one concluding that there is little evidence of effectiveness.[20, 779]

- *Red clover* has shown some minor promise, short term, for menopausal symptoms.[215, 369] But randomized trials have been less than stellar.[32, 33, 264, 359] Red clover acts beneficially like estrogen in *some* tissues, increasing the synthesis of nitric oxide,[712] but not in other tissues.[32]

Natural Is Not Innocuous

It's one thing if an herbal remedy doesn't help relieve symptoms; then you've only lost money. But what if a remedy actually has a negative effect? Adverse effects from taking phytoestrogens and other herbal remedies have also been reported in several studies.

- **Endometrial hyperplasia.** In a randomized trial of 400 women taking 150 milligrams daily of isoflavone or a placebo, 6 cases of endometrial hyperplasia all occurred in the phytoestrogen group. The authors concluded that these supplements should be viewed negatively.[790]

Two researchers reviewed 18 randomized trials of black cohosh, red clover, kava, dong quai, evening primrose oil, ginseng, and combinations of these, and the following adverse effects were found.[369]

- **Gastrointestinal complaints, hypotension, headache, and dizziness** were listed for black cohosh. But another researcher who extensively reviewed black cohosh concluded that favorable safety data for short-term use had been provided.[215]

- **Breast tenderness and weight gain** have been linked to the use of red clover.[369]

- **Insomnia, diarrhea, vaginal bleeding, and mastalgia** (swollen, tender breasts) resulted from the use of ginseng. Women should be cautioned about using these supplements if they are also on estrogen therapy.[369]

- **Breast cell changes.** *Si-Wu-Tang* is a basic Chinese medicinal herb that was tested in the lab and found to have potent dangerous effects on cell proliferation. The researchers concluded, "To our knowledge, information about the pharmacokinetics of Si-Wu-Tang or related herbal remedies remains lacking." In other words, taking this herb may be dangerous.[129]

The Foods and Nutrients We Eat: Learning from Scientific Research

Separating myth from scientific data is complicated when it comes to eating. So-called "folk wisdom" is not always wise.

Is Tofu Toxic to Your Brain? It May Be, in Midlife

That probably got your attention. Tofu, a staple of vegetarian diets, is widely touted for its "healthful" attributes. An unsettling report from the Honolulu Heart Study suggested that habitual consumption of tofu in midlife might be responsible for poorer cognitive function in later life.[839] The study surprised its own authors, who tested cognitive function in 4,631 surviving members, 70 to 93 years old, of a group that was originally enrolled about 30 years earlier (in 1965).

The researchers were trying to detect why age-related dementia was so common in older persons. They concluded that "20 to 25 percent of the cognitive impairment observed in this population appears to have been attributable to tofu consumption." In other words, tofu was accelerating brain aging! Potential mechanisms were unknown, but speculation pointed to the known antiestrogenic effects of tofu.[839]

As is shown in chapter 11, the brain loves estrogen and progesterone, so any substance that negates the effects of estrogen could be a problem. If you love tofu, however, it seems unlikely that *moderate* consumption would hurt you.

The Power of Whole Foods for Good Health

You may have heard of free radicals, those unstable oxygen molecules that can damage your cells. A large body of research suggests that certain foods might beneficially "scavenge" or mop up free radicals and inactivate them. Free radical damage contributes to many disease processes, including certain cancers, asthma, rheumatoid arthritis, stroke, and cataracts. Since your body regularly produces free radicals when you exercise or experience prolonged stress or a compromised immune system, you should ask whether eating certain protective foods might be relevant.

Does "nature's design" include an ideal garden filled with foods to protect you? Apparently, yes.

Apples

In Finland, a 1967 national registry enrolled 10,054 men and women and studied them for 28 years. By 1994, 21 percent (2,085 people) had died. The habitual food habits, flavonoid analyses components, and disease records of the entire 10,054 were examined. Several foods stood out as being significantly protective in reducing the risk of death or suffering from chronic disease. Apples and onions were the main foods that were responsible for the protective effects. Grapefruit and berries were close contenders. But the habitual apple consumers had the lowest incidence of heart attacks, lung cancer, asthma, cataracts, type 2 diabetes, thrombotic strokes, and cancer at all sites.[406]

What magic substances do apples provide? It remains unproven, but a different study suggested that the nutrients contained in apples offer the best antioxidants available. (*Oxidation* is the word used to describe a chemical reaction in which oxygen is added to an element or a compound, generating a process that "ages" tissue. Antioxidants are substances that inhibit the destructive effects of oxidation.) Using chemical methods detailed in their scientific paper, researchers tested how much oxidation could be prevented by various known antioxidants.[27] The apple source of antioxidants was the winner. Next best was estrogen. An apple a day may well keep your doctor away, with no side effects, only good eating.

Whole Grains

A whole grain consists of the bran, the germ, and the endosperm. The bran and the germ contain many nutrients and phytochemicals (plant chemicals that affect metabolism), whereas the endosperm is largely starch and provides mostly energy (calories).[742] When you buy packaged cookies, crackers, bread, cereal, or pasta, the chances are good that you are buying a "refined" grain. A refined grain contains only the endosperm and so provides fewer nutrients and phytochemicals than the whole grain does. Use the label to identify the healthier options. The label should start with the word *whole*, not *enriched* or *multi*. Enriching a product removes the whole grain and adds preservatives, artificial colors, sugars, and salt to restore flavor and extend shelf life. Although enriched grain will enrich the seller, it may not enrich your health.

In the United States, adults typically consume 5.7 servings of refined grains each day and 1 serving of whole grain; the *reverse* is best to maintain good health. People in experiments who increased their whole-grain consumption over 4 to 8 weeks experienced beneficial outcomes. They significantly lowered their fasting insulin, their total and low density lipoprotein (LDL) cholesterol, and their blood pressure.

Another benefit to decreasing your consumption of processed foods and increasing your intake of fresh fruits and vegetables is that you'll guard against developing a potassium deficiency.[323] The refining process removes potassium, a vitamin that's vital for bones, the cardiovascular system, and kidney function. Currently, for people in most Western countries, their average potassium levels are less than one-third of what is needed for good health. Replace processed foods with whole foods, and you will benefit.

What else are whole grains good for?

- *Weight loss:* A woman's weight gain over a twenty-year period can be predicted simply by knowing what kind of grains she regularly consumed. This was reported in the huge Nurses Health Study, which enrolled women (registered nurses) who provided continuing information about their health and habits from 1976 on.[460] You probably won't be surprised that overall, the women gained weight as they aged. What was intriguing was the degree of gain. The higher the level of whole grains in the diet (see table 4.1), the lower the body mass index; the converse was also found. The higher the *refined* grain grams per day, the greater the weight gain.[460] (Eight grams is "high.") The old distinctions of soluble and insoluble fiber, however, have turned out to be less important.[98, 680]

- *Longevity:* Other large groups of women have provided similar data for specific diseases that are now associated with being

Table 4.1 Great and Not-So-Great Grains

Food	One Serving	Fiber Assignment (grams/serving)
Whole Grain—Life Giving		
Bran	1 tablespoon	1.5
Brown rice	1 cup	3.3
Cooked oatmeal	1 cup	4.0
Dark bread	1 slice	1.1
Popcorn	1 cup	1.1
Whole-grain breakfast cereal	1 cup	≥3.0
Wheat germ	1 tablespoon	0.9
Other grains (e.g., bulgur, kasha)	1 cup	3.2
Refined Grain—Life Depleting		
English muffins, bagels, or rolls	1	1.3
Muffins or biscuits	1	2.0
Pancakes or waffles	1 serving	2.0
Pasta	1 cup	2.2
Pizza	2 slices	5.2
Refined-grain breakfast cereal	1 cup	≤2.5
Sweets/desserts		
Cookies	1	0.6
Brownies	1 usual piece	0.7
Doughnuts	1	0.8
Home-baked cakes	1 slice	0.5
Pie	1 slice	2.2
Ready-made cakes	1 slice	1.1
White bread, including pita bread	1 slice	0.6
White rice	1 cup	1.0

Adapted from D. R. Jacobs, M. A. Pereira, K. A. Meyer, and L. H. Kushi (2000): Fiber from Whole Grains, but Not Refined Grains, Is Inversely Associated with All-Cause Mortality in Older Women: the Iowa Women's Health Study, *American Journal of Clinical Nutrition* 19(3):326S–330S.

overweight. In the Iowa Women's Health Study, after eight years of following 42,000 women's health outcomes, it was found that habitual consumption of whole grain foods was associated with a reduced risk of mortality from any cause. Also, living with and suffering from cancer and coronary heart disease were much less likely in the group that had a habit of eating whole grains. In contrast, these causes of death and disease tended to increase in people whose diets were high in refined grains.

- *A healthier heart:* In the Iowa study, to qualify for the highest whole-grain consumption a woman needed to consume only about three servings per day; the lowest category contained women who reported eating only one serving every five days. Death from ischemic heart disease was half the rate in those who ate the highest versus the lowest amounts of whole-grains.[376] Women eating adequate amounts of whole grains tended to have other healthier behaviors, too. Table 4.1 shows the whole grains and the refined grains that are typically available in supermarkets.

Your intake of whole grains can make a difference in your health. Pizza may have lots of fiber, but it's also a refined grain, so don't eat it every day—and tell your teenager!

Dairy Products

Your nervous system thrives on calcium. Adequate calcium in the colon helps sop up dangerous chemicals and with adequate habitual use appears to help prevent colon cancer.[326] Adequate dietary calcium can cut the risk of breast cancer, too.[700]

The amount of calcium you need depends on your hormone condition.

- *If you have the estrogen levels of a fertile, nonpregnant woman* (see table 3.1 in chapter 3), you need at least 800 milligrams per day.

- *If you are a postmenopausal woman who is taking hormones* so that you circulate fertile levels, then your calcium need would be about the same, 800 milligrams per day.

- *If you are postmenopausal and your estrogen levels are low* because you're not on hormone therapy (see table 3.1, in chapter 3, to compare yours), you need much more calcium—between 1,200 and 1,500 milligrams per day.

Calcium from Food Is Better Than Calcium from Pills

Getting your calcium from food seems to offer better health benefits than getting your calcium from supplements.[877] Why? Apparently, milk contains bioactive substances that are not found in the supplements. Perhaps the whey (the watery liquid that separates from the solid part of milk when it turns sour) augments the effects of calcium. Table 4.2, "Calcium Values of Common Food Sources," shows some good food sources of calcium.

Table 4.2 Calcium Values of Common Food Sources[168]

Food	Portion	Calories	Calcium (milligrams)
Cereals, Cooked			
Barley or rice cereal	¾ cup	108	188
Oatmeal or mixed cereal	¾ cup	110	188
Dairy Products			
American cheese	1 ounce	107	195
Cheddar cheese	1 ounce	112	211
Cottage cheese, creamed	1 cup	239	211
Edam cheese	1 ounce	87	225
Swiss cheese	1 ounce	104	259
Ice cream (chocolate)	1/6 quart	174	131
Ice milk (vanilla)	1/6 quart	136	189
Buttermilk, from skim	1 cup	88	296
Skim milk	1 cup	89	303
Whole milk, 3.5 percent fat	1 cup	159	288
Vanilla pudding	½ cup	139	146
Yogurt from skim with nonfat milk solids	1 cup	127	452
Goat milk	1 cup	163	315
Eggs			
Scrambled, with milk and fat	1 medium	112	52
Fish and Shellfish			
Flounder	3 ounces	61	55
Mackerel, canned	3½ ounces	192	194
Oysters, raw	5–8 medium	66	94
Sardines, canned	8 medium	311	354

(*Continued*)

Table 4.2. (*Continued*)

Food	Portion	Calories	Calcium (milligrams)
Scallops, cooked	3½ ounces	112	115
Shrimp, raw	3½ ounces	91	63
Fruits and Seeds			
Figs, dried	5 medium	274	126
Orange	1 medium	73	62
Sunflower seeds	3½ ounces	560	120
Syrups and Sweets			
Blackstrap molasses	1 tablespoon	43	116
Maple sugar	4 pieces (2" × 1")	348	180
Chocolate candy	1 bar (2 ounces)	296	52
Beans			
Lima, green, cooked	6 tablespoons	111	47
Snap, green, cooked	1 cup	31	62
Wax, yellow, cooked	1 cup	22	50
Vegetables			
Artichoke	Edible part	44	51
Beet greens, cooked	½ cup	18	99
Broccoli, raw	1 stalk (5" long)	32	103
Broccoli, cooked	2/3 cup	26	88
Cabbage, Savoy, raw	2 cups, shredded	24	67
Chard, cooked	3/5 cup	18	73
Chicory	30–40 inner leaves	20	86
Collards, cooked	½ cup	29	152
Endive	20 long leaves	20	81
Escarole	4 large leaves	20	81
Fennel, raw	3½ ounces	28	100
Leeks	3–4 (5" long)	52	52
Lettuce, romaine	3½ ounces	18	68
Mustard greens, cooked	½ cup	23	138
Parsley, raw	3½ ounces	44	203
Parsnips, raw	½ large	76	50
Rutabagas, cooked	½ cup	35	59
Sweet potatoes, baked	1 large	254	72
Watercress, raw	3½ ounces	19	151

What Dairy Can Do for Your Health

Dietary calcium also decreases your risk for developing hypertension. The Dietary Approaches to Stop Hypertension (DASH) Study showed that by increasing their consumption of low-fat dairy products, fruits, and vegetables, people could often reduce their elevated blood-pressure levels. Adding low-fat dairy was substantially better than having the same diet without the dairy component.[875]

Eating *adequate* amounts of foods that contain calcium is also great for weight control, according to the results of a series of experiments reported by various researchers. Unfortunately the calcium in spinach and other green vegetables binds tightly to the fiber and does not absorb well. But calcium-fortified milk (which doubles the amount of calcium naturally found in milk) is even better than regular milk.[586] The basic idea is this: If you include abundant low-fat dairy foods in your otherwise healthy daily diet, you will be trim, as well as healthy.[327] And if you are overweight, you will find that by adding three servings a day of low-fat dairy foods to your daily reduced-calorie regimen, you are headed for substantial weight loss without pain.[327, 330, 874, 876]

Although high-calcium supplemented cereal and calcium carbonate pills were somewhat helpful in a reducing diet, adding real milk to the supplements doubled the rate of fat loss. This led researchers to suggest that milk proteins contain a yet-to-be-identified bioactive compound that may act synergistically with the calcium to lower the storage of fat in the body and increase fat burning.[874] I think this makes sense. Most women gain weight as they age, but those who have the habit of maintaining a high-calcium diet do not.[327]

Dr. Heaney found in his review of the role of calcium and weight management that a calcium habit keeps the weight down.[330] In other words, the more calcium a woman consumed, the trimmer was her body.

Not every study finds the benefits of calcium, but most of them do. An exception was the Honolulu Heart Study described earlier. Five years after that report on tofu, other scientists reviewing the data reported that heavy milk drinkers more than doubled their risk of developing Parkinson's disease.[591] But the authors concluded that neurotoxins from pesticide-laden food had affected the milk they were drinking (so perhaps this was also the case for tofu).

The risk of developing breast cancer was *much* lower in women who had a daily habit of ingesting at least 800 milligrams of calcium *from dairy sources* in the Nurses Health Study. They had one-third the risk, compared to those who consumed the least amount of calcium each day. Of 88,691 nurses, breast cancer had been diagnosed in less than 3 percent of them over the 16 years they were analyzed.[700] Cancer is reduced in women who drink skim milk, eat yogurt, and enjoy a high-dairy calcium habit. Vitamin D is also involved in these outcomes.

The foods I've just highlighted should be part of every woman's diet, her complementary health practices. But those are simply individual foods. How should a health-minded woman eat on a daily basis?

The Upside of Lactose Intolerance

Lactose intolerance is an enzyme-deficiency condition in which the milk *sugar* cannot be digested. The majority of adults who have not recently been drinking milk will experience digestive distress (gas, bloating) when they first resume. If this happens to you, know that the distress eventually vanishes if you start slowly. (Or eat yogurt instead of drinking milk; the problem does not occur with yogurt.) But the digestive gassiness you may experience has a health benefit: while you may be feeling inner turmoil, the calcium is being beaten into the walls of the intestine and is absorbed better than with an undisturbed intestine.[168] Sometimes chaos generates good results.

Wholesome Eating Plans

The Mediterranean diet represents a healthful way to eat that helps you feel good and age slowly, while preventing many common devastating diseases.

What's on the menu? This pattern of eating includes a high intake of vegetables, legumes, fruit and nuts, cereals, and olive oil; a low intake of saturated lipids; a moderately high intake of fish; a low to moderate intake of dairy products (mostly in the form of cheese and yogurt); a low intake of meat and poultry; and a regular moderate intake of alcohol, primarily in the form of wine and generally with meals.

News about the benefits of adhering to a Mediterranean diet and its effect on longevity in a Greek population was reported in the prestigious *New England Journal of Medicine* in 2003.[783] Starting in 1994, researchers assessed adherence to the Mediterranean diet using a 10-point scale in 22,000 people. They found that the higher the degree of adherence, the lower the total mortality rate. The health advantages were shown by the decrease in deaths due to both coronary heart disease and cancer. All ages that were studied saw benefits within four years. The study discovered that no individual food was responsible for the improvement in health. A pattern of well-rounded eating was necessary to produce the benefits.

The Healthy Aging Study found similar results in its ongoing study, which followed 1,507 men and women 70 to 90 years old, in 11 European countries. When the researchers analyzed the 935 people who had died versus those who were still alive after 10 years, they found that the group with a healthy lifestyle had less than *half* the death rate of the other group. Their healthy habits included adhering to the Mediterranean diet, engaging in moderate physical activity, having moderate alcohol use, and not smoking. People who followed these behaviors most closely had a little over one-third (35 percent) the likelihood of succumbing to any disease, including coronary heart disease, cardiovascular disease, and various cancers, in comparison to people who did not adhere to the behaviors as faithfully.[407]

Other studies, testing specific diseases, point to the same conclusions as those from the Healthy Aging Study. Let's review them:

- Maintaining a healthy blood pressure. In 40- to 75-year-olds, blood pressure was shown to dramatically drop (without use of drugs) within two weeks of changing from an unhealthy diet to the combination diet, which was rich in fruits, vegetables, and dairy products that were low in saturated and total fats.[323]

- Protecting your eyesight. The Nurses Health Study of 121,700 registered nurses and the Health Profession Follow-Up Study, which enrolled 51,529 male health professionals ages 40–75, found that "neovascular age-related maculopathy" (leading to loss of vision) was significantly reduced by the habit of eating at least three fruits a day.[141] The study is important because it establishes that long-term regular fruit intake can help preserve good eyesight in both women and men. The study also tested whether pills or supplements would show similar findings, and it reported a clear "no."

Eating well is only part of the healthy living equation for women.[142] The other major factor is regular physical activity. Let's look at what fitness can do for you.

Exercise: The Real Fountain of Youth

Regular appropriate physical activity is safe and effective in promoting good health.[530] It makes you feel good and happy. It increases muscle and bone strength and lowers the proportion of body fat. And it lowers the risk of death from diabetes, hypertension, and colon cancer.[477] Although moderate-intensity aerobic exercise of 30 minutes a day did not reduce the severity or the frequency of hot flashes in a randomized controlled trial, it did reduce memory lapses in postmenopausal women 50 to 75 years old who had been sedentary and overweight.[7] And it also reduced the likelihood of developing memory problems by 88 percent in older (ages 85 and older) people.[756] Sitting on your couch can't do that for you.

Increasing your physical activity is an important goal, regardless of your current state of health. It improves your capacity to take in oxygen, which increases your lifespan. Technically, this is measured as "VO2 max" or maximum volume of oxygen.[477]

What ultimately ends an undiseased life is inadequate VO2 max. In other words, when you cannot deliver adequate oxygen (VO2), your body will expire. You should exercise every day to maintain a healthy VO2.

One study showed greater elasticity in the large carotid artery of postmenopausal women who were without obvious cardiovascular disease and who habitually exercised compared to sedentary women.[530] This finding is especially important for *pre*menopausal women because it suggests that it is possible to prevent the postmenopausal loss of elasticity of this large artery.

An active life is always better than a sedentary life. Even for people who had cardiovascular disease, CDC data revealed that those who were active had 40 percent lower annual medical expenses than did inactive people: $3,784 versus $6,313.[814] (This analysis was done in 2003, reflecting 2003 prices; the totals would be much higher today.)

What Physical Activity Can Do for You

Many studies have been published showing that one or another type of regular physical activity produces extraordinary benefits.

It makes you happier. About 30 minutes a day of any combination of activities, such as walking, swimming, wielding a broom, or raking leaves produced a healthier and happier life among a group of 249 women who were 59 to 84 years old.[506] That's a relatively small investment for such an important payback.

Regular exercise helps you battle the bulge. Unfortunately, two-thirds of adult American women are overweight (with a BMI of 25 or higher), with half of these being obese (having a BMI of 30 or higher).[567]

Table 4.3 lets you calculate your own body mass index. To use the table, first find your height in the far left column. Then move right across the row until you find your weight. The magic number is lower than 25, because 25 marks the beginning of "overweight" scores.

The good news is that you absolutely can prevent weight gain during menopause. When 500 women were enrolled in a healthy lifestyle project over 5 years to test whether weight gain was inevitable, the answer was a resounding "no." Contrary to the general U.S. trend of weight gain with age, more than half of the group had a *lower* weight 5 years later than when they enrolled.[710]

Where You Should Start

If you've never exercised before, take it easy and start slowly. Avoid injury by listening to your body and not pushing it harder than it wants to go. Make a small investment in a fitness evaluation at your local gym or YMCA. Two activities that are very accessible and user friendly are walking and tai chi. (Personally, I am a big fan of walking, tai chi, and swimming, and I do some of each activity almost every day.)

Walking is easy, needs no special equipment (aside from a supportive pair of shoes), and can be done anywhere. Walking is a great way to get into the exercise habit. You'll feel and see results rapidly. Among 27 sedentary postmenopausal women, only 6 weeks of walking, 5 days a week, 30 minutes a day, improved their psychological health, as measured in attitude, depression scores, fear of illness, and sense of well-being.[28]

You'll probably stick to it. Walking 5 days per week for 15 weeks at 65 percent of maximal aerobic power proved effective in a Scandinavian

Table 4.3 The Body Mass Index Table

	BMI								
	22	23	24	25	26	27	28	29	30
				(overweight)					(obese)
Height				**Weight** *(lbs)*					
5'0"	112	118	123	128	133	138	143	148	153
5'1"	116	122	127	132	137	143	148	153	158
5'2"	120	126	131	136	142	147	153	158	164
5'3"	124	130	135	141	146	152	158	163	169
5'4"	128	134	140	145	151	157	163	169	174
5'5"	132	138	144	150	156	162	168	174	180
5'6"	136	142	148	155	161	167	173	179	186
5'7"	140	146	153	159	166	172	178	185	191
5'8"	144	151	158	164	171	177	184	190	197
5'9"	149	155	162	169	176	182	189	196	203
5'10"	153	160	167	174	181	188	195	202	209
5'11"	157	165	172	179	186	193	200	208	215
6'0"	162	169	177	184	191	199	206	213	221
6'1"	166	174	182	189	197	204	212	219	227
6'2"	171	179	186	194	202	210	218	225	233
6'3"	176	184	192	200	208	216	224	232	240
6'4"	180	189	197	205	213	221	230	238	246

This table translates the units used to calculate BMI (cm and kg^2) into the units familiar to Americans (feet, inches, and pounds). To use the table, first find your height in the far left column. Then move right across the row until you find your weight. The number at the top of the column indicates your BMI.

study of 134 postmenopausal women. Again, it also had a high completion rate: 130 of these 134 women completed the 15-week program. There were only 4 dropouts in 15 weeks! *Amazing.*

You can do it your way. You don't have time to walk 30 minutes continuously? Then break it up into two 15-minute or three 10-minute bouts. The Scandinavian study also showed that it did not matter how the woman chose to break up her exercise assignment. Exercise improved the maximal aerobic power and the body composition equally when the exercise was done either all at once or divided into two daily sessions.[29]

Tai chi has its origins in martial arts. It is slow-moving (it's been called "poetry in motion") but powerful. The practice emphasizes correct form—no slouching!—and involves shifting weight from one leg to another, flexing joints, and extending your arms and legs, all of which improve your strength and balance. Again, you'll find you want to stick with it. Women enjoy these classes. (I have!)

You'll see benefits fast. People see good results as early as three months after starting, with continued improvements at six months. Tai chi produces a clear improvement in physical functioning, especially in balance control. If you can keep your balance, you prevent falls and breaking a bone. Tai chi is a marvelous and inexpensive activity whose tested low-intensity motions enhance your life quality and independence without your risking injury.[450]

How much exercise do you need? For how long do you need to work out? Set a goal of 210 minutes a week for your exercise requirements, and break it up any way you like. Half of all causes of mortality in the United States are linked to social and behavioral factors, such as smoking, diet, alcohol use, accidents, and a sedentary lifestyle.[726] This means you have enormous power to choose behaviors that could prevent such a chain of events.

One Habit to Kick

Various methods have been studied to help people learn how to correct bad habits.[800] As with exercise, whether you get started on your own or in a group that meets on a regular basis, you can learn what your bad habits are and can change them. People who enroll in tailored diet and exercise intervention programs that employ willpower and energy, rather than a drug, are highly successful.[800] People can choose good habits. Reject bad ones, especially the worst habit of all: smoking.

Lung cancer is now the leading form of cancer deaths among women. And 90 percent of all cancer deaths are attributed to smoking.[625] But did you know that smoking also increases your risk for developing cervical cancer? That's the case whether you are a smoker or are exposed to passive "secondary" smoke in your home or workplace.[784] Other bad news about smoking and health: If you smoke and take oral hormone therapy (HT), your blood levels of estradiol will be lower, even inadequate. So, if a woman is a smoker and is taking HT, she should not take it orally.[79, 769]

By now, we all recognize smoking for the painful addiction it is. But you can fight it yourself. Studies comparing the widely marketed nicotine patches did not find better long-term outcomes than those produced by a placebo; the relapse rate was the same.

Instead of feeling as if you are giving up smoking, think about how you are giving a gift to your body by gaining oxygen, energy, strength, and life.

A Trick to Quit Smoking

Every time you feel a craving, you can use this trick to fight back: Slowly inhale the air just as you used to inhale the tobacco. Take a deep breath (a deep drag) as you draw the oxygen into your lungs. Hold the air in your lungs for a count of 5, and then slowly let it out. Take as many "drags" as you need, and feel the craving vanish temporarily. Then drink 3 to 4 ounces of tart grapefruit juice or eat half of a small grapefruit. This will help convert the feeling of intense irritability and anger (caused by withdrawal from the addiction) into an amazing burst of energy. Use that energy to clean up a room or clean out a closet as you simultaneously "clean out" your blood. Doing so will help you fight the cravings, which will subside in time, and you'll begin to feel as clean inside as your home is.

Two Supplements to Consider

Vitamin D is extensively reviewed in chapter 8 because of its essential role in maintaining strong bones. But, like all other nutrients, what is good for one part of the body is often good for many other parts, and it's worth going into here. Vaginal dryness and painful intercourse often accompany hot flashes. Vitamin D can make a vital difference.

Vitamin C also has many benefits in 500 milligram maximum doses. This amount appears to be the limit that your body can absorb per hour when you're under stress or to promote rapid healing.[168, 344]

Its antioxidant power has long been recognized, and it is reviewed in chapter 9.

The D Difference

We have to ingest other vitamins, but D is a vitamin that your body makes. In nature, sunlight shining on bare skin starts the manufacturing process. On a summer day, if you expose your whole body to the sun for 15 minutes, and you are younger than 60 years of age and in good health, your skin will absorb the ultraviolet B (UVB) radiation. After age 60, the process becomes less efficient; so we probably need even more UVB. For all ages, sunlight will jump-start the body's chemical manufacturing process, which converts its own cholesterol into a substance that travels through the bloodstream and stops at the kidneys for additional metabolic conversion. Ultimately, the pre–vitamin D becomes the active form, which attaches to receptors to do its work. This biologically active form is called vitamin D3, or vitamin D for short. Sunlight is life giving!

Apparently, estrogen and vitamin D work together to maintain healthy vaginal tissue. If you're lacking in either the hormone or the vitamin, your vaginal tissue is likely to be dried out and easily torn or bruised.[866]

Unfortunately, serum vitamin D inadequacy is pervasive in the United States, putting women at risk for developing diseases such as osteoporosis, diabetes, and breast and colon cancer. The Framingham Study, which followed thousands of healthy people in Massachusetts for many years, found that those who had deficiently low levels of serum vitamin D had three times the risk of developing osteoarthritis—a common problem for large numbers of people.[37]

The same study did not report on vaginal atrophy, but I think it likely they would have found it among the women with osteoarthritis. The take-home message for now is that you should probably be taking a vitamin D3 capsule or tablet every day, and at least 1,000 IU is the minimum effective dose for women over the age of 40. There are no adverse effects (at levels even 4 times higher) but many benefits.

Taking glucosamine sulfate to reduce the progression of osteoarthritis has been proven to be effective and safe. As an example, 319 women (over age 45, all postmenopausal, not on HT, and with primary knee osteoarthritis for 2 years) orally took either a placebo or a once-a-day formulation of 1,500 milligrams of a glucosamine sulfate powder solution. Results showed that this formulation was effective at reducing the joint space and (in consequence) the severity of pain from progressing.[99] A different researcher summarized the results of 15 studies that had altogether enrolled 1,775 patients: 1,020 people took glucosamine sulfate and 775 took chondroitin sulfate.[646] As quickly as 2 weeks after treatment was initiated with both supplements, an improvement in symptoms (versus a placebo) had been objectively demonstrated. Both substances are well tolerated and are widely sold over the counter with apparent safety.

If you suffer from joint stiffness and pain and are not allergic to shellfish, which is the source of these supplements, you should discuss them with your doctor and consider trying them.

Other Complementary Practices

Acupuncture has begun to show some promise in treating hot flashes, in university-based research conducted at Stanford and Harvard. Women suffering from more than six hot flashes per day underwent individualized acupuncture treatment. As a control, half of the group underwent a "sham" acupuncture procedure where needles appeared to be inserted but did not penetrate the skin. Genuine acupuncture performed better than sham acupuncture. The severity of the hot flashes was modestly reduced (28 percent reduction), and this was significantly better than the outcome from the sham procedure.[364] No other acupuncture benefit over a placebo was demonstrated in quality of life or sleep improvement, only for hot flashes. This very modest improvement was confirmed by another investigator, but it is in direct contrast to the near-perfect results from estradiol treatment.[859]

Sedatives and antidepressants are not recommended to treat menopausal symptoms. The first actual randomized controlled trial of these drugs in 150 women showed results no better than those of a placebo.[759]

Behavioral Programs

You can also join a group under the guidance of a learned leader who helps you evaluate and improve your health habits. You can find such programs locally at health centers, health clubs, and YMCAs or through group affiliations you may have at work or in your community. A good example of a successful program is the Mediterranean Lifestyle Program (which, as its name implies, focuses on the eating habits of the Greeks). The program was tested with 279 postmenopausal women.[780] They enjoyed it so much, they kept coming after the study ended. And once they were engaged, their health inevitably improved. The program enrolled women in waves (groups) and began with a two-and-a-half-day nonresidential retreat, then weekly four-hour meetings to cycle through one hour each of physical activity, stress management, Mediterranean potluck meals, and a support group. The program consistently reduced risk factors for coronary heart disease by addressing stress management, weight loss, and physical activity, and this improvement translated to better health, both physically and mentally.

Mindfulness-Based Stress Reduction programs for hot flashes are now widely available in the United States and have shown about a 40 percent reduction in the severity of flashes compared to a placebo. This is a small effect, nothing like the 95 percent benefit of hormones. Mindfulness is defined as a state of sustained attention to ongoing mental contents and processes (physical sensations, perceptions, affective states, thoughts, and imagery). Mindfulness is also an essential part of cognitive-behavioral therapy, but unlike this therapy, no attempt is made to change or modify thoughts. Women who had more than six hot flashes per day, of moderate to severe intensity, showed a 40 percent reduction in the overall severity of their hot flashes, which was slightly greater than the 20 to 30 percent placebo effect that was expected.[115] Your state of mind *is* relevant to your health.

Conclusion

It is rewarding to take action to promote your good health. Become responsible for your journey. When you face decisions about complementary health products and practices, you do it *alone*—without your physician, who is licensed to practice medicine. So be skeptical when you read claims of product ads that are not rational. If the use of the product or the practice seems clearly invasive, it would be wise to consult a physician before you try it. If it's noninvasive, such as yoga-type breathing or stretching exercises, try it. See how it feels. Listening to your body and the signals it sends is a high art that can promote your well-being. Pay attention to how the exercise and the foods you choose affect your body, and you will learn how to get moving and choose life-giving habits.

5

Pelvic Problems: Bleeding and Pain—Hyperplasia, Cervical Cancer, and Endometriosis

W HAT DOES IT MEAN WHEN YOUR uterus or pelvic organs send out distress signals, such as unexpected bleeding or pain with intercourse? It means you must take action to find the cause.

Unexpected Vaginal Bleeding

For every menstruating woman, bleeding is a fact of life; it's healthy, functional bleeding—it has a purpose. Bleeding that is *not* expected is labeled dysfunctional. Dysfunctional uterine bleeding (DUB) is also called abnormal uterine bleeding, excessive menstrual bleeding, or menorrhagia (heavy menstrual bleeding). The good news is that abrupt changes in the length of the monthly cycle are often normal. Sudden changes in your sex life (ending a relationship or starting one after a time of celibacy) can cause hormonal and bleeding changes, but that has to do with the rhythm of your sex life, not with an underlying pathology.[169]

Aging can also bring changes: hormonal secretion from your ovaries triggers a variety of normal changes in blood flow, timing, duration, and character, beginning around age 43 until menopause. All are part of the expected pattern of the change of life. And hormonal

77

therapy regimens themselves generate their own patterns of "normal withdrawal bleeding." But unexpected bleeding can also be a signal of disease and/or endocrine dysfunction. When you don't know why you're experiencing the bleeding, you need to consult your doctor.

As women approach menopause, their last 60 menstrual cycles normally contain a wide variety of cycle lengths.[104] It is not unusual for the last cycles to range from 10 days to 20, 30, or even 60 days from the onset of one bleeding sequence to the onset of the next. Again, most unexpected bleeding is not caused by any pathology. A prescription for sequential HRT can often regularize this pattern.

How much blood loss is abnormal? You would have to lose at least 80 millileters (5.3 tablespoons) per cycle. Frankly, you won't be measuring your flow, but you'll know that it's too much or too heavy if you have accidents in public, can't leave the house, or otherwise lose control of your personal hygiene.[657] Schedule a thorough medical evaluation and screening to rule out four potential causes. All of them need to be checked because more than one cause can coexist.

- Anatomical causes, such as fibroids, polyps, or endometrial hyperplasia

- Systemic (bodywide) causes, such as blood disorders or thyroid, liver, or renal disease

- Iatrogenic causes, the inadvertent result of your current medical treatment. Anticoagulants, tamoxifen, glucocorticoids, intrauterine devices (IUDs), certain herbal remedies. and steroid regimens can all trigger bleeding

- Hormonal causes, which are usually due to your ovaries not producing enough progesterone to stabilize the lining of the uterus

Fibroids occur in 80 percent of women and are a common cause of bleeding. They're discussed in chapter 7.

Blood disorders can cause abnormal bleeding. The most common is Von Willenbrand's disease, which is found in 13 percent of women who experience heavy uterine bleeding.[544] Symptoms that suggest this disease include easy bruising, frequent gum bleeds when flossing, one or two nose bleeds per month, and excessive bleeding at childbirth, tooth extraction, and/or surgery.[416]

If you have any of these symptoms along with abnormal vaginal bleeding, you need to locate a specialized center that has expert knowledge of blood disorders. It has been well documented that many analytical errors have been made by medical offices that do not specialize in blood disorders, so you will want to avoid the possibility of a misdiagnosis.[383, 416] Your gynecologist should be able to recommend a specialized center.

Insist on a thorough screening for any blood disorders. Recent evidence indicates that in a group of women diagnosed as having "ovulatory dysfunctional uterine bleeding," as many as 10 to 15 percent actually have a systemic blood disorder.[248] Other rarer blood abnormalities include:

- Platelet abnormalities
- Thrombocytopenias (abnormal decrease in platelet numbers)
- Thrombocytopathies (deficient function)
- Leukemias
- Coagulation factor deficiencies, such as vitamin K deficiency
- Congenital disorders
- Effects of using anticoagulants[248]

Other systemic problems that are associated with heavy bleeding include:

- *Thyroid anomalies.* These can be evaluated with blood tests for the thyroid hormone screening (TSH screening) that may reveal abnormal thyroid hormone levels. A reproductive endocrinologist can help you.
- *Anovulation (absence of ovulation).* This is identified when blood tests reveal an absence of progesterone in the 4 to 10 days before menses. An appropriately timed prescription for progesterone helps normalize such bleeding if you are still premenopausal.
- *Vitamin A deficiency.* This can cause heavy menstrual bleeding. Vitamin A supplements of 25,000 IU twice daily resolved problems within 2 weeks in 37 of 40 bleeders after blood tests revealed deficiencies.[457] Supplementation of this magnitude should not be done without a physician's guidance.

Medical Evaluation of the Uterus

Assess any hormonal influences on your body. Endometrial hyperplasia (*hyper*, "excess tissue," that is showing *plasia* or "growth") is a common uterine response to imbalance in estrogen-progesterone levels. It is a condition that you want to resolve. This is diagnosed under a microscope with an endometrial sample, taken either during an office biopsy or an operative D&C (dilation of the cervix and curettage).

Endometrial hyperplasia can occur during the menopause transition years if progesterone levels diminish *before* estrogen begins its menopausally related decline. Similarly, unbalanced HRT regimens can do the same. If progesterone is rebalanced, the hyperplasia will almost always "revert" to normal tissue. Unfortunately, after a number of years of uncorrected hyperplasia, a small percentage (estimated at 3 to 7 percent) of the tissue will become dangerously plastic and can subsequently develop cancer.[168]

Your First Meeting with Your Gynecologist: What to Expect

Dr. Millicent Zacher, of Thomas Jefferson University, noted that before procedures are done to determine the causes of worrisome bleeding, the first step is undergoing a good exam by your gynecologist. Given the limited amount of time with your doctor, you want to use it efficiently. Before the exam, prepare:

- A short list of concerns; a calendar clearly noting when and how much bleeding has occurred
- Copies of any previous records, laboratory reports, and write-ups of other procedures you have had done
- Written histories of your past medical, surgical, and gynecological care
- Relevant family history, such as cancers

Expect a complete gynecological exam, including a Pap smear (even if you've just had one) and possibly an office ultrasound. A complete blood count and a thyroid evaluation will be done. At the conclusion of the visit, you and your doctor should have a brief discussion of possible treatment. You may also be given Internet sites or reading materials for further clarification. Occasionally, your doctor will take an endometrial biopsy (a sample from the lining of the uterus) at this visit if she concludes that immediate treatment is needed.

Transvaginal ultrasound is a pain-free method of seeing into the uterus. The clinician inserts a wand vaginally to slowly scan the tissue. She views the uterus lining (endometrium) and the muscular walls (myometrium). If the lining appears too thick for the time in your cycle or menopause, then an endometrial sample can be biopsied. Biopsies tested in women with normal bleeding and using HRT sequential regimens showed ultrasound thickness between 3 and 10 millimeters deep, and all typically revealed normal cells.[173]

Saline-infused ultrasound, also called a sonohysterogram or SIS (saline-infused sonography), is often the next step in evaluating abnormal bleeding. The procedure images the uterus and the uterine cavity using vaginal ultrasound after sterile saline is used to inflate the uterine cavity. It can often be done in your gynecologist's office with minimal discomfort. (See www.ASRM.org, the American Society for Reproductive Medicine, for more on this procedure.)

A hysteroscopy may follow the SIS if more data are needed. A hysteroscopy visualizes the cervical canal and the uterine endometrium (*endo* for "inside" or "within"; *metrium*, "the womb"). The fiber-optic instrument is inserted vaginally, then channeled into the cervical canal. A tenaculum, a grasping tool, is used to grip the cervix and to hold the uterus still so that the hysteroscope can get into the cervical canal.

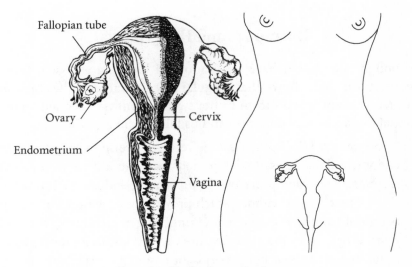

Figure 5.1. The female reproductive organs.

What You Should Know about Hysteroscopy

- There's an ouch factor. The tight grasping by the tenaculum is intensely painful for women who are estrogen-rich, probably because of numerous nerve endings located in the cervical tissue.[81] Postmenopausal women who are low in estrogen do not feel such severe pain.[663] If you are estrogen-rich and plan on having this procedure done, you should ask for a painkilling drug.

- A hysteroscopy can be pain free. In a 2006 publication, a newer *flowing saline* method was advocated. Basically, saline replaces the tenaculum. Dr. Ron Sagiv and his colleagues reported on 130 procedures that compared this new method *without* anesthesia to the original procedure using Novocain. The new flowing saline procedure was significantly less painful *without* anesthesia than the tenaculum-grasping procedure *with* Novocain.[663]

Once bleeding is diagnosed, it can often be corrected with a hormone therapy prescription. A helpful resource, "When Disease Strikes," from my book *Hysterectomy: Before and After* provides extensive information to help women avoid unnecessary hysterectomies.[168] Unfortunately, the regrettable situation in the United States as late as 2005 was that only half of the cases of excessive bleeding were diagnosed *before* a hysterectomy was undertaken to stop the bleeding.[473]

Hormones and Hyperplasia

Although you should have any abnormal bleeding assessed, several recent studies have shown that irregular bleeding, amenorrhea (absence of menstruation), and spotting after twelve months of sequential hormonal therapies were common and usually without pathology.

Sequential HRT regimens. One research group in Italy tested the endometrial thickness and reported that four different sequential regimens were each protective in preventing endometrial hyperplasia.[211] These varied regimens each provided a progestin for ten days per month and an estrogen daily, mimicking nature during the fertile years. When the ultrasound measure was this low (6 millimeters), the result showed *normal,* nonhyperplastic tissue (it revealed normal proliferative or secretory cells when studied under the microscope.)[173]

Another group in Italy examined different regimens among its patients. "Abnormal bleeding" occurred in 119 of the 585 women. For continuous-combined regimens where progestin is taken every day with estrogen, *abnormal bleeding* was defined as *any* bleeding after six months. For a sequential regimen, *abnormal bleeding* was defined as bleeding occurring at the wrong time: either before or more than seven days after taking the last progestin for that cycle. Biopsy results were reassuring. Subsequent ultrasounds measuring the thickness of the lining and the biopsy analysis revealed that *simple hyperplasia* occurred in only 13 of these 119 "abnormally bleeding" women. Biopsy revealed *complex hyperplasia,* the more dangerous version, in only 4 of the 119. No evidence of cancer or atypia (precancerous cells) was found among any of these abnormal bleeders.[574] So, biopsies showed no demonstrable pathology in 96 percent of the women with abnormal bleeding. "Abnormal" rarely meant "diseased."

Different progestins, the same estrogen. A third group, in California, randomly assigned 596 women (45 to 65 years old) into different regimens to compare unexpected bleeding among sequential versus continuous-combined regimens. The study tested different progestins but used only conjugated equine estrogen (such as Premarin).[452]

The fewest cases of unexpected bleeding (2 percent) occurred in the sequential users of bioidentical micronized progesterone. Next lowest (7 percent) were the sequential users of a synthetic progestin MPA (medroxyprogesterone acetate) with their Premarin. Unopposed estrogen caused unexpected bleeding in 40 percent of the women, and continuous-combined Prempro caused unexpected bleeding in 37 percent of women in this 36-month study. That's one of many reasons that I believe women are best served by sequential hormone therapy regimens, rather than continuous-combined regimens.

Some hormonal regimens are better able than others to prevent hyperplasia. Consistent results have appeared for more than twenty years since the discoveries pioneered by Dr. R. Don Gambrell. Placebo users experienced more endometrial hyperplasia than did women using well-balanced, sequential hormone regimens. The optimal regimens had daily estrogen, balanced with progesterone or a synthetic progestin hormone used daily for only the last two weeks of each monthly cycle.[173, 313]

Short-term study: The first effort to conduct a randomized controlled investigation for short-term treatments of DUB was reported in 2006.[545] These were temporary, very high doses of either MPA (medroxyprogesterone acetate) or an oral contraceptive pill containing norethindrone and ethinyl estradiol.

The results: Within two weeks, both hormone regimens stopped unwanted bleeding in more than 75 percent of the forty women. The oral contraceptives (OC) group looked a bit better with a *cure* in 88 percent versus the MPA *cure* in 76 percent. Unfortunately, the oral contraceptives seemed to cause more side effects, such as nausea.

OC also can stop chronic abnormal bleeding. One study of women who had failed to experience benefits from the first OC they took showed that relief *could* be obtained by testing other OCs. According to researchers, "For women wishing to avoid a hysterectomy, continued efforts at medical treatment may bring substantial improvement in pelvic pain, pelvic/bladder pressure and stress incontinence with fewer days of restricted activity."[439]

Long-term study: Beginning in 2001, researchers in Japan tested an *intrauterine system* (IUS) containing a progestin (levonorgestrel) for long-term control to stop unwanted bleeding caused by various benign (noncancerous) conditions.

The results: Women could obtain relief from recurrent heavy bleeding associated with both fibroids and ingrowths of the endometrium into the uterine musculature (a benign condition called adenomyosis).[295, 435, 498] The hormone restored apoptosis (i.e., cell death, which stops runaway growth and proliferation).

The breast cancer drug tamoxifen produces a high incidence of endometrial hyperplasia.[782] In fact, 90 percent of the postmenopausal women who were taking a 20 milligram per day dose (and agreed to be evaluated) developed endometrial hyperplasia. If you are taking tamoxifen for breast issues, you need to discuss this with your physician.[125]

Surgical Management of Unwanted Bleeding

There are several competing technologies that do stop bleeding—in varying ways—by destroying the tissue. After an evaluation, a biopsy of the tissue to determine the presence of disease, and a diagnosis of your condition, your doctor can plan an effective treatment.

If you have simple hyperplasia, adenomatous (a more advanced stage of) hyperplasia, or endometrial cancer, you need to obtain a clear diagnosis. Otherwise, you might find yourself agreeing to a hysterectomy, only to discover later that your uterus had no disease.

"Endometrial ablation" technologies preserve the muscular (myometrial) portions of the uterus, while destroying the endometrial lining. This is done either with hot water contained in a balloon that shapes itself to the uterine cavity or by microwaves, electrical cautery, a laser, or cutting out the lining altogether. Left behind is a sealed-off scarred endometrial surface. No studies have examined whether these procedures alter the communication between the uterus and the ovary. A procedure that removes polyps can be followed by ablation. If you are not at risk for uterine cancer, it offers a good alternative to getting a hysterectomy.

What You Should Know about Endometrial Ablation

- Ablation destroys the uterine lining. It is not used if there is any cancer present. It doesn't work for uterine fibroids.

- It's not risk free. It requires local or general anesthesia, so factor in their potential side effects. It takes only twenty minutes and offers a fast recovery but can cause vaginal discharge for several weeks.[88]

- There are many ablation tools, but they have not been systematically compared to see which method is most effective with the least adverse effects.[383] Your doctor is likely to offer you the method that is available to her in the hospital where she operates and the one she is most experienced and comfortable with. Ask for published success rates of the method she uses and her own results. Here are your choices:

  Thermal balloon endometrial ablation is one method with a 90 percent success rate in one study, but it is not so good for women with blood disorders like Von Willenbrand's disease.[383] The first report of an acute hemorrhage treated this way appeared in 2002.[558]

  Microwave endometrial ablation, roller ball, and *resectoscope* are other ablation tools. These terms describe the energy source or tool.

A randomized controlled trial among fertile-age women with heavy menstrual bleeding compared 129 women who underwent microwave ablation to 134 who had a resection via electrocautery. Both methods successfully averted hysterectomies for close to 90 percent of the women. Menstrual symptoms were much improved at the follow-up two years after either procedure. Both procedures diminished pain in the pelvis and during menstruation, and caused no urinary deterioration or new symptoms of urinary incontinence.[43] These benefits are in direct contrast to a hysterectomy, which is known to increase the risk of incontinence. The microwave procedure under general anesthesia is computer-guided, with instantaneous feedback directing your surgeon where to obliterate endometrial tissue without damaging the uterine wall.

- There are potential side effects from the procedure. "Adhesions" are defined as connections between opposing surfaces of the internal organs and the abdominal wall at sites where there should be no connection.[311] They can cause pain and other problems. A research group found that 36 percent of 22 women had intrauterine adhesions 6 months after an endometrial ablation.[447] They also noted that relatively few long-term follow-up investigations had been conducted. Those follow-ups would be useful to help women and their physicians make good decisions about the risk of recurrence.[447]

Try the least-invasive procedure first, and only move to more drastic steps if the less-invasive ones fail. Ablation is less drastic than a hysterectomy.

Endometriosis: Pain in the Pelvis

One of the most common causes of pelvic pain is endometriosis, an estrogen-dependent disorder. It is the presence of uterine endometrial tissue (the tissue normally found lining the inner cavity of the uterus) growing outside of the uterus. Chronic pelvic pain that lasts for more than a year afflicts an estimated 15 to 20 percent of women between the ages of 18 and 50, while 6 to 10 percent of women in this age group are estimated to have endometriosis.[261] So pain does not necessarily indicate endometriosis, and endometriosis does not always cause pain. But for women suffering from long-term pelvic pain, a diagnostic search finds this disease in up to 50 percent of the cases.[35]

The causes of pain are elusive and can be mimicked by diseases other than endometriosis.[776] But pain (with intercourse, ovulation, or periods) drives women to seek help. For many women who subsequently were diagnosed with endometriosis, their pain had been incorrectly considered normal by family doctors.[46]

What Causes Endometriosis?

The origin of endometriosis is not known, but there are some good theories. One is that endometrial cells, regurgitated through the fallopian tubes and out into the spaces around the uterus, cause implantation of the endometrium onto tissue outside the uterus.[61] Take a look at figure 5.1 on page 81. When a uterus contracts during menstruation or orgasm, substances inside can exit in only three directions: down toward the vagina or up through the two fallopian tubes and then flowing out into the spaces around the ovaries, the surface of the uterus, and the outer membrane of the colon.

These endometrial cells can embed themselves where they do not belong. They can grow, shrink, and bleed just as endometrial cells within the uterus do under the influence of the ebb and flow of estrogen and progesterone each month.[9]

Studies have recorded rhythmic myometrial contractions ascending at ovulation and descending during menstruation.[501] I suspect that the purpose behind this part of nature's design is to drive sperm up the uterus during orgasmic contractions, into the fallopian tubes, where fertilization of the egg occurs. And muscular energy in reverse, down during menses, will drive the blood down and out through the vagina. You don't want the muscular contractions to move up when you are menstruating.[169] Orgasmic uterine contractions or penile thrusting against the cervix might drive the menstruating endometrial tissue the wrong way—up the fallopian tubes.[169] Compared to women who abstained from sex, women who engaged in it while menstruating had a significantly higher incidence of both endometriosis and unexplained heavy bleeding.[169] Coitus during menses is associated with endometriosis.[240] It would be good to avoid this behavior.

If you have endometriosis, you will need to see a gynecologist. The treatment of endometriosis accounts for 25 to 35 percent of all laparoscopies and 10 to 15 percent of all hysterectomies each year.[1]

Diagnose or Treat First?

In 2006, the Royal College of Obstetricians and Gynecologists recommended that patients with chronic pelvic pain (including those who are suspected of having endometriosis) receive medical therapy without a preliminary diagnostic laparoscopy.[261] The American Society for Reproductive Medicine stated, "Endometriosis is common and is found in 70 percent of patients who suffer from chronic pelvic pain. It can derive also from other disorders: GI, urinary, neurologic, musculoskeletal, psychological."[776] So, they say, treat first. For women who can safely take oral contraceptives, powerful arguments support trying them first. If the pain is relieved, it may be best not to look further because of the invasive nature of the diagnostic process and these surgical risks.[397, 776] The levonorgestrel-intrauterine system (IUS) has also been reported to provide significant relief from pain without the known side effects of stronger drugs.[276]

Passionate arguments in the scientific journals are being made for diagnosis first. For example, Ray Garry, MD, of King Edward Hospital in Western Australia, said, "It is a fundamental principle of medicine that an accurate diagnosis should be achieved as rapidly as possible before instituting the most appropriate therapy. . . . The diagnosis of endometriosis is a histologic one (i.e., diseased tissue is studied under the microscope)."[261] Therefore, diagnosis can only be achieved *after* surgical excision of the suspect lesion. The least-invasive surgery employs the laparoscope.

Diagnosis involves some risk. Unfortunately, diagnostic laparoscopy and excision biopsy are invasive procedures with distinct adverse effects and even (rarely) mortality. Regrettably, one-third of all diagnostic laparoscopies reveal no visible pathology. Vaginal ultrasound won't do the job unless the disease causes ovarian enlargement and cysts. Noninvasive rectal ultrasound with an MRI can improve the success rate only when the endometriosis is confined to the deep pelvic and rectal regions. And treatment, especially surgery, is not a guaranteed cure.

One out of every three surgically treated patients does not improve.[740] But women with deep dyspareunia (painful intercourse) were well served by laparoscopic full excision, combined with postoperative hormonal-suppression drugs to prevent new growth. One year after surgery, 50 percent no longer had deep dyspareunia, 35 percent reported less pain, and only 19 percent had no benefit.[237, 238] Other experts describe a clear downside to long-term hormonal suppressive therapy: a more rapid aging in all of the functions of the body.[84]

Unfortunately, surgical treatment by excision may not help for long, either. The first study to report on the effectiveness of excision of all stages of endometriosis in a blind, placebo-controlled trial found that surgical excision produced short-term gain, with 80 percent of the women reporting improvement at six months after surgery.[1] Compared to 22 percent who improved in the placebo group (these women underwent a laparoscopic look but no excision), the 80 percent figure *seemed* very good. Unfortunately, six months later, 43 percent of those who had undergone the excision now had biopsy-proven disease during the second surgery and only 31 percent had no evidence of any disease.[1] By 2007, sadly, a clear confirmation of how limited these gains were was provided by an analysis of 1,000 women's lifetime experiences with their own surgically confirmed endometriosis.[713] The conclusion: "The disease has a profound effect on the health of these women and effective therapies are urgently needed."

New Drugs: The Aromatase Inhibitors

Routinely used in breast cancer patients, aromatase inhibitors appear to be the first breakthrough in the medicinal treatment of endometriosis since the 1980s. These new drugs, anastrozole and letrozole, suppress local estrogen production. Side effects of aromatase inhibitors are said to be "reasonably benign: mild headache, nausea, and diarrhea. Unfortunately, long-term use carries the potential risk of osteoporosis and osteopenia."[35] Many clinical trials are needed before this becomes standard treatment.

Stay Informed

Endometriosis is a difficult disease to diagnose and treat successfully.[504, 751] Women who suffer with it must take it upon themselves to

stay informed. The Endometriosis Association (www.endometriosis
.org) is a self-help group that provides an accessible resource. There
are no clear answers, but since you are the one who bears the risk and
enjoys the benefits, you owe it to yourself to make decisions based on
your own best judgment.[45] Good judgment might well include choos-
ing the least-invasive treatment first.

Some women resort to having a total hysterectomy for endometriosis. Sadly, even after surgery, the pain may remain in up to 17 percent
of women.[35] And for those left hormonally deficient due to the surgery,
logical arguments have recently been made for hormonal-replacement
therapy to provide an important benefit versus a small risk for the
overall health or longevity of the patient.[724]

Another Cause of Unexpected Bleeding

Conditions and diseases of the cervix, or entrance to the uterus, may also
be the cause of abnormal bleeding. Chief among these is cervical cancer,
the second-most common cancer in women worldwide (400,000 cases
per year).[360] The main risk factor for developing cervical cancer is infection with the human papillomavirus (HPV) through sexual intercourse.

There are no blood tests for cervical cancer. Currently, cancer is
detected via Pap smears, a visual exam of the vaginal issue, and a cervical biopsy. If you have a sex life, you should have a gynecological exam
at least once a year.

In the United States, 13 percent of the female population age 65 and
older account for 25 percent of the new cases and 41 percent of the
deaths from cervical cancer.[862] Although HPV is detected in 20 to 65 percent of Pap smear specimens (the highest rate occurs in women in their
teens and twenties), there are at least 200 subtypes. The lifetime risk of
acquiring an HPV infection is estimated to be 80 percent. The good news
is that despite the widespread incidence of the HPV virus, only a small
proportion of cases have the high-risk subtypes that become cancerous.
In most women, these viruses clear up on their own. The few women in
whom this does not happen are at risk for developing cervical cancer.

Cases of invasive cervical tumors that are diagnosed after the age of
45 are often due to previously undetected HPV. Death rates are greatest
for women over 45. From 1995 to 2001, the CDC (Centers for Disease

Control) databank showed that 13 percent of U.S. women had an HPV infection.[66] The new HPV vaccine, along with regular Pap tests, offers the potential to prevent this disease.

Once you have cancer of the cervix or of the uterus, no drug regimens that are currently available can be used to adequately treat it safely. Yes, progestins and other hormonal drugs (GnRH analogs) at high continuous doses did reverse 57 to 75 percent of the cases of endometrial cancer and 83 percent to 94 percent of the precursor stage (atypical complex hyperplasia).[377] This is not safe enough. A hysterectomy and perhaps subsequent radiation therapy appear to be the most rational options for a woman's future health in these cases.

Avoid a Hysterectomy

The incidence of unnecessary hysterectomies varies throughout the world. In the Netherlands, half of the women who are referred with excess bleeding have a hysterectomy within the next five years. But more than one-third of these hysterectomies are unnecessary: the women have anatomically normal uteruses removed.[88]

"When in doubt, take it out" is a bad idea. A joint statement from the Women's Hemostasis and Thrombosis Clinic, Duke University, the Royal Free Hospital in London, the University of Milan, and the University of Rochester says it all: "Guidelines are needed for the gynecologist because so many plausible disorders were not being ruled out before removing a healthy uterus."[473]

Unexpected bleeding is rarely serious. It can usually be resolved without rushing into surgery. Granted, bleeding stops with a hysterectomy, but the adverse effects of using this "ultimate" resolution are severe:[383]

- Accelerated aging[621]
- A shorter lifespan[236, 573, 579]
- The lifetime presence and pain of adhesions
- A more difficult time with fatigue,[195] depression,[201] maintaining healthy bones,[176] and cardiovascular health (see chapter 9)
- Problems with
     The control of urine and the bowels[301]
     Marital and sexual well-being[443]

Abdominal hysterectomy procedures are the most common cause of iatrogenic (brought on unintentionally by a doctor) femoral (to the front side of the thigh) nerve injury, at 11 percent of these surgeries.[371] A more serious problem is urinary tract and bladder injuries. Fortunately, these are much less common, but they do produce serious problems. For every 1,000 procedures, about 15 injuries to the ureter and 30 injuries to the bladder are documented.[270]

Conclusion

The general principle for managing your good health when faced with pelvic problems that include bleeding and pain is to try the least-invasive procedure first, and only move to more drastic steps if the less-invasive ones fail. Doing so would reduce the current hysterectomy rate by at least 75 percent!

6

Declining Pelvic Muscle Tone: Pelvic Prolapse and Urinary Incontinence

WITH AGE, INACTIVITY, AND SOMETIMES disease, muscles throughout your body may become flabby, weak, and unable to support your body structures. The muscles of your pelvic floor are no exception. Pelvic muscle weakness can result in incontinence (an inability to control your bladder or bowels) and/or prolapse (the dropping of the uterus, the bladder, and/or the rectum within the vagina or past the vaginal opening). Vaginal vault prolapse is the descent of the top of the vagina, which typically occurs after a woman has had a hysterectomy.[156] Prolapse may be caused by inadequate muscle tone. This sometimes results from childbirth, but there may be other causes.

Pelvic organ prolapse generates between 200,000 and 300,000 inpatient surgical procedures annually in the United States.[106, 165, 566] The Pelvic Organ Prolapse Quantification System that was developed in 1996 by the International Continence Society provides a uniform method of scoring the degree of prolapse in order to monitor change in the condition. Table 6.1 on page 94 lists the stages, which are defined by how protruded beyond the vaginal hymeneal ring (or entrance to the vagina) the leading edge appears on examination.

Notice that the degree can range from invisible to visible. If you're assessed with one stage, though, it may not get worse. According to

Table 6.1 International Continence Society Stages of Pelvic Organ Prolapse Determined by Pelvic Organ Prolapse Quantification System Measurements

Stage 0. No prolapse; measured from the hymeneal ring, the anterior and posterior points are all −3 centimeters; and cervix or posterior fornix is between −TVL (total vaginal length) and TVL −2 centimeters. The *fornix* is the recess formed between the vaginal wall and the vaginal part of the cervix; *proximal and distal* refer to near and farther from the center; *anterior and posterior* refer to front and back.

Stage I. The criteria for stage 0 are not met, and the most distal prolapse is greater than 1 centimeter above the level of the hymen (less than −1 centimeter).

Stage II. The most distal prolapse is between 1 centimeter above and 1 centimeter below the hymeneal ring (at least one point is −1, 0, or +1).

Stage III. The most distal prolapse is greater than 1 centimeter below the hymeneal ring, but no farther than 2 centimeters less than TVL.

Stage IV. Represents complete vault eversion; the most distal prolapse protrudes to at least TVL −2 centimeters.

This list is adapted from I. Nygaard, C. Bradley, and D. Brandt (2004): Pelvic organ prolapse in older women: Prevalence and risk factors. *Obstetrics Gynecology* 100(3):489–497.

Dr. Anne Weber, prolapse is dynamic, rather than progressive. In fact, it often regresses.[823] In other words, you can have the condition one year and not the next.[92] Obesity is one of the few modifiable risk factors that have been identified as a cause. As usual, it helps to watch your weight.

Prolapse: Fairly Common, but Not Deadly

No population wide data have been gathered in the United States, but investigators estimate that 30 to 93 percent of mobile women will experience prolapse.[566]

Examinations of 270 Iowa participants in the Women's Health Initiative Study revealed that 65.2 percent were at least at stage II or beyond and 25.6 percent had the leading edge of internal structures protruding outside the vagina. The investigators concluded that pelvic organ prolapse is common and some degree of prolapse is *normal*, especially in women in their mid-60s.[566] Neither hormone therapy, nor the number of pregnancies, nor vaginal delivery were associated with the occurrence of prolapse. But for women who did have prolapse, those with more than two vaginally delivered babies were more likely to experience further descent over time.[92] Those most at risk were in poor health status overall.[652] African American women have less than half the risk of Caucasians.

What Is the Cause of Prolapse?

There are theories, including a stretching of the vaginal tissue, the thinning of tissue, aging with estrogen deficiency at menopause, and breaks in the fascia of the vagina. But the theories have not been supported by facts.[824] Very little is known about the physical and biological manifestations of prolapse. A potential cure at the molecular level appears unlikely.[526]

The majority of women who undergo pelvic floor reconstructive surgeries have previously had hysterectomies in each of the studies that list prior surgeries.[709] Probably, surgical removal of the uterus further weakens the supporting structures that are needed to hold the pelvic anatomy in place.

Do you need to do anything about prolapse? It really depends on you. Although some authors state that women with prolapse suffer from chronic pelvic pain and pressure, urinary and fecal incontinence, sexual dysfunction, and social isolation,[526] other experts assert that pelvic pain is not associated with prolapse and, frequently, prolapse is not a problem that requires surgery.[823] A stage IV prolapse with internal structures protruding outside the body will obviously be a problem, as well as a medical emergency if the woman is unable to urinate. Fortunately, this is relatively rare,[823] occurring in less than 7 percent of women.[652] Moreover, the actions you take with stage II or III prolapse may prevent the further descent of the prolapse.

There is no inevitability that the problem will worsen, and prolapse does not demand treatment (or surgery) unless you are currently suffering.

Nonsurgical Approaches

The actions you control—like engaging in judicious exercise, maintaining or restoring a healthy weight, and wearing a medically prescribed support device—can often solve the problems without any adverse effects.

Kegels

For women suffering from significant effects of prolapse, pelvic floor rehabilitation through Kegel exercises—pelvic floor muscle training—may be helpful.[823] (It certainly can't hurt!) The American Physical Therapy Association (www.apta.org) can help you locate local practitioners.

Exercise Modifications

Apparently, no studies have addressed the questions I asked my mentor, Dr. Garcia, more than thirty years ago. I wondered whether aging bodies could safely endure jumping-type sports. If ligaments were losing their elasticity, was it sensible to play tennis or volleyball or run? Wouldn't low-impact fitness regimens such as swimming, dancing, tai chi, walking, and weight lifting better serve the woman? Dr. Garcia agreed that the idea was rational. I feel that women can use their own wisdom to guide their choices.

A Support Device

A pessary is a plastic device, such as a ring, placed in the upper vagina to keep the uterus in position when ligaments are too weak to support it. According to Dr. Anne Weber, if a pessary is properly fitted and placed, a woman should be unaware of it and unrestricted in her activity. Pessaries can be removed, cleaned, and reinserted as needed. Vaginal ulceration and irritation can result when routine hygiene is ignored. A properly fitted pessary can help a woman delay or avoid surgery.

Hormones

Vaginal estrogens are often prescribed, because they are beneficial in restoring atrophic tissue and reducing the likelihood of ulceration, especially in conjunction with pessaries.

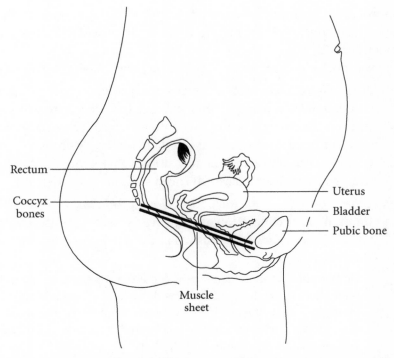

Figure 6.1. The pelvic floor muscles that form the complex sheet of support are indicated by two bold lines from the pubic bone, to the coccyx (spinal) bones. It helps to see the enormous job this sheet of muscles must perform to support and suspend the uterus, bladder, and other internal tissue well above the openings of the rectum, the vagina, and the urethra.

Surgical Repair

Take your time when making a decision about surgery. Unfortunately, the surgery itself can predispose women to future prolapse, painful intercourse, incontinence,[709, 823] and adhesions.

Do the surgeries that are available actually work? According to 80 published studies, the recurrence rates of prolapse ranged from 9 percent (a good result) to 55 percent, with more recurrence likely as longer amounts of time have elapsed since the surgery.[824]

In 1997, experts argued that current information in anatomy textbooks was not accurate and that surgeons who believed that they were repairing the distention-type problem reported using procedures with "surprisingly few effectiveness studies for anterior vaginal prolapse."[824]

Only recently have studies begun to explore the outcomes of these surgeries, and only one study has followed up to provide data five years after surgery.[709]

If your doctor recommends prolapse surgery, you should know:

- Rates of success are not uniformly predictable. Surgeons cannot with certainty inform patients whether the procedure will yield beneficial or detrimental results on their sexuality, urinary function, and general satisfaction with their surgery. Moreover, surgical skill is not uniform. The few studies that show good results involve surgeons who have advanced skills and experience.

- Surgery doesn't mean the end of your problems. Consider this comprehensive conclusion after a lengthy analysis of the current state of the art that was published in the *Journal of Obstetrics and Gynecology.*

  > Despite the fact that transvaginal [accessed through the vagina rather than through laparotomy via the abdomen] colporrhaphy [a surgical procedure in which the vagina is sutured to narrow it] has been the preferred surgical procedure for rectocele (protrusion of rectum into the back wall of the vagina) repair among gynecologic surgeons for over 100 years, long term data are not available on outcome and there is a suggestion of a high incidence of painful intercourse from this surgery. . . . In summary, the traditional surgical procedure provides moderate relief of functional symptoms [of prolapse] and a high rate of de novo dyspareunia [new onset of painful intercourse]. Surgeons [and patients] should be aware that restoring structure [from prolapse] with surgical repair may not restore defecatory or sexual function.[165]

  This is a sad situation because this comprehensive clinical expert review from MDs at Johns Hopkins Medical School and the University of Michigan Ann Arbor represents the opinions of high-level academics.[165] Surgeons who recommend surgery for a prolapse have difficulty proving that successful outcomes will occur. Worse yet, women have rarely been systematically asked for their opinions to measure their satisfaction.[651]

- Recurrence is a risk. One report of 152 consecutive patients who reported noticing a vaginal bulge found that their average age was 62 and that 68 percent had previously had hysterectomies, and 33 percent had previously had prior surgeries to repair their prolapse. So the authors acknowledged a greater than 30 percent failure rate for prolapse surgery.[335]

Although it is of important academic interest to watch for improved results from certain procedures, an individual woman may be hard-pressed to locate one of the more highly skilled surgeons who has a lower likelihood of surgical failure.[709] Therefore, if you can prevent surgery with exercise, pessaries, or weight loss, logic suggests that this be your first course of action. But if a prolapse is blocking your bowel or urinary function, then you might be wise to choose surgery. The good news, according to Dr. Anne Weber, is "Virtually all women with prolapse can be treated and their symptoms improved even if not completely resolved."[823] My review of the scientific literature suggests that for women with prolapse, surgery should be a last resort. Try the least-invasive route first.

Uterine prolapse should not be confused with another condition that may also result from the loss of tone in pelvic region tissues. Cystocele (dropped bladder) occurs when the vaginal wall is forced down by the bladder pushing down. Rectocele is a condition in which the vaginal wall is forced down by a protrusion (herniation) of the rectum. Both conditions can produce some difficulties with continence.

Urinary Incontinence (UI)

The term *stress urinary incontinence* denotes involuntary leakage during physical effort or exertion, during sneezing or coughing, or when a doctor observes it in a medical exam. Urinary urge incontinence is another condition: the involuntary contraction of and emptying of the bladder. Epidemiological data in the United States show that incontinence peaks in old age; by middle age, 1 in 3 women report leakage at least weekly, and approximately 1 in 4 women with UI consults a health-care professional for help. Prolapse increases the risk.[515]

As shown in figure 6.2 on the following page, the ureters carry the urine from the kidneys to the bladder, which serves as a holding tank.

UI makes women anxious, embarrassed, and unwilling to undertake a wide range of activities. This can be logically expected to diminish their quality of life.[253] Expert researchers recommend avoiding surgery, if at all possible, since many gaps in current medical knowledge hinder

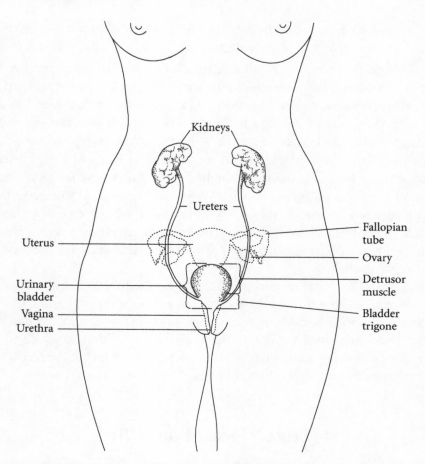

Figure 6.2. This frontal view allows you to see the physical relationships and should be viewed along with figure 6.1, which shows the side view of the same anatomical structures.

women from objectively selecting the best therapy. And surgery can have serious adverse consequences.[568]

More than 1,000 postmenopausal women who were generally healthy members of an HMO participated in a two-year follow-up study that provided some compelling information. More than 60 percent of the women in this group, ages 55 to 75, acknowledged that they had UI. Prior hysterectomy increases the incidence of a new onset of severe problems. Yet having UI during one year does not mean that the woman will have it the next year.[374] Each year 19 percent of continent women developed incontinence, and 14 percent of the incontinent become continent. So the data suggest that incontinence progressively increases into old age, even in well-functioning older adults, but that women *can* overcome incontinence.[374, 537]

What causes UI? We don't know yet.

Pregnancy (or the lack of it) is not necessarily a risk factor. Contrary to the conventional wisdom that never having a baby protects a woman against UI, a careful study of sisters clearly found that rates in 143 postmenopausal nulliparous women (those who never had a baby) and their 143 parous (those who have had a baby) biological sisters were similar. This strongly suggests that familial factors play a greater role than vaginal delivery does in the development of urinary incontinence. The majority of parous women *are* continent.[101] But parous women have a greater likelihood of showing a visible defect in the pelvic muscles of continence on an MRI exam: 20 percent of the group of primiparous (those who have given birth to one child) women versus 0 percent of nulliparous women.[198]

In the United States, more than 50 percent of women are overweight (with a body mass index [BMI] ranging from 25 to 30). Heavier women suffer greater problems with UI and a greater frequency of nocturia (a nighttime need to wake up and use the bathroom).[31, 198] One study of 180 morbidly obese women (with a BMI of 40 or higher) showed that young age was not protective; 67 percent of women ages 16 to 55 acknowledged having UI. And 32 percent of these unfortunate women also suffered from anal incontinence.[645] Presumably, weight loss would help.

Nonsurgical Treatments of UI

Weight loss and postural changes (such as crossing one's legs) help, but reducing fluid intake does not help. Smokers suffer more nocturia (getting up at night to urinate) and more UI than nonsmokers do.[31, 568] Moderate physical activity clearly reduces the likelihood that a woman will develop UI, according to a 2007 analysis of the 2,352 women in the Nurses Health Study who developed new "leaking" problems in their mid-60s. Women who had the highest levels of moderate physical activity per week, such as walking, were most immune to a new onset of UI.[184] So keep moving!

Pelvic floor muscle training is highly effective and should be done first. If you practice this, it is likely you won't need to do anything else. If you can stop a stream of urine without grimacing or contracting any muscles that show on the surface of your body, you are probably engaging the correct muscles.

All of the regimens show good results, but some are easier to do.[105, 277, 535] Behavioral training programs require that you learn the basic anatomy of your body, then discover which muscles need strengthening and identify the relevant muscle group. These programs are very easy to do. Simply place a (clean) finger in the vagina to learn whether the correct muscles are contracting; you'll feel the pressure. Some teaching regimens are that simple. Others use a tool linked up to a computer screen. The tool contains a tamponlike instrument that you insert vaginally, then look at the feedback screen to see your compression strength as you squeeze around the tool. Women owe a debt of appreciation to Dr. Arnold Kegel, a physician who invented the technique for strengthening the pelvic floor.

Dr. Kegel published his pioneering "Physiologic Therapy for Urinary Stress Incontinence" more than fifty years ago (1951) in the *Journal of the American Medical Association* (*JAMA*). By 2002, it was well confirmed that properly taught Kegel exercises are effective in curing UI for most women.[535] (These exercises have been widely used for more than twenty-five years; for a more complete description, the reader can find them in *Hysterectomy: Before and After* by W. B. Cutler.[168]) Women who do the exercises at least three times a week can expect a high probability of curing themselves by rebuilding their muscle strength. As you strengthen your pelvic floor muscles, your prolapse problems should also diminish. Like prolapse, UI is a dynamic mechanical condition. Neither problem inevitably worsens.

Here is the proof that these programs work: One research group conducted a randomized, controlled clinical trial to test whether women could be trained to build the muscles to control continence. To qualify, the women had to be basically healthy, 54 years or older, with at least one occurrence of incontinence per week. Half were assigned to a control group, half to the test group. The 75 women in the control group were told to keep a urinary diary for 6 weeks. They did no exercise and underwent no training. The other 77 women attended an initial 45-minute training session that included education on urinary anatomy and physiology. The women were provided with a verbal and a written set of instructions for doing Kegel exercises.[755] They were not given physical examinations and did not undergo invasive pelvic measures. Then the behavioral training group attended weekly 20-minute sessions in groups of 3 to 5.

The results were good. After 6 weeks, the treatment group had a 50 percent reduction in the average number of incontinence episodes per week. One-third of the treatment group was 100 percent improved (dry), but 28 percent had no improvement. At 6 months, 33 percent said that the program had helped them a great deal, and only 12 percent felt that it had not helped them at all. The group that did not engage in the behavioral modification training did not show any improvement. I agree with the authors' conclusion: "Our trial results support the Agency for Health Care Policy Research guidelines that 'the first choice should be the least invasive treatment with the fewest potential adverse outcomes.'"[755]

Do drugs help? The research shows that some "effective" drugs work no better than keeping a bathroom diary![568] Paying attention to your bladder by keeping the placebo diary seemed to be about as good as taking a drug (duloxetene) and keeping the same diary. But the diary by itself has no adverse effects.

According to a recent systematic review, the urogenital effects of selective estrogen receptor modulators (SERMs) have not been positive.[12] Although occasional benefits can be demonstrated,[275] this result is not supported by other studies.[12] SERMs were originally developed to treat breast cancer and were initially categorized as antiestrogen.[12]

Do hormones help? Too few studies have been published to provide a clear answer.

An increased risk for developing UI in women who are taking hormonal therapy versus a placebo was observed in the Women's Health Initiative trial. The hormone tested was Premarin, and the women were overweight. Similar results were reported in the much larger Nurses Health Study.[297] The number of hormone users was higher among nurses with UI than the nonusing nurses. The hormone Premarin or its generic equivalent, conjugated equine estrogen, was used by 73 percent of the hormone users.[151] And having a hysterectomy did not explain these results, because the outcome was similar for both the intact women and those who had undergone a hysterectomy.

Premarin also led to more UI in a third study of 619 women with prior hysterectomies.[275] Either the choice of hormone preparation or the nurses' overweight condition may have been a factor here, and the results may not apply to women who are trim or to those who time the start of their hormones to the early transition years before estrogen levels have been depleted.

Hormones Do Help with Aging Changes in the Urogenital Tract

Postmenopausally, the female genital and lower urinary tracts undergo similar effects with aging and estrogen depletion. Decreased blood supply leads to atrophy (shriveling up) of the tissues of the lower urinary tract. Estrogen therapy has been used for many years to reverse these urogenital aging symptoms. To demonstrate this, a group of investigators evaluated changes in urinary symptoms and the introital Doppler velocimetry (measurements of blood flow in blood vessels using real-time ultrasound images) of the lower urinary tract. Their study of 73 women showed that estrogen therapy (Premarin) alone could increase blood supply to the lower urinary tract in women with prior hysterectomies. Symptoms appeared to improve after three months, but the size of the improvement did not reach statistical significance. There was no increase in UI among these estrogen users from either the oral or the vaginal cream route.[468]

What You Should Know: Hormone Therapies and UI

The results of the Women's Health Initiative have been reviewed by experts on hormone therapy and UI. Dr. Cheng-Yu Long and colleagues noted that women under age 60 did not show this increased risk of UI after starting the hormones. They also reviewed other published studies and reviews of 23 articles, which found self-reported improvement in rates of UI ranging from 64 to 75 percent in hormone users.[468]

- Hormone therapies are varied. We must keep in mind that all hormone therapies are *not* alike. Estrogen has been used since 1995 in the management of UI. The way I see it, the healthy functioning body, metaphorically, is like a cruising train with good momentum on a clear track. When that momentum slows—with declining health and advancing age-related maladies, it is much more difficult for you and your physician to regain a healthy momentum. Despite valiant medical efforts to restore good health, it is less fruitful to administer hormone therapies after women have developed age-related ailments; most benefits occur when women take hormones *before* they develop age-related ailments.

- With hormones, timing may be key. I suspect that for hormones and UI, the data will eventually reveal a pattern that is similar to hormones and general aging of the body. Namely, as we age, there is a window of opportunity to prevent the loss of muscle tone and keep the blood circulating to support the muscle. Hormones play a key role when that window is wide open. Maintaining a reasonable body mass index also helps keep strong pelvic muscles and the resultant good urinary function. Once the window closes and the muscle tone becomes lax, it *can* sometimes be recovered, but it takes much more work to get that train to regain its healthy momentum.

- The increases in UI in hormone users in the Women's Health Initiative applied to the older women, most of whom were overweight and atherosclerotic. I wonder whether there is a message here, as in the cardiovascular health research, about beneficial results if HT is started early enough. There are insufficient data for a conclusion in 2008, but logic suggests this is likely.

- Hormones may improve the outcome of surgery, should you opt for it. For women who already have UI, one researcher reported that estrogen was beneficial if it was started immediately after a TVT (tension-free vaginal tape) procedure (see the following section) and if the estrogen preparation chosen was estriol vaginally inserted.[878]

Surgical Treatments for UI

More than 20,000 women older than 70 undergo surgery for UI each year in the United States, but research studies in this age group are lacking.[537] Recent reviewers of the literature conclude that fewer than

10 percent of the published 943 studies meet required standards for providing valid information that other surgeons and patients could effectively use to determine their procedures' success rates.[568]

The operating surgeons' skills and training are varied. None of the studies through 1996 described the women's quality of life after surgery, and few obtained any information about the patients' perceptions. Only 31 were prospective (gathering information like a prospector, as he goes, rather than from memory, looking back later), and 28 of these 31 studies were conducted at a single medical center, which may not be generalizable to other situations and groups of women. Incontinence is a long-term problem for women, but most studies covered only short-term outcomes.[545, 565]

Laparoscopic Colposuspension

This procedure was introduced in 1991 as a minimally invasive surgical approach to UI. But recently the Cochrane Incontinence Group concluded that laparoscopic colposuspension may have only short-term benefits, such as quicker recovery (it's minimally invasive, so there's less of a wound to be closed and to heal).[568] The group found more postoperative complications, though. And the laparoscopy procedures are more costly, due to the fact that this highly skilled surgery takes longer to perform. The quicker, but more invasive, methods that don't involve the laparoscope can be completed in less time, but with longer recovery.

Tension-Free Vaginal Tape (TVT)

Tension-free vaginal tape (TVT) is a polypropylene midurethral sling that quickly gained worldwide use because of its simplicity. It was easy for surgeons to learn how to perform this surgery faster than they could do laparoscopic procedures. Very effective marketing by the TVT purveyors also helped make the procedure popular. Unfortunately, it became impossible to recruit enough women into randomized trials to compare TVT to Burch (laparotomy, that is, an incision through the abdomen) colposuspension; hence, the trial was stopped before enrollment was completed. Subjectively, in one large multicenter trial, only 43 percent of the women in the TVT group and 37 percent of the women in the open colposuspension group reported that their stress leakage had been cured.[568]

What You Should Know about Surgical Devices and Therapies

FDA approval doesn't mean risk free. The FDA does not generally require that clinical trials be conducted before surgical devices for incontinence, such as the implantable meshes and vaginal tapes, are marketed. The complex "Premarket Approval Application" of devices, once it is completed with studies and approved, does assure the public that the devices are safe and effective if used in the intended way. Most legally marketed devices, however, bypass this rigorous screening. "The Premarket Notification 510(k)" is a short-cut: a submission process to the FDA that demonstrates that a new device is "substantially equivalent" to a legally marketed device. If the new medical device is so approved, it may be legally marketed and distributed in the United States.

Unfortunately, this shortcut exposes consumers to certain risks. For example, hernia-repair surgeons have made great strides through innovations in the type and the design of mesh products, which were inserted during surgery to hold tissue in place. This led to government approval for these mesh products for hernia repairs.[565]

The mesh products were then approved as devices for vaginal slings using the 510(k) shortcut. According to experts,[87, 562] this usage, and its FDA approval, was a mistake. Unlike the sterile field of hernia repair surgery, vaginal surgeries are not sterile. Instead, they involve a clean but not sterile region that potentially introduces bacterial infection where the sling is placed.

In 1996, the ProteGen sling, made from mesh used in cardiac surgery, received FDA approval through a 510(k) Premarket Notification. Other slings, including the TVT, rapidly followed.

Long-term safety studies are not required. Although manufacturers are not required to demonstrate long-term safety before bringing these devices to market, the FDA does have a Web site where people can report adverse reactions. Called MAUDE (Manufacturers and Users Device Experience: www.fda.gov/cdrc/maude/html), it is voluntary for physicians but required for manufacturers, and it's not being used as it was intended.

In 1995, there were 9,000 new devices and then in 2000 13,000 devices introduced in the marketplace, and these outpaced the FDA's ability to inspect them (3,602 inspections were performed in 1995 and 1,841 in 2000). This is very dangerous for the woman who is considering surgery using a new device. One such UI device yielded a 30 percent erosion rate in the sling after five months.[568] The erosion of inserted material causes major health problems as the tape breaks apart, embeds into human vaginal tissue, and produces scars, internal bleeding, pain, and infections.

You can't assume that the lack of reported adverse effects means there aren't any. Even if you do a background check on the technique or the device you're considering for UI, you may not run across any adverse effects. Don't assume this means that the device or the technique has a high rate of success. Dr. Peggy Norton, a gynecological surgeon whose main practice involves surgical repair of these mesh erosions, published shocking conclusions about problems with these tapes. She presented a lecture to about 150 doctors at a recent continuing medical education seminar held at the annual clinical meeting of ACOG (American College of Obstetrics and Gynecology).[87, 562] She described her personal three-hour ordeal to remove one set of eroded tapes and said that many women have come to her with such problems. She related how these distressed women had been stonewalled by the original surgeon, who falsely claimed that each was the only patient in whom this unfortunate circumstance had occurred. Dr. Norton knew that these were lies because she was treating multiple patients with the same problems from the same set of surgeons.

As perhaps the only biologist in her audience, I was amazed to see the show of hands from surgeons who said yes, they too had experienced adverse reactions in their patients' mesh erosion repairs, requiring additional surgery after other surgeons had inserted these tapes. I counted about 50 of the 120 attendees who raised hands; only one surgeon raised a hand to the second question, acknowledging that he had also reported it to MAUDE.

Dr. Norton explained that filing the report is tedious, time-consuming, and not obligatory for surgeons. Doctors can tell the manufacturer's sales representatives, who should report them on MAUDE, but Dr. Norton found that they don't "get around to reporting" what is conveyed to them. She likened this to asking the fox to protect the hens in the henhouse.

It is a dangerous world for consumers who seek pelvic surgery. Case reports of problems (bladder erosions, dyspareunia, dysuria, bacterial infection) with the tape procedures have also recently been published.[15, 589, 626, 757] Unfortunately, unlike the MAUDE Internet site, these are even more difficult for the consumer to find.

Conclusion

After reviewing some of the recent scientific literature, I find myself agreeing with Drs. Nygaard and Michael Heit: "Stress urinary incontinence is common and may impact women's quality of life. Conservative management of confirmed UI should precede surgery. There are many gaps in knowledge about the disorder and likely heterogeneous etiology may ultimately lead more sensibly to better selected therapy."[568]

Take ownership of the health of your body. Learn how to do the Kegel exercises, and do them every day to keep your muscles strong. Avoid surgery if you can. And if you must have surgery, get and check both short- *and* long-term references that show the effectiveness of the procedure and the products by the surgeon you are considering. Ask the person who proposes surgery for a way you can confirm what proportion of his or her patients with similar procedures felt satisfied that they had chosen surgery, after two years had passed. When you are told to sign an informed consent form, you will be best served if you have done your homework.

7

Diagnosis Fibroids: The Top Four Treatments and Why They May or May Not Work for You

UTERINE FIBROIDS ARE A COMMON cause of unexpected bleeding and pain. They are technically tumors, which can make you feel as if you have to rush to treat them and get rid of them. Perhaps that's why fibroids are the single most common reason for 180,000 of the 600,000 hysterectomies performed on women each year in the United States.[727, 836] The overwhelming majority of fibroids in Europe and North America "are still managed surgically and with hysterectomy rather than myomectomy."[621] But careful studies confirmed that even very large uterine fibroids can be successfully removed with a myomectomy, a procedure that conserves the uterus.[621] There are now even better, less stressful, and more effective competing alternatives available.

By 2006, editorials in medical journals were addressing the turf battle for patients that these competing "remedies" for fibroids have provoked. One scholar wrote, "Treatment of uterine fibroids should be focused on the patient's needs and not a 'turf' problem of gynecologist vs. radiologist. Patients, not the physician, should choose among options based on being presented the data from which to make a rational choice."[363] Find your best option by using your own careful research and good judgment.

Large studies published in 2005 and 2006 demonstrated that hysterectomies result in more deaths, more disabling side effects, more loss of work, more cost to patients, and longer recovery times compared to all other fibroid remedies. In 2002, Dr. Alan DeCherney (later the Editor in Chief of the journal *Fertility and Sterility*) noted, "Of all postoperative symptoms . . . fatigue interfered with the patient activities the most, impairing the ability to undertake a wide range of daily activities and responsibilities or producing consequent feelings of frustration regarding this impairment in the majority of patients."[195] I want to help you make the best-informed choice so that you will avoid a hysterectomy.

What Are Fibroid Tumors?

Fibroids are about as common as freckles: smooth muscle-cell lumps that form in the wall of the uterine muscle. They are benign and occur in 70 percent of reproductive-age women.[124, 379, 787] They grow and shrink in response to specific sex hormone signals.[27]

Fibroids should not be confused with cancer or a risk of developing cancer. Both scientists and clinicians point out that the development of fibroids and their growth have no features in common with cancer.[787, 813]

A Fibroid by Any Other Name . . .

Is still a fibroid. Fibroids are called by many other names, all interchangeable: uterine leiomyomata, myomas, fibromyomas, leiomyofibromas, and fibroleiomyomas. The tumors consist of both smooth muscle (myo) and fibrous (fibro) tissue. These benign tumors originate from smooth muscle cells of the uterus, although in some cases the smooth muscle of uterine blood vessels may be their source. They range from seedlings to large sizes, from solitary to multiple. Their location in the uterus determines the medical label.[813]

- *Intramural:* within the muscle wall itself, the myometrium (they do not reach the outer or the inner wall of the uterus)
- *Subserous:* extending to the serosa (the outer wall)
- *Submucous:* internally impinging on the uterine cavity

Usually, they are painless and harmless, unless their bulk creates pressure on some other tissue.[379] (But pain that leads to the detection of a fibroid does not prove that the tumor is causing the pain.[685] So the cause of the pain can be complex and requires a good medical evaluation.) And, usually, fibroids remain undetected unless an ultrasound examination reveals their presence. Their incidence increases with age across all races.[208, 316, 456] By the time women reach age fifty, ultrasound scans will find fibroids in 70 percent of white women and 80 percent of black women.[543] Either two- or three-dimensional ultrasound can accurately identify the fibroids more than 98 percent of the time.[760] They often remain the same size for many years.

Sometimes fibroids cause trouble. They can cause heavy menstrual bleeding, which can lead to the fatigue of anemia, pelvic pain or pressure, and abdominal distention. Decisions about treatment should be made slowly and carefully. Since fibroids shrink after menopause, sometimes it's best to take no action.

Estrogen is believed to be very important in the occurrence of fibroid tumors, but only progesterone—in the presence of estrogen—causes

---

Fibroids and Sex

The sexual lives of women with fibroid tumors have not been well studied, but they should be. These tumors involve the pelvic region, which is richly filled with nerves and which becomes engorged with blood during the various phases of sexual response.

A study of Italian women and a second one of North American women have each reported that women with fibroid tumors are as sexually active as those without.[178, 239] According to one study, self-reported sexual sensations appeared to be heightened by the presence of fibroids. Compared to volunteers who were having a health assessment, women with fibroid tumors more often enjoyed cervical tapping, as well as vaginal stimulation, which led to orgasms during sexual intercourse.[177] Dr. Millicent Zacher, the gynecological surgeon who coauthored the study, suggested that the excess blood flowing to the pelvis in women with fibroids might explain these enhanced sexual sensations.

the cells to multiply, as measured by increased mitotic activity that can be seen under magnification.[124]

In 1989, Japanese researchers first demonstrated a monthly cyclic variation in the growth and shrinkage of fibroid tumor cells of fertile-age women.[727] The tumors were observed to grow after ovulation and shrink when menses started. This implicated progesterone, which was well documented to circulate in the blood for only half of each fertile cycle.

Still, it was not so simple. Two clinical studies showed that high-dose synthetic progestin could shrink the uterus, although maybe not the tumors.[727]

Researchers put myometrial and fibroid tissue into lab dishes and added different hormones to their "baths." In an estrogen-rich bath, progesterone stimulated a cascade of chemical changes that increased the growth of fibroids. Overall, progesterone stimulated fibroid cell growth but not normal uterine muscle cell growth.[259, 499, 699, 857] These discoveries and others led to a flurry of research that was designed to treat fibroids medicinally.[123, 251, 351, 429, 503, 605, 788, 815, 816] If surgery could be avoided, through the development of pharmaceuticals, then women could be spared the stress, the cost, and the risks.

The levonorgestrel intrauterine system (IUS) is a hormone-administration system for a particular synthetic progestin, delivered locally (within the uterus), that is useful for women who experience excess bleeding due to fibroid tumors. The device was described in chapter 5. One study reported benefits that began to appear within three months in women who had been suffering from sizable (one inch or larger) fibroids that caused moderately enlarged uteruses. There was a 6-fold reduction in menstrual blood loss after 12 months, among 17 of the 20 women who had been anemic. They experienced a full recovery from iron deficiency that the blood loss had caused.[295]

Hormone Therapy and Fibroid Growth

Can using hormone therapy spur fibroid growth? Apparently not. The first evaluation of hormone therapies on fibroids in peri- and post-menopausal women used the records of a health cooperative of 256 women with fibroids and 276 others for a "case-control" study. (But they excluded women who were sequential hormone therapy users.) Hormone therapy use was clearly not a key factor.[638]

Why a Hysterectomy Should Be Your Last Choice

Having a hysterectomy impairs the blood supply to the ovary, reducing its hormone output. That accelerates aging. Although a few studies have reported that after women had hysterectomies, the onset of ovarian failure was not advanced and hormonal levels were not influenced,[126] other studies have shown that a hysterectomy does hasten the onset of menopause and that after having hysterectomies, women have more severe menopausal symptoms at a younger age than intact women do.[201, 394, 705, 761] The confirming proof was published in 2006. See the box on page 116 ("The Proof That Hysterectomy Causes Deterioration of Ovarian Function").

If a medical treatment with an IUS fails to work, surgery can offer benefits that are worth considering. The medical societies now list seven "indications" for which surgical treatment of fibroids may be appropriate:[370]

- Abnormal uterine bleeding that doesn't respond to conservative treatments
- Iron-deficiency anemia that is related to abnormal uterine bleeding
- A high level of suspicion that the fibroids are malignant
- The growth of fibroids after menopause
- Infertility with a distortion of the endometrial cavity or tubal occlusion
- Pain or pressure that interferes with quality of life
- Urinary tract obstruction

According to Dr. Gloria Bachman, an expert gynecologist, researcher, and medical educator, only in the last decade have alternative treatments flourished, giving women options that allow them to have successful outcomes while avoiding major surgery for fibroids.[40]

If you decide on surgical and other procedures, you must choose among different specialties. A specialist will probably prefer the procedure she's most skilled in and is extremely unlikely to have skills in all of the available procedures.

If you are going to have surgery, review chapter 11 and take action to prepare for a calm postoperative state. Healing is fastest when you have peaceful social connections with friends and family members.[206] Investigators reported that environmental stress that causes high ambient glucose (sugar in the blood) will increase the development of adhesions during the critical first few days after surgery.[662] Diabetics and people whose postsurgical stress responses produce high levels of cortisol—which elevate the ambient glucose level—are at greater risk of developing adhesions.

Stress delays the wound-healing process and increases the likelihood of bacterial infection. Even modest delays in healing may have profound consequences for individuals who are recovering from surgery or other wound-healing conditions. Plan before the operation—rally loving family members and supportive friends around you and avoid emotional stress—and this should help you reduce the risk of adhesions. The surgeon cannot offer this critical care. Your loved ones can, if they know you need it. Even your dog can help.[593]

Invasive Treatments

The options available are listed in the order they should be considered, from least to most stressful to the patient, because if you can solve the problem with a newer, less costly procedure, your recovery will be faster, less painful, and simpler.

- *Uterine artery embolization* involves blocking the tumor's blood supply without cutting any tissue out or making incisions to expose the pelvic region.

- *Myomectomy* removes fibroids from the uterus, sparing the woman from having a hysterectomy.

   Hysteroscopic resection removes tissue through the hysteroscope; the tissue is accessed through the vagina, and the procedure requires no cutting.

   Laparoscopic myomectomy is the removal of tissue via the laparoscope (a periscope into the lap region), through which surgery is conducted.

Laparotomy-accessed myomectomy is achieved through an abdominal cut.

- *Thermoablative techniques* use temperature to destroy tissue; they include myolysis with heat, cryomyolysis with cold, and laser ablation. These methods have not been widely adopted and have been mostly supplanted by uterine artery embolization.[749]

- *MRI-guided focused ultrasonic ablation* involves zapping the tumors via ultrasound without any surgery; this technique was newly approved in the United States in 2007.

- *Hysterectomy* is the removal (*ectomy*) of the uterus (*hyster*).

The Proof That Hysterectomy Causes Deterioration of Ovarian Function

Using color Doppler ultrasound imaging techniques, Dr. Xiang and colleagues in China examined 50 women before and after they underwent hysterectomies or myomectomies. Each woman was examined three times: once before surgery, then exactly one month after surgery, and finally two months later. Blood was tested each time to measure the reproductive system hormones: estrogen, progesterone, FSH, and LH. At each examination, the ovaries were scanned with the ultrasound equipment, which can "see" whether the ovary is preovulatory, ovulatory, or postovulatory.

The results: There is a clear decline in ovarian function after a hysterectomy but no loss after a myomectomy. A hysterectomy reduced the ovarian blood supply and ovarian hormone production.[860] The authors' rational conclusion was:

> The present study indicates a deterioration effect on ovarian function. Thus it is better not to remove the uterus in patients for whom other conservative treatments may be available. And for the patients needing hysterectomy, a more effective method should be introduced such as removal of portions of the uterus, or keeping as intact an artery network as possible among the uterus, oviduct and ovary. Thus, the function of the ovary would be kept as fully as possible and patients would have a better quality of life, especially in young women.

These researchers deserve our thanks for their elegant, sophistic-
ated work.

Uterine Artery Embolization

Uterine artery embolization (UAE) or uterine fibroid embolization
(UFE) to treat fibroids was introduced in 1995 by French physicians
led by Dr. J. H. Ravina. They reported that tumors will regress when
their blood supply is blocked by tiny *embolizing* particles that are
instilled into blood vessels that supply blood to the tumor.[632, 634] The
procedure was also used at Yale-New Haven Hospital even earlier to
stop postpartum hemorrhage in women to help them avoid having
hysterectomies.[577] It was called "pelvic arterial embolization" (which
internally blocks the artery).

Embolization is fast and simple for the patient, but it results in
about two days of postprocedure pain that usually can be controlled
with prescription painkilling drugs. It is highly effective. Although
technically invasive, it is not considered surgery because there is no
cutting and stitching. It is administered by interventional radiologists.

The result: starve the tumor and save the uterus. Much like an intravenous drip, a catheter is inserted on each side of the pelvis between
the navel and the hip bone to gain access into the artery that supplies
blood to the uterus. Then the catheter is snaked into the uterine vessels until it reaches the tumor region. Once the catheter is installed,
tiny particles are dripped slowly through it, into the arteries. The IV
drip stops when the blood flow has been clogged by the tiny particles.
Blocking the blood flow to the tumors deprives the fibroids of nutrients. The tumors starve, shrink, and atrophy. Sometimes this leads to
an atrophied fibroid that passes out of the woman's body (in a process
that is much like giving birth). This may occur weeks after the procedure. At other times, the body seems to absorb the shrunken tumor, or
it remains behind as a tiny inoffensive mass.

The UAE is one of the newer uterine-conserving procedures that
spares women from having hysterectomies while getting patients out
of bed, healthy, and ready to work dramatically faster than any other
currently proven procedure.[621, 880]

The first series reported on 16 patients, ages 34 to 48, with symptomatic fibroids, who were scheduled for surgery, but first the UAE was attempted in hopes of preventing surgery. This study provided early positive findings that the procedure worked and could prevent invasive surgery.[632, 634] Two years later, the same authors reported on 88 more women.[631]

Overall, the results were remarkable: 89 percent of the women experienced a return to normal menstrual periods. On average, the volume of each tumor shrank by about 70 percent, and 71 of the 80 women were able to avoid surgery after undergoing a UAE. In 1999, Dr. Ravina again reported on a larger group of 99 women who had undergone the procedure between 1991 and 1997. These women provided data to show that 90 percent of the procedures were successful and the 10 percent that failed were largely those that were observed when the method was first being developed.[598, 633, 635]

Consider undergoing the UAE as a pretreatment.[632] By 2005, even for women who were going to have myomectomies to remove fibroids, having a UAE before the operation significantly reduced the pre- and postoperative bleeding and reduced blood loss during surgery (50 ml versus. 250 ml); having a UAE before the myomectomy also prevented the recurrence of fibroids (0 versus 19.4 percent recurrence) at 16 months.[461] And after 5 years of follow-up, for women who had UAEs in addition to myomectomies, this had not compromised their fertility rates.[462]

For years, the UAE procedure was considered "investigational,"[4] but the procedure evolved as more women were studied.[4] Different particle sizes were tested. The need for and the timing of administering painkillers were worked out. Different races and age groups were evaluated.[278]

For example, at Georgetown University Hospital, from 1997 to 2001, a questionnaire was sent out at 3 months after women had undergone UAEs and then at 12 months.[733] The results were good: there were no complications in 90 percent of the women. The low rate is comparable to or better than the rates for a myomectomy or a hysterectomy in other studies. After a 5-year follow-up, 76.4 percent of the women consistently reported real satisfaction with the procedure.[732] By 2005, investigators could predict which UAE procedure would likely fail to prevent a hysterectomy. (Women with symptoms that had not improved at the 12-month follow-up were 5 times more likely to require further interventions.) Also, if the volume (size) of the dominant fibroid (the biggest one) shrank, it helped predict good long-term benefits.

Similar evolving improvements in the UAE were reported from the Ontario Uterine Fibroid Embolization Trial.[622] Satisfaction was very high, with 85 percent of the women saying they would be willing to undergo a repeat UAE if needed and only 7 percent expressing strong dissatisfaction. The first large voluntary registry, from 72 different radiology sites in the United States, showed good results from the initial postprocedure data. More than 95 percent of the women had no major problems during the first 30 days after their procedures.[850] Because these registries were voluntary, it was assumed that only the centers with the best skills had registered.

The ACOG (American College of Obstetricians and Gynecologists) has recently recognized the UAE as an acceptable therapy, acknowledging that the procedure reduces fibroid size and improves menstrual bleeding in the short term.[279]

Are you a candidate? Not everyone can undergo a UAE. About 3 percent of patients have arteries that are so curled up that the interventional radiologist cannot gain access. Large fibroids, greater than 10 centimeters, may disqualify you because complications are much worse in these cases and may not be worth the risk.[598] For women older than age fifty, the procedure tends to produce amenorrhea (absence of menses).[278]

As in all procedures, a small percentage of women experience adverse effects. These have been described in medical journals.[36, 212, 594, 765, 786, 863] They seem to be rare and curable.

The UAE has been investigated in more than 50,000 patients and for more than 90 percent of the women shows excellent results.[362, 363, 621] As always when seeking help, you need to find a highly skilled medical professional with a good track record.[880]

Myomectomy

Removal of the fibroids, via an abdominal incision or vaginally, is another option that may help a woman avoid having a hysterectomy. Despite its benefits, the myomectomy is neither well known nor widely performed. In the United States, ten hysterectomies are performed for each myomectomy for fibroids.[373, 836]

Is your doctor's recommendation based on fact or perception? The excessive rate of hysterectomies is largely due to doctors accepting certain ideas, some of which are not based entirely on facts.[373] Despite a lack of supporting data, medical students are studying a textbook that asserts that myomectomy is associated with greater disease. That textbook is *Telinde's Operative Gynecology*, 7th edition (1992). Further criticism revolved around the interpretation of data within this textbook. The critics state, "Where the textbook above said a recurrence rate of 15 to 30 percent [as a reason to do hysterectomy instead of myomectomy], it fails to state that only 1/3 of those require further treatment." [373] In other words, only 5 to 10 percent of the women who undergo myomectomies to remove their fibroids and conserve their uteruses need any further treatment. If medical students and surgeons were taught inaccurate information, no wonder more of them prescribe hysterectomies than myomectomies.

Know your facts: one study compared 103 equivalently healthy women around 45 years of age who underwent myomectomies to 89 others who underwent total abdominal hysterectomies without the removal of their ovaries or tubes.

The results: the hysterectomy group was worse off, experiencing

- More blood loss (796 ml versus 464 ml)
- More surgical injuries (2 uretal, 1 bladder, 1 bowel, and 1 femoral nerve injury versus zero for the myomectomy group)

All surgeries were performed by senior residents and supervised by a small group of experienced surgeons. Outcomes of the two procedures are more comparable than previously thought.[373] I would suggest that the myomectomy is less stressful than the hysterectomy.

You may be told that you are not a candidate for having a myomectomy. If you hear these reasons from your doctor, discuss the facts:

"Your fibroid is too big." The size of the fibroid does not rule out your having a myomectomy. Five studies have shown that large fibroids can be successfully removed, while sparing a woman from having a hysterectomy.[836] But despite this evidence, many women are told that their large fibroids require hysterectomies.

Arguing that this practice should change, in 2006 the authors of the study made some strong statements: "Women may be informed by their gynecologist that myomectomy is not indicated because hysterectomy is safer or associated with less blood loss or that sarcoma may be present"; these statements are disproved by recent evidence. The 2006 reports pointed out that as far back as 1931, Dr. Victor Bonney, an early advocate of myomectomy, concluded that "the restoration and maintenance of physiologic function is or should be the ultimate goal of surgical treatment."[836]

"You risk losing too much blood." Manage your blood loss during surgery with the Cell Saver. This device is used during surgery to collect the blood that is lost when vessels are cut. Rather than the hospital discarding this blood, the device allows the red blood cells to be collected and subsequently returned to the body. Since one argument against the myomectomy had been that it can produce blood loss greater than from a hysterectomy, the use of a Cell Saver was particularly relevant in a 2006 report that advocated the benefits of a myomectomy.[836] According to the author of the study, "The device suctions blood from the operative field. If [the] patient requires reinfusion, the blood is processed by centrifugation and filtered, mixed with saline, and reinfused." This reduces or avoids the need for either a preoperative blood donation or a blood transfusion. If you are contemplating surgery, ask about the Cell Saver.

"You'll need pretreatment with drugs." There was a time when women were advised to take the powerful gonadotropin-releasing hormone drugs (GnRH) to inhibit estrogen and temporarily shrink the tumor in hopes of limiting blood loss during surgery. Actual randomized controlled trials, however, have confirmed that the practice should be abandoned.[801]

Recurrence of fibroids was significantly higher in women who had pretreatment with GnRH before their myomectomies, compared to those who did not: 37.5 percent versus 14.8 percent.[655] Since GnRH has many side effects and no benefit has been shown for its use before a myomectomy, the evidence is now against its routine use.

The Myomectomy Has Been Proven to Be Effective

If you decide to have surgery to remove your fibroids, find a surgeon who has the expertise to perform the procedure you choose or discover you need. Recurrence rates were low and about equal for either a laparotomy (an abdominal incision) or a laparoscopy (the use of a periscope to avoid making an incision). This was shown both in randomized controlled trials and in hospital reviews over a 40-month period in an academic hospital in Rome.[655] Various technical details that were presented by authors who had specialties in one or another technique all show that a myomectomy is effective for close to 90 percent of women, regardless of the tumor size, the patient's age, or her BMI (body mass index).[312, 451, 768]

Adhesions: A Risk of the Myomectomy

The rate of adhesions developing, however, appears to be consistently lower for a laparoscopy (where a tiny incision is made)—between 17 percent occurrence of adhesions for anterior and 33 percent for posterior incisions—versus a laparotomy (which creates a major wound) (adhesions developed in more than 90 percent of patients).[370] Laparoscopic surgery is more expensive because it takes longer, uses more hospital resources, and requires more advanced training.

So if you decide you want your fibroids removed, take comfort in knowing that if you find a surgeon with a good track record in performing myomectomies you will be 90 percent likely to avoid a hysterectomy.

By 2006, strong arguments for myomectomies were appearing in gynecological journals, such as this one in *Fertility and Sterility*: "Increasing uterine preserving treatment options and new perspectives on myomectomy might both help to reposition hysterectomy as the last, not the first, line of treatment for symptomatic fibroids."[621] This is good progress, I think.

Myomectomy versus Uterine Artery Embolization (UAE)

How should you choose between a myomectomy and a UAE? Read this proof: By 2007, a number of different studies had provided the first evidence that the UAE seemed to be a better option.[97, 226, 279, 850] The women's hospital stay was shorter (24 versus 61 hours, on average), her return to work was faster (20 versus 62 days' delay), there were fewer adverse events (22 percent versus 40 percent), and symptoms didn't recur as often. The UAE was significantly cheaper than a myomectomy, caused much less pain after the procedure, and did not expose women to the risks of surgery and general anesthesia.

The bottom line: Every study revealed the benefits of the UAE over a myomectomy. It was cheaper, faster, and less painful, and women could resume their lives much sooner.

High-Intensity Focused Ultrasound (HIFU)

The HIFU is a new method that uses a high-intensity beam focused on the target fibroid via a vaginal wand; it was originally tested in animal studies.[401] Now a gynecologist with special equipment can "see" what is happening in "real time."

In China, HIFU treatment of liver cancer, breast cancer, bone tumors, and soft tissue sarcoma is being successfully reported. In Europe and Japan, the HIFU is in clinical use for benign prostatic hyperplasia in men. In the United States, clinical trials for the treatment of fibroids have recently been approved.[773, 773]

Although ultrasound has been successfully used for noninvasive treatment, it has been limited. A method to precisely target and "zap" only the tumor, not the bone, the muscle, or the blood vessels, was first tested in 2003 using an MRI (magnetic resonance imaging) in ultrasound surgery. The first studies reported on 9 women with fibroids who were scheduled for hysterectomies, but they agreed to try treatment with ultrasound first. These studies showed that the procedure was technically feasible and safe.[773] Confirmation of its safety soon followed.[748]

MRI-Guided Ultrasound Ablation: A Quicker Recovery

By 2006, the authors who pioneered this technique reported successful outcomes in more than 100 women. Dr. Elizabeth Stewart and her colleagues concluded, "In well trained hands, the procedure is safe and for a substantial proportion potentially effective. There is a rapid, 1 day, return to work compared to UAE which is 13 days and myomectomy or hysterectomy 72 days."[749]

I suspect that the widespread use of this new procedure is inevitable, once the results are confirmed with further studies and trials. Maybe by 2010, women will be able to undergo this procedure as easily as they can have a UAE in 2008.[747]

Hysterectomy

The term *hysterectomy* means just what its two parts say: *hyster* is the "uterus"; *ectomy* means "removal." A total hysterectomy means the total uterus is removed. A subtotal hysterectomy means only part of it is removed, usually conserving the cervix and the back part of the vagina and thereby sparing the pelvic floor. Ovariectomy describes the removal of the ovary. Bilateral ovariectomy means the removal of both ovaries.

The United States has three times the rate of hysterectomies that Sweden and Norway have. From 1990 to 1997, the abdominal (laparotomy) route was the most common hysterectomy performed, with the longest hospital stay.

A hysterectomy removes fibroids but may cause other serious conditions. During a hysterectomy, any anatomical distortions of the uterus increase the risk of damage occurring to adjacent structures, such as the urinary tract and the bowels. If the woman has had prior surgery, any existing adhesions may increase the technical difficulty of the procedure and heighten the chance of bowel injury.

A Good Mind-Set: Absent Cancer, Refuse Hysterectomy for Fibroids

In 1997, Dr. Anne Weber analyzed the data from hundreds of premenopausal women with fibroids to determine what predicted their having hysterectomies. She found that the main determinant was the specialty of the provider, not the disease of the patient. Patients of oncologists were more likely to undergo hysterectomies; patients of fertility specialists were much less likely to undergo hysterectomies.[822]

Post-Hysterectomy Complications

- About 10 percent of the women developed stress incontinence after having hysterectomies.

- Additional long-term problems that women experienced after undergoing hysterectomies for fibroids include the development of vaginal vault prolapse.[156, 813] Postoperative consequences should be recognized and considered before deciding on surgery. The other treatments for fibroids do not risk a prolapse.

- Women who have undergone hysterectomies have a higher risk than intact aging women do of developing hormone-related deficiencies.[216] Even when a woman's ovaries are retained, the ovarian lifespan is still diminished, and, consequently, lower bone density, increased risk of cardiovascular disease, and more severe estrogen-deficiency symptoms have been reported.

- A hysterectomy is a major operation with serious morbidity (sickness) in 3 per 100 women; mortality (death) in 3 per 1,000 women; and risks of long-term complications, such as fatigue, pelvic pain, and urinary and sexual problems.[337, 383]

- A hysterectomy, with or without an ovariectomy (castration), is associated with women experiencing a greater frequency and severity of hot flashes, cardiac symptoms (e.g., angina, Syndrome X), migraine headaches, urinary tract symptoms, depression, diminished bone minerals, and osteoporosis.[670] It also causes a more rapid decline in bone density.[176] For this reason, hormonal therapies are particularly essential for menopausal women who have had hysterectomies.

- Adhesions are another complication from a hysterectomy.[250, 661, 662] At McGill University, a review of medical records from three major Montreal hospitals showed 322 cases of bowel obstruction (over a 7-year period) and concluded that the laparotomy-accessed hysterectomy (using the abdominal route) plays a major role in the occurrence of adhesion-related small bowel obstruction. It was noted that this rarely occurs after a hysterectomy that is performed via a laparoscope.[10]

- By 2006, the McGill surgeons advocated for this more technically advanced procedure (through a periscope) so as not to open the abdomen. Unfortunately, these methods have their own risks, which were detailed earlier. Women who agree to abdominal surgery should seek surgeons who are familiar with ways to reduce the risk of adhesions.

If you must have a hysterectomy, keep this in mind: less cutting is better. The general trend in the last ten years has revealed that the least amount of surgery possible produces the least amount of damage. And if any other procedure short of a total hysterectomy can be done that will solve your problems, this should always be the first choice. The examples that follow point the way to this general conclusion.

Ask your doctor about the possibility of your having a subtotal hysterectomy. The procedure of removing the body of the uterus but not the cervix or the back part of the vagina has become more widespread. In fact, the rate tripled over the seven-year period from 1990 to 1997, but subtotal hysterectomies still represent only 2 percent of all hysterectomies that are performed.

To compare the subtotal versus the complete hysterectomy, one investigator recruited 125 women from Alabama, Tennessee, and Detroit who were scheduled to undergo hysterectomies via a laparotomy. Obese women comprised about a third of those studied. The outcomes were equal. There was no difference in cost between the procedures, suggesting that no more complications occurred in one procedure than in the other.[702] This finding is important. One reason women have been told to choose total, rather than subtotal, hysterectomies was the mistaken idea that a complete hysterectomy would cause fewer problems for them. This is not true!

A comparison of subtotal abdominal hysterectomies and total abdominal hysterectomies in two London hospitals over a five-year period showed that the subtotal type had better outcomes. The subtotal type required less operative time, caused less blood loss, resulted in significantly less fever, and needed fewer antibiotics (meaning that there were fewer infections), and the women had shorter hospital stays.[774] The authors stated that a subtotal abdominal hysterectomy is easier to perform than a total abdominal hysterectomy, with fewer risks to the urinary tract.

Be prepared to use facts to counter perceptions. Your doctor would not willingly mislead you, but remember that your doctor's perceptions may motivate him or her to recommend a particular procedure. When researchers surveyed 1,647 gynecologists in Maryland, Virginia, and Washington, D.C., regarding total versus subtotal hysterectomies, 770 responded.[873] Most of them said that they routinely perform total, not subtotal, hysterectomies: 45.1 percent said they always do them; 55 percent do so to remove the risk of cervical cancer or to prevent the women from needing any future Pap smears, even though 92 percent of the gynecologists felt that the risk of the women developing cervical cancer was small to negligible, even if the cervix was left intact. Studies show that the facts are inconsistent with the recommendations being made for women to undergo hysterectomies.[873] Women should be ready to make choices that their doctors may subtly oppose, because the physicians are using "viewpoints," rather than evidence-based reasoning, to make their recommendations.

Comparing the Vaginal to the Abdominal Hysterectomy

A hysterectomy can be performed by opening the abdomen (called a laparotomy) or through the vagina, where it's not necessary to make a large incision.

A 2004 study tested whether the vaginal compared to the abdominal approach to hysterectomy in obese women would produce more complications. The reverse seemed to be true in a review of 369 obese patients. The outcomes were better for a vaginal hysterectomy, which avoids cutting open the abdomen. A vaginal hysterectomy had:

- One-fifth the incidence of postoperative fever or urinary tract infection
- Less than one-tenth the incidence of wound infections[372]
- A shorter operating time and hospital stay

Since this study was not a randomized, controlled trial, it acknowledged that selection bias might have skewed the results. But even so, less cutting seemed to generate less damage.

The Total Laparoscopic (No Abdominal Cut) Hysterectomy

The laparoscopic approach to surgery described in chapter 5 avoids cutting open the abdomen.[101] The surgeon blows gas into the belly region to distend the area and separate the organs so that they can be reached surgically through the tube using fiber-optic instruments.

Again, be prepared to use facts to counter your doctor's perceptions. The laparoscopic hysterectomy was first reported on in 1989, the same time that a study was conducted of the laparoscopic cholecystectomy (gallstone removal). Although the laparoscopy for gallstone removal has virtually replaced the earlier open surgery, gynecology has not evolved in kind. With more than 500,000 hysterectomies being performed per year, medical schools have failed to encourage the laparoscopic hysterectomy, which is a safer, quicker procedure. In 2004, Dr. Tommaso Falcone, a professor and the chairman of the

Department of Ob/Gyn at the Cleveland Clinic Foundation, argued that medical school leadership has failed to recognize, recruit, and afford status to surgeons who teach these modern skills.[233]

The most challenging procedures are often better for you. German researchers concluded that compared with an abdominal hysterectomy, a laparoscopic or laparoscopic-assisted vaginal hysterectomy provides many advantages but takes more skill.[19] Patients recover more quickly and have shorter hospital stays and a faster return to work. Surgeons need more practice—performing at least thirty procedures—to be competent in their training experience.

What this means to you: No surgery is simple, and you want to find someone who is skilled in the chosen procedure. A laparoscopic procedure in skilled hands seems better for the patient who is undergoing a hysterectomy.[570]

So why aren't women being offered these procedures? One author, putting it delicately, explained that the different routes are used because of doctors' conflicting goals and skills.[130] In one study at the National Taiwan University Hospital, researchers compared hospital record data over two years from 452 patient records to develop guidelines for the future. For women who had large uteruses at the time they were to undergo hysterectomies, the procedure that required the most technical skill, the laparoscopically assisted vaginal hysterectomy (LAVH), produced the best outcome: it caused about one-fourth the loss of blood (66 ml) as a transvaginal hysterectomy without a laparoscope (242 ml). There were no injuries to the ureter or the bowels on either procedure. Researchers concluded, therefore, that the LAVH is safe for most patients and offers a more rapid recovery and a quick return to normal activities. But it is technically more demanding, is more expensive (consisting of two separate simultaneous procedures), and requires greater skill and more experience.

Other researchers reported on 437 patients undergoing supracervical vaginal hysterectomies with laparoscopes in rural northwest Alabama.[536] They explained that this method is initially challenging for surgeons to learn but is better for the patient.

Hysterectomy Type and Risk of Death

Call it the ultimate side effect, but a hysterectomy, like all surgeries, carries a risk of death. Dr. Anne Weber evaluated the Ohio Hospital Association database to study the risk of death occurring from various gynecological procedures.[821] Overall, of 179,307 patients, 274 had died in the hospital during or immediately after having hysterectomies. For cancer-related hysterectomies or those performed on pregnant patients, 89 women died for every 10,000 hysterectomies performed. In comparison, for noncancer hysterectomies, 7.5 per 10,000 died. Since more than 500,000 women in the United States undergo hysterectomies for noncancerous reasons each year, this would translate into 375 women dying per year from the hysterectomies they underwent, if Ohio were similar to other states. This is not a huge number overall, but it is nevertheless very sad!

What You Should Know

The death rate was highest for the abdominal hysterectomy and lowest for the laparoscopically assisted vaginal hysterectomy. The rate was cut in half for the vaginal route. Although an abdominal hysterectomy seems to be riskier, Dr. Weber pointed out that the abdominal route tends to be chosen for procedures that are expected to be more difficult. Costs may be a factor, too. Hospital charges for an abdominal hysterectomy were the cheapest and those for a laparoscopic-assisted vaginal hysterectomy were the most expensive (adding a 75 percent cost to the base price).

Conclusion

There is a high incidence of hysterectomies being performed on women, often unnecessarily. Take steps to avoid one, if possible. If you have troublesome fibroids, find an expert who can offer an IUS, a UAE, or an HIFU. If these experts convince you that your condition disqualifies you for these procedures, then consider a myomectomy. Follow the path of least-invasive treatment, and you are unlikely to need a hysterectomy to resolve your problem with fibroids.

Recognize that a hysterectomy is rarely your best choice, and whether your doctor recommends it may depend on where you live. Hysterectomy is the second-most frequently performed surgical procedure on women (the first is cesarean section).

- Twenty million U.S. women have had one.
- In just five years (from 1994 to 1999), 3,525,235 hysterectomies were performed on women older than 14.

- More than half (52 percent) were done on women under 45.

- The highest annual rate occurs in the South, with 6.5 hysterectomies per 1,000 women; the lowest rate is in the Northeast, at 4.3 hysterectomies per 1,000 women; almost as low are rates in the West, with 4.8 hysterectomies per 1,000 women, and in the Midwest, with 5.4 hysterectomies per 1,000 women.[400]

- By age 60, more than 40 percent of all women in the United States have had hysterectomies.[670]

Using CDC data, one analyst showed that the annual U.S. rates of the surgery revealed a dramatic drop in 1988 that has lasted as the greatest decline to this day.[446] This is the copyright date of my book *Hysterectomy: Before and After*,[168] which I recommend to readers who want more information specifically about this procedure, as well as on how to prepare for surgery and postoperative care. At the time it was published, it made many statements that shocked the established members of the academic gynecological community. Eventually, it became widely recommended to patients because of its careful explanation of the cited facts.

At Least, Keep Your Ovaries

Reflecting entrenched perceptions about proper "clinical art," an oncologist argued that 3 to 4 percent of women who undergo hysterectomies will need to be operated on again for subsequent ovarian pathology.[718] No reference was provided to support this assertion. The castration of healthy ovaries during a hysterectomy is performed on 75 percent of women ages 45 to 54 and on fully 40 percent of those who are 15 to 44 years old.[246] The most recent, careful analysis of large bodies of data, however, showed that women who have endured hysterectomies, with their ovaries left intact, have a 40 percent lower risk of developing ovarian cancer than do women who never had hysterectomies. Castration (the removal of both ovaries) of women who do not have ovarian cancer cannot withstand scrutiny.[592, 593] Yet not all experts agree.[190, 692, 752]

Surgeons once routinely convinced women to accept ovariectomies because of the difficulty of detecting ovarian cancer before it reaches an advanced stage. Such a practice never was reasonable because ovaries are important for a woman's overall health all through her life, and ovarian cancer is *very* rare.[170] And the outlook is beginning to improve even there.[127] Imagine considering the removal of other healthy organs to preempt a rare devastating disease that is unlikely to happen. This is not rational. Just say no!

Choosing Treatment Options If Fibroids Are Causing You Trouble

You can now seek options that may make better sense for you than those suggested by the particular physician who offers your diagnosis. Just a few years ago, you had only two options: surgical removal and GnRH, an unpleasant hormonal suppressive agent.[351] Now that radiologists have developed technologies to shrink tumors without surgery, these procedures appear to offer a better choice than either a hysterectomy or a myomectomy for most women. And the HIFU procedure looks extremely promising as well and might be even better than the UAE. None of these have been systematically compared,[316, 547, 813] which is not surprising given the turf battles and competing economic interests of the specialists involved.

Your options may also be limited by your doctor: different treatments are offered by various specialists who may not want to refer you out of their field of practice. Each woman needs to determine her best course of action.

Take Command

If you are having a problem with fibroids, I hope you will seriously study the information presented here. Your informed, objective and dignified command of the facts can *profoundly* affect the solutions you seek and find. Don't be in a rush to get the process over with. Every surgery provides fodder for future medical problems. Surgery is dangerous. Reject the attitude of "when in doubt, cut it out."

Hospital infection rates expose women to danger, independent of their reasons for seeking treatment in a hospital. Pennsylvania is the first state to publish, hospital by hospital, the rates of opportunistic infections that were recorded. The data are organized by peer groups because some hospitals take on tougher problems, which make weakened patients more vulnerable to illness and/or death from infection.[273]

These data reveal the infection rates in Pennsylvania hospitals in 2005 and expose a risk that is independent of the other risks of surgery (see the *Philadelphia Inquirer*, November 15, 2006, pages 1 and 12). Unfortunately, the data do not provide information about how many of these cases of infection were specifically after gynecological surgeries (see www.PHCc4.org).

Opportunistic staph infections that you acquire during a hysterectomy, a myomectomy, or an endometrial ablation (which are common surgeries for bleeding or fibroids) can incapacitate you for months or years and may require extensive and expensive recovery. These are mainly caused by inconsistent (or no) hand washing. The issue is not trivial for a woman who is considering whether to accept her physician's suggestion that she undergo a "little" surgery for her fibroids.

8

Protect Your Bones—with Exercise, Posture, Vitamin D, Calcium, and Hormones

YOUR BONES FORM YOUR SKELETON—the scaffolding of your body and the protective shield for your internal organs. Their strong outer structure, composed of calcium and other minerals, is interlaced with tiny blood vessels and nerves. Their inner, more liquid portion (marrow) is rich in blood vessels and is the manufacturing site of your red blood cells. When you reached your full height, the lengthening of your bones stopped, but for the rest of your life they dynamically change in *thickness*.

Imagine an architectural-design firm that is commissioned to keep a posh apartment complex attractive and functional. Similarly, a lifelong renovation process continuously remodels your bones. Your "remodeling units" work throughout your skeleton.[91, 265, 350, 514] Thousands of tiny manufacturing "job-sites" are set up, removing and re-forming the skeleton as materials are supplied in your diet and new bone tissue is deposited. This massive reconstruction project is directed by your hormones using the materials you have supplied in your diet along with the recycled components. Around age 35 to 40, as your progesterone levels begin to decline, the bone *removal* activities tend to outstrip bone *formation*, and adult bones begin to decrease in density. If your body cannot maintain enough new bone formation, your bones will continue to lose density and become increasingly fragile as you age. That architectural firm is slacking off. Eventually, this fragility results in osteoporosis.

Let me explain the magic of bone structure and function. I will show you how to keep your bones strong your whole life long.

Bank on Your Bones

Like a bank where you deposit money to cover future expenditures, healthy bones act as a bank for calcium. Your lifetime dietary practices exert major influences on how solvent your bank account stays. The more calcium and vitamin D that you can deposit before age 35, the greater your peak bone mass. Osteoporosis rarely develops before menopause; that much was known as early as 1941.[14] It took 40 more years to discover the reason: the decline of reproductive (sex) hormones around menopause. If you haven't had a hysterectomy, your perimenopausal transition beginning around age 40 sets in motion a change in hormonal patterns that initiates the "withdrawal" of these calcium savings, typically about 1 to 2 percent per year. The richer your bone bank and your sex hormones, the better off you will be. If you're an African American woman, you will likely have much more bone mass than if you're a white American. In one study, African American women had quadruple the average testosterone level and double the average estrogen level as their white counterparts before menopause.[600]

Hysterectomy and Bone

It's hardly surprising that having a hysterectomy is bad for your bones. A hysterectomy disrupts the sex hormone symphony. Surgical menopause (removal of the uterus and the ovaries) triggers a dramatic loss of bone. Unchecked, a hysterectomized woman can lose more than 60 percent of the bone she had as a young woman. In 1988, my colleagues and I published evidence showing that a hysterectomy (even when the ovaries were retained) accelerated the loss of bone in comparison to bone loss in intact women of a similar age.[176] Until a post-hysterectomy woman takes aggressive action with a combination of nutritional, hormonal, and exercise regimens, she is at extreme risk of developing osteoporosis.

Weak bones break; 40 percent of white women at age 50 can expect to eventually suffer a bone fracture.[89] Without preventive action, most women by age 80 will have weak bones, with only 40 percent of the total body bone mass they had at age 40. Unfortunately, the diagnosis of osteoporosis is generally made only after the fractures reveal that profound losses of bone have already occurred. Take action *before* you have a fracture.

Bone Tests: Keep It Simple

Your bone strength depends on how much microdamage exists: the collagen and the textural quality; the geometry of the bone (its shape, its tendency to bend or break under pressure); and its mass, or bone mineral density.[265, 386]

There are inexpensive and very useful measures to test your wrist and heel bones. If your heel or wrist bones have good density, your hip and spine bones should be fine. One of my discoveries in 1988 was that your *spinal* bone density could be efficiently and inexpensively tested by measuring your wrists with "single photon absorptiometry" if you were correctly categorized as either "intact" (nonhysterecto-mized) or "hysterectomized."[176] Testing bone in the heel (calcaneus) also works. These two-minute tests have very low radiation, using either single-photon absorptiometry or ultrasound, and are widely available. A DEXA test, using a dual-energy X-ray absorptiometry, is expensive and can measure hip and spine bones. But the risk of hip fracture among more than 9,700 postmenopausal women was predicted by the bone mineral density in the heel or the forearm.[54, 164] Keep it simple with easy, low-radiation tests.

Defining Osteoporosis

Osteoporosis was originally defined by the World Health Organization in 1994 as a disease characterized by low bone mass and microarchitectural deterioration of bone tissue, the combination of which would lead to an increased risk of fractures.[199] A score, the t-score, of −2.5 or lower was considered quantitatively representative of osteoporosis.

The T-Score

If you never had or don't remember your elementary statistics course in college, picture 100 women standing in a line, evenly distributed from the shortest on the left to the tallest on the right. A bad –2.5 t-score (in height) would place you right between the second- and the third-shortest. Likewise, bone density can be measured by an X-ray type machine, and a score provided and scaled. The –2.5 t-score on bone mineral density would put your score between the second- and third-lowest bone mineral density score of 100 young, healthy women. This is pretty bad!

In 2000, osteoporosis was redefined by the National Institutes of Health (NIH) as a skeletal disorder characterized by compromised bone strength predisposing people to an increased risk of fracture.

The National Osteoporosis Risk Assessment Study enrolled 200,000 postmenopausal women in their early 60s and found a clear correlation between bone mineral density and the number of fractures within the next year. But not all women with fractures had low bone mineral density, and not all women with low bone mineral density had fractures. Hip fractures tend to occur after age seventy-five and are difficult to predict based on spinal measures that cannot take into account the woman's behavioral habits, slippery stairs, and sense of balance. For both younger and older women, spinal fractures are much more common and can be predicted and often prevented.

Fear of Fractures

These are not minor issues. By age 80, more than half of all women show deformities of the spine that are consistent with a fracture.[683] Vertebral fractures are two to three times more prevalent than hip fractures and can be extremely painful and debilitating and can produce postural deformities, as shown in figure 8.1 (see page 140). But any fracture is serious: Half of those who fracture a hip will have a permanent long-term disability; 25 percent will require long-term nursing-home care. And additional complications after a fracture include pressure ulcers, pneumonia (from low oxygen capacity caused by a person's lack of mobility), urinary tract infections, and depression. Fractures are well worth preventing.

Fear of Falling

Falls are the precipitating trigger for 90 percent of the hip fractures, 50 percent of the vertebral fractures, and 99 percent of the wrist fractures.

If it's hard for you to rise from a chair without using your hands and if your gait is poor, you've got the two significant traits that are associated with falls. Other risk factors are taking sedative hypnotics or having impaired vision and neuromuscular function.

For people who face such risks, the household environment should be reconfigured to reduce "booby traps" that can be tripped on. Loose area rugs, uneven floors or shallow steps, inadequate lighting, debris on the floor, and pet accessories all cause falls.

Among older women, falling appears even more likely in those with vitamin D deficiency. Vitamin D deficiency is rarely obvious because it requires a blood test that many labs are *not* able to perform accurately. By 2005, scholars at the National Osteoporosis Foundation were in consensus that vitamin D_3 supplementation at a minimum of 800 IU per day is strongly recommended. By 2007, the data clearly showed that 800 IU per day is not enough.

What's a woman to do to protect her bones? Fortunately, there are actions you can take:

- Engage in appropriate and regular physical exercise.
- Hold yourself erect with dignity (i.e., maintain good posture).
- Eat intelligently—nutritionally rich foods that provide the essential nutrients your bones require.
- Avoid unhealthful habits such as smoking,[404] excessive drinking, couch potato sitting, and eating junk food.
- Take nutritional supplements such as calcium and vitamin D_3 right after eating (to enhance absorption) when you don't get enough either through your food or exposure to sunlight.

Such a disciplined approach will reward you with basic joie de vivre and good bones. The great thing about the actions you take to prevent disease is how great you feel once you make them part of your daily routine.

How Exercise Affects Bones

If you exercise appropriately, you are less likely to trip and fall because your "balancing muscles" will be in strong condition.[556] Can you change your socks and underpants gracefully from a freely standing position? Without using walls or chairs? If yes, you probably won't fall. If no, ten minutes of gentle leg exercises twice a week with ankle weights can dramatically improve your balance.[556]

Very Vigorous Training Builds Bone

The verdict is unanimous: your bones benefit when your muscles are exercised. For example, one experiment studied 260 postmenopausal women, 40 to 65 years old, for 12 months. All were given calcium supplements (800 mg per day). The 260 women were divided into 4 groups and measured to note changes in bone density.

Group 1 did not exercise and took no hormone therapy (HT).
Results: No increase in bone density.

Group 2 did not exercise but did take HT.
Results: Increase in bone density.

Group 3 engaged in regular, vigorous exercise but took no HT.
Results: Increase in bone density (like group 2).

Group 4 did regular vigorous exercise and took HT.
Results: Increase in bone density (like groups 2 and 3).

The vigorous exercise, let's be clear, was no stroll in the park. The rigorous regimen included weight lifting, stretching, and additional resistance exercises for balance and flexibility.[271] The women worked out at an intensity that was 60 percent of their maximal heart rate—hard enough to be working, but not excessively stressful. They also engaged in regular stair climbing, while they wore 10- to 28-pound weighted vests. (Imagine carrying a couple of bags of groceries up 300 steps, and you'll get the idea.)

The researchers were comparing benefits to bone density brought about by HRT, with and without exercise. Women who took a placebo and did no exercise did not show any increase in bone mineral density. But either exercise *or* hormonal therapy worked about the same.

What you should know: Get—and keep—moving. Bone mineral density improved if the woman took hormones or if she exercised vigorously. But if she neither exercised nor used hormones, bone density did not improve. For your bones, as well as the rest of your health, choose an exercise program you will stick to.

Good Posture Helps Your Bones

Regular exercise for maintaining balance and muscle tone will prevent falls and help promote an erect, graceful, and dignified posture.[455, 623] Kyphosis (the hunchback posture) typically becomes noticeable in the early sixties of an intact woman and reflects the characteristically low-estrogen and low-progesterone years after menopause. One study that my colleagues and I did surprisingly showed that 35 percent of healthy women executives were already kyphotic in their late thirties.[172] *This is alarming!*

Figure 8.1 shows the kyphotic posture, which leads to the hunchback that is characterized by the loss of muscle tone combined with the crushing of thinning bones, as osteoporosis progresses within the spines of aging women.

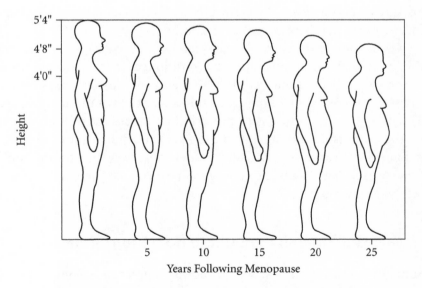

Figure 8.1. Postural change associated with osteoporosis without HRT.

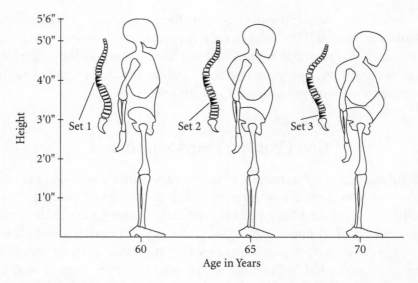

Figure 8.2. Spinal osteoporosis—location of bone fracture with resulting postural change.

Not everyone becomes kyphotic. I think you *can* prevent kyphosis. Buy a mirror to get started. If you are able to keep the muscles of your back and midframe taut and tight through regular exercises, and if you stand and sit erect, your own muscles will hold your spine erect. Good posture takes practice and will start to "feel" right, compared to slouching. As the twig is bent, so grows the limb.

Take a look at the three skeletal regions (figure 8.2) that are under the greatest stress because they are positioned at the natural curves of the spine. If the bones are thinning and the postural muscles are too weak, these regions experience the greatest gravitational pressure. This is why erect posture is so powerful; it reduces the pull of gravity on these "pressure" points. If you use a particular chair most often, try hanging a mirror where you can routinely observe your posture. You'll find yourself "sitting up." See how good posture *looks* better, and it will feel better as you practice.

Get Enough Sunlight to Boost Your Bones

Sunlight is the trigger that sets in motion a great many physiological processes that maintain and enhance life. Just as green plants need sunlight to thrive, so do women. Sunlight's ultraviolet radiation warms and penetrates your skin, and its creamy molecules of cholesterol are converted into a "pre" vitamin D. These particles of previtamin D travel in the bloodstream to the kidneys, where further conversion renders them into a usable form of vitamin D.

By 2007, cellular receptors for vitamin D had been found just about everywhere that scientists had looked: in the skin, the gonads, the brain, the vagina, the pancreas, the stomach, and the heart muscles. Vitamin D helps prevent or reduce the risk of osteoporosis. It also fights breast and prostate cancer, hypertension, and cardiovascular disease.

Bones in the Buff

In Benjamin Franklin's 1729 autobiography, he revealed that he understood the importance of sunlight when he described his daily habit of sitting naked in a window to allow sun on his skin every day for at least fifteen minutes.[247] (Apparently, he found a private location to do so!) It is stunning to consider that in the middle of the eighteenth century, Franklin's genius extended from discovering the geophysical forces of electricity to developing public libraries, founding the University of Pennsylvania, making major contributions to the fledgling U.S. democracy, and recognizing the need for sunlight on his own skin. Fifteen minutes a day, when the sun can penetrate your skin through ultraviolet B radiation, is probably just about right. You may be able to "try this at home" with judicious care.

Vitamin D Absorption: Skin Shades Matter

The paler your skin, the greater its capacity to respond to the sun and convert its cholesterol precursor product into the vitamin D that is essential for so many of our bodily functions, such as calcium absorption and cancer prevention. The darker your skin, the higher its content of melanin, a substance that absorbs the UVB and thereby blocks the beneficial action of UVB that generates previtamin D. So the darker your skin, the more exposure to sunlight it needs to do its job: forming previtamin D. Even the elderly, with their reduced levels of previtamin D_3, still have a large capacity to make adequate vitamin D if they get enough sunlight!

The Dark Side of Sunblocks

A sunscreen with a sun protection factor of 15 that is applied to sun-exposed skin absorbs more than 99 percent of the ultraviolet B radiation. Unfortunately, using a sunscreen blocks the very site where sunlight is converted into vitamin D. If you have tanned skin, this also blocks the sun's capacity to deliver vitamins. So I'm not advising you to get a *tan*, just get *some* sunlight on your bare skin. Like Ben Franklin. (See chapter 10 regarding dermatology concerns.)

Vitamin D terminology is confusing in the literature and inconsistently defined in dictionaries. For the purposes of this book, refer to figure 8.3.

Vitamin D: How Much Is Healthy?

The medical evidence about vitamin D is recent. In 1941, the recommended dietary allowance (DA) for vitamin D was set at 400 IU.[841] This was the amount that was recognized as essential (for example, one teaspoon of cod liver oil) to prevent the bone-deformity disease known as

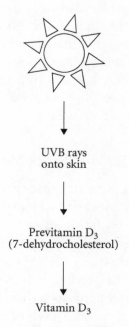

UVB rays
onto skin

Previtamin D₃
(7-dehydrocholesterol)

Vitamin D₃

Figure 8.3. Sunshine ideagram for vitamin D.

rickets. Since then, a large body of research revealed that rickets was not the only disease that can occur if a person does not have enough vitamin D.

Vitamin D insufficiency can lead to osteoporosis, muscle pain and fatigue, hypertension, cardiovascular disease, and other physiological debilities that then progress to cancer of the breast, the colon, and the prostate; diabetes; multiple sclerosis; and lupus.[331, 355] These are serious problems you don't want to face.

For example, more than 25 percent of breast cancer deaths in European women can be attributed to a lack of exposure to ultraviolet B from sunlight.[290, 291, 355]

Now, evidence shows that women over the age of 70, or those who don't have enough reproductive hormones, either need regular sunlight on exposed skin or should ingest at least 1,000 IU per day of a supplement. For people who suffer from fragile bones or poor health, most expert scholars in the field of vitamin D research recommend much higher levels.[328]

Table 8.1 Vitamin D: Short- and Long-Latency Diseases[841]

Short-Latency Diseases (these appear quickly):

- Rickets
- Osteomalacia

Long-Latency Disease (these appear slowly):

Loss of calciotropic effect:

- Osteoporosis
- Muscle pain and fatigue
- Hypertension or cardiovascular disease

Loss of antiproliferative effects:

- Cancer (breast, colon, prostate)

Loss of immunomodulatory effects:

- Diabetes
- Multiple sclerosis
- Lupus

Measuring Vitamin D in Blood

Only in the last few years have researchers had the capacity to reliably measure blood levels of the circulating vitamin D and then only in highly specialized research laboratories.[326] So while reliable blood tests are not available, your need for adequate blood levels of vitamin D requires your action now.

Can You Get Enough Vitamin D from Food?

There are a few—very few—food sources that naturally contain high doses of the form of vitamin D that our bodies need. These include cod liver oil, sardines, and salmon. Unfortunately, the amount of vitamin D supplement that is currently added to milk is trivially low.[355]

Which Supplement Is Effective?

By 2004, researchers had evidence from enough scientific studies to show that vitamin D_2, the supplement most commonly sold then, was ineffective. Vitamin D_3, cholecalciferol, was the most effective form.[25] In 2004, it was difficult to find vitamin D_3. Now, you should be able to find, or place an order for, vitamin D_3 (cholecalciferol) supplements in health food stores and supermarkets.

So, How Much Vitamin D_3 Is Enough?

The amount of vitamin D_3 you need to achieve or maintain a given blood level of vitamin D concentration is not yet known, but investigations have approximated the answer.[841] Dr. Robert Heaney works in Omaha and conducted research studies there during the winter months of two successive years. Using the experimental data that they obtained, the study's authors concluded that for a 70-year-old person, the recommended levels of 600 IU per day are far too low and would produce a serum level of vitamin D that is inadequate for bone maintenance and calcium absorption.[331] Studies show that supplementing with less than 700 IU of vitamin D per day failed to produce the exciting and very beneficial results that were shown in studies of higher levels: 800 to 1,000 or more IU per day.[77, 78, 132, 191, 785, 803]

How Much Is Too Much?

The upper limit for vitamin D has not been set. Each study seems to suggest an even higher level than previously studied, so we can approach the limit from the question of toxicity. That result is pretty clear. You'd have to have a continuing daily intake of more than 10,000 IU per day (250 mg/day) to risk toxicity.[329]

Vitamin D Requirements for Bone Health: Research Examples

Study #1: Vitamin D reduces falls. About 90 percent of hip fractures involve falls. Fractures that are caused by falls occur in about 5 percent of elderly people every year. Vitamin D has benefits on muscle strength, as well as on the preservation of bone. Nutritional scientists tested whether 800 IU per day of vitamin D_3, when added to a calcium supplement (1,200 mg/day), would reduce falls and improve bone health measures in elderly women.[77] Elderly women, in long-stay geriatric care units in nursing homes, took the nutrients or they took a placebo. Within a 3-month period, vitamin D_3 combined with calcium supplementation had reduced falls by 49 percent in frail, elderly women with vitamin D deficiency at baseline.

Study #2: Vitamin D improves lower body fitness. Following up on that theme, Dr. Bischoff and her colleagues next studied a representative sample of noninstitutionalized U.S. women by testing how their baseline circulating blood levels of serum vitamin D compared to lower-extremity function; that is, the ability to rapidly walk 8 feet or quickly rise from and sit down in a chair 5 times in a row. The results were quite clear. Those with better walking ability and faster sit-to-stand speeds showed significantly higher levels of circulating serum vitamin D in their blood.[78]

Study #3: Vitamin D lowers the rate of fractures. Other ways of examining relationships produced similar conclusions about the benefits of vitamin D.[78, 803] In a study conducted at the Cambridge School of Clinical Medicine in the U.K., men and women who participated swallowed 1 capsule of vitamin D_3 at 100,000 IU per capsule, or a placebo, every 4 months (3 capsules per year or 300,000 IU per year). After 4 years of the regimen (12 capsules), lab tests were done to confirm compliance by measuring serum vitamin D in the blood. The results showed that people in the group taking vitamin D_3 did much better than those in the group taking a placebo. They had a 33 percent lower rate of fractures in the hip, the wrist, or the forearm. Even better outcomes might have occurred if the vitamin D levels achieved in the blood had been higher because the vitamin D group had plasma levels that were only 40 percent higher than those for the placebo group.[785]

Study Conclusions Explained

Not every study finds these positive results. A close examination of the studies that fail to find a benefit of vitamin D, however, also shows that the participants had poor compliance; that is, a large majority did not take the vitamin as prescribed.[609, 637] This means it never had a real chance to work or fail. Current statistical methods require "intention-to-treat" analysis, which includes all participants, despite the fact that some did not follow the regimen. In other words, noncompliant people who didn't take the vitamin are included in the treated group.[665] Some researchers believe that this methodology generates distorted conclusions.[489] I agree with these objections to treating *nonparticipants* as if they were participants. They are "ghosts," rather than volunteers who made it to the finish line. Scientific reports in which intention-to-treat research methods are used should be viewed with skepticism. I believe one must look at how the questions were analyzed before drawing conclusions from them. That is what I have tried to do for you throughout the book.

Vitamin D: What's a Smart Woman to Do?

It seems prudent that every woman should take a vitamin D_3 supplement of 1,000 IU per day if she doesn't do a "Ben Franklin" daily. Ideally, the supplement should be taken after, not before, a meal to enhance the absorption.

Calcium: It Does Your Body Good

Calcium is the "stuff" of bones but also serves many key roles throughout the body. It regulates nerve impulses, influences hormonal levels, and reduces hypertension. Every day, through sweat, urine, and feces, the body disposes of more than 700 milligrams of calcium, whether or not you consume any. That's about the supply in a pint of skim milk or yogurt. These must be replaced, or the mineral will be withdrawn from your bone bank.

Back to the Bank: Deposits for Good Health

Bones hold 99 percent of the calcium in your body. How much calcium your bones contain is regulated by two hormones produced in your parathyroid gland: parathyroid hormone (PTH) and calcitonin. When we ingest calcium, some of the nutrient gets absorbed from the intestine into the bloodstream, and some of what is absorbed becomes "a deposit" into the bone bank. If you don't get enough calcium, the PTH will signal your bones for a "withdrawal" to supply it into the blood. If the deficiency continues long enough, you will experience some serious effects.

Age and PTH

PTH (parathyroid hormone) tends to increase with age. PTH promotes the resorption of bone by osteoclasts (bone-chewing cells), thus thinning your bones. What does this mean? High calcium in the diet is beneficial, if the serum level of vitamin D is adequate. Consuming at least 1,200 milligrams per day of calcium lowers the harmful age-related elevations of PTH that cause bone to become porous.[132, 398, 511]

Too Little Calcium: The Overall Risks

A continuing low intake of calcium causes deficiency diseases by three separate mechanisms.[326]

1. *Skeletal wasting.* The skeleton has so much calcium that in extreme deficiency, in a year it loses only about 3 percent of its bone. After ten years, insufficient calcium could lead to 30 percent of your bone being wasted away.

2. *Kidney stones and colon cancer that could have been prevented.* Intestinal calcium absorption is very inefficient. Of the calcium we consume, less than 40 percent is absorbed into the bloodstream. The "inefficient absorption" appears to provide benefits that Dr. Heaney believes reduce the risk of both kidney stones and colon cancer. These unabsorbed calcium ions attach to unabsorbed food crystals or particles ("oxalates"), as well as to fatty and bile acids, which are then excreted. If your kidneys are protected from this load of excess bile and fats, they are at less risk for developing kidney stones.

   The same is true for colon cancer. Dr. Heaney believes that a person who has a long history of adequate calcium in the diet is much less likely to ever experience colon cancer. It makes sense to me, too.

3. *Hypertension.* Abundant calcium also serves to reduce hypertension or high blood pressure. While hypertension is a "disease with many parents," according to Dr. Heaney, you can effectively manage it by increasing the amount of calcium in your diet and reducing your fat intake, as well as making other nutritional and behavioral modifications in your lifestyle. Although antihypertensive drugs are effective, they are expensive and have side effects. Calcium is inexpensive, has no side effects, and needs no medical prescription. But you should never discontinue your antihypertensive medications and switch to calcium on your own. Consult your physician.

Increasing Bone Density: Reducing Fractures

The evidence suggests that calcium will reduce your risk of suffering from bone fractures as long as you take enough vitamin D with it.[191] As you've seen, this is because vitamin D_3 increases the absorption of dietary calcium. And vitamin D has other powers in muscles. It helps prevent falls.

Calcium and vitamin D work! The graph on page 149 (figure 8.4) comes from a study published by Dr. Dawson-Hughes and colleagues in 1997. It shows that, compared to a placebo, elderly women who took daily vitamin D_3 (at 700 IU with 500 mg of calcium) for 36 months

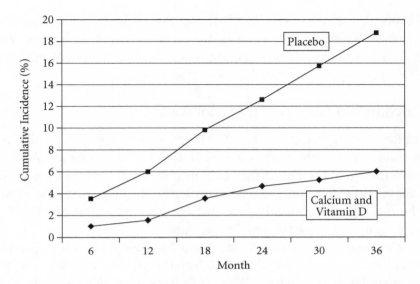

Figure 8.4. Supplementing with calcium and vitamin D: reduced nonvertebral fracture incidence.

showed protection from fractures. Note how the placebo users suffered from breaks in their bones and how the cumulative rate climbed within 36 months to include 20 percent of the group. At only 500 milligrams per day of calcium, combined with 700 IU of Vitamin D$_3$, which was considered relatively high for its time, participating women did not gain bone mass, but at least their bones were protected from further age-related and age-expected loss. Would higher quantities of vitamin D and calcium have been even more beneficial? It appears likely.

Vitamin D and Calcium: Striking the Right Balance

The research shows that not only do you need both calcium and vitamin D, you need them in the right ratio.

High Calcium, Low Vitamin D (Not Right)

A 2004 study compared the regimen of 1,000 milligrams per day of calcium, which is pretty high, combined with 400 IU per day of

Vitamin D_3, which is too low.[398] Under this regimen, there was only a partial benefit. Within 4 weeks, the PTH levels did decline, as was expected from higher calcium in the blood, but blood levels of markers of bone resorption did not decline as hoped.

Calcium, but No Vitamin D (Not Right)

Similarly, an investigation in 1999 tested 800 milligrams per day of calcium citrate without any vitamin D as part of a regimen.[659] After 2 years, there had been no change in bone mineral density for those who took the nutrient and a 2.3 percent decline in bone mass for those who took the placebo, but there had been no reduction in PTH. So once again, only a partial benefit was shown.

What you should know: To meet your changing needs for optimal bone health, you should combine adequate levels of vitamin D_3 with adequate levels of calcium. What is "adequate" varies with age and with the level of reproductive hormones (estrogen, progesterone, testosterone). At least 1,000 IU per day of vitamin D_3 combined with 700–1,500 milligrams per day of calcium seems rational.

How Much Dietary Calcium (or Its Supplement) Is Beneficial?

By 2003, it was clear that the amount of calcium absorption varies with the blood level of vitamin D found in a postmenopausal woman.[332, 338, 339] Dr. Heaney's team proved that if you have enough vitamin D, supplemental oral calcium pills will be adequately absorbed. The choice then has to do with cost and whether the pill is easy or difficult to swallow.[332] Some pills are gigantic, while others are small.[338, 339] They all work. So vitamin D_3 is the key. Take it with your calcium. See chapter 4 to review why calcium from food is better than from pills.

Don't Swallow Claims about Soy

Genistein, one particular isoflavone in soy, has been the subject of many published studies. It shares some chemical properties with estrogen, and it is known to bind to the estrogen receptors in human beings.[137, 534] The only study to evaluate synthetic isoflavones over the long term found no significant changes in bone density from baseline.

In summarizing the research in this field, one expert (2004) stated that it is doubtful that short-term use of dietary or supplemental isoflavones is good for skeletal health in postmenopausal women. A year later (2005), the effect of pure genistein on bone markers and hot flashes in 100 postmenopausal patients was published in the *International Menopause Society*'s journal.[13] In comparison with a placebo, high doses, 99 milligrams per day of pure genistein, did not alter the bone markers of resorption or formation at all.

The downside of soy: There were negative side effects to taking this high a dose of genistein. Both back pain and bloating were significantly more likely to occur in the genistein supplement than in the placebo participants.[13] I do not recommend that you rely on genistein to help your bones.

Instead Swallow This

Don't waste your money on soy; instead, buy some prunes. An animal study suggested that dried plums (prunes) reverse bone loss in ovariectomized rats who had sustained the (expected) postovariectomy bone losses.[210] The results suggest that dried plums can completely reverse the loss of both tibial and femoral bone density that is due to ovarian hormone deficiency in ovariectomized animals.

Since prunes offer other health benefits (such as preventing constipation that can increase small bowel diseases), there seems to be no harm in any woman adding them to her diet if she is concerned about maintaining her bone strength after surgical menopause or a hysterectomy. On days that you add one serving (three or four prunes) to your daily diet, this one food would supply both part of your fruit and part of your dairy need that day. No rigid data are yet available to quantify units, but hopefully you like prunes. They're great for you.

How Sex Hormones Protect Bones

A woman's sex hormones—her estrogen, progesterone, and testosterone—can be thought of as the Executive Management Team in the lifelong remodeling process of her bone.

Progesterone as a Bone-Preserving Hormone

Progesterone protects your bones. Dr. Jerilyn Prior, a preeminent progesterone researcher, showed that bone remodeling is closely related to the ovarian cycle of the fertile years.[614, 617, 618] Her studies provided good evidence that estrogen by itself offers only part of the sex hormone requirement of healthy bones.[51] Dr. Prior believes that to deter postmenopausal bone loss, estrogen is better than no hormone, but *progesterone plus estrogen* is best, resulting in a large gain in bone.

After a woman has a premenopausal ovariectomy, the bone resorption in her body greatly overshadows the formation.[619] This is not good. Bone turnover is increased dramatically above normal premenopausal levels after surgery. Dr. Prior appears to be on target. She describes the benefits of sequential progesterone that mimics the pattern of the ovulatory cycle of bone-replete fertile women. Nature's design seems to work best for hormones and bone health. Take progesterone half of the month and estrogen every day.

Hormone Therapy and Bones

When a postmenopausal woman stops taking estrogen and has *not* previously been taking progesterone, bone loss is accelerated twofold higher than it is in women who were taking progesterone with estrogen.[613] It is essential for women and their physicians to understand the importance of estrogen and progesterone,[292] as well as the difficulties that are likely to occur with their abrupt cessation.

Many women, in response to the Women's Health Initiative and its media blitz, were advised to stop taking hormones altogether. The "sky is falling" reaction that ensued was regrettable. Suddenly stopping hormones hurts the bones of intact women—although less severely than it hurts the bones of a woman who had an ovariectomy or a hysterectomy. If you are one of the women who stopped taking hormones, get your bone health tested.

Studying Hormone Regimens and Bone

The evidence has continued to confirm unequivocal benefits of hormonal therapies for the bones of women after their fertile hormone cycle has ended. Our bones are stronger when we're young and deserve more attention as we age.

What you should know: Hormones help bones. Scientific literature makes it clear that any sex hormone regimen will help bone density, whether estrogen alone,[230, 294, 484, 563, 804] estrogen and a progesterone or a progestin,[95, 122, 294, 542, 608, 820] or estrogen with an androgen, such as testosterone or DHEAS (dehydroepiandrosterone sulfate).[187]

It's never too late to start hormone therapy.[54, 681] Frail women over age 75 who started estrogen and progestin experienced an increase in bone mineral density on the total body, the lumbar spine, the hip, and the trochanter region (the upper thigh-bone) joining the hip. They also showed better results on their bone metabolism: more building, less breakdown.[804] Although the earlier you start, the better, your bones will always appreciate HRT.[54, 681]

Which Hormone Regimens Are Best?

Most often in the United States, a woman who has had a hysterectomy is prescribed estrogen without progesterone. I think this should change. This U.S. pattern contrasts with studies published from Europe, where progesterone is recognized by many researchers as an important component to balance the estrogen.

Estrogen by Itself Does Benefit Bones

What you should know: More estrogen is better. The more estrogen that is provided in the regimen, the greater the increase in, or the more secure the maintenance is of, bone.[173, 229, 230, 294, 563, 597] There is a clear dose-dependency. (But estrogen overdoses cause breast pain and other problems, so you need to balance estrogen with progesterone appropriately.)

The Benefit of Adding Progesterone or Progestins to Estrogen

This is also dose-dependent. The higher the amount of progesterone, the better. For example, in 2005, a study tested 1 milligram per day of estradiol orally taken by pill combined with norethisterone (NET), a synthetic progestin drug widely used in Europe. With the estrogen level held constant, the higher the levels of NET that were added to the estrogen, the better the spinal bone mass improvement.[294]

Progesterone combined with estrogen: The opposite experiments were also performed. The higher the level of estrogen that was added to the steady dose of progesterone, the more bone was gained.[95, 122, 820]

Sequential Regimens Are Better Than Continuous-Combined Regimens

In a continuous-combined regimen, a single pill provides a combination of estrogen and a progestin. This regimen does not mimic the natural reproductive cycle of a woman. It is not nature's design. Sequential regimens provide the progesterone only half of the time and appear to be more beneficial.

For example, an 18-month, double-blind, placebo-controlled trial found that women taking a placebo lost 4.5 percent of their bone mineral density, but either sequential or continuous-combined regimen users *gained* 4 percent in their bone mineral density over the same 18-month period.[542] The sequential regimens allowed a more economical use of hormones because a better effect could be achieved at a much lower total dose.[608]

But if you have heart disease, your bones may not benefit from Prempro. The results from the bone studies of the healthy women that were just described may not apply to women with heart disease. The HERS study tested 2,763 intact women with coronary disease, treating them with either a placebo or the continuous-combined estrogen and progestin, Prempro.[366] More Prempro than placebo users experienced fractures during the 7 years of treatment, but the difference was called "statistically non-significant"; that is, no better than would happen by chance.

What you should know: The longer you take hormones, the better your bones will be as you age. As long as hormones are providing good benefits for you, keep using them.[564]

Osteoarthritis and Hormones

People with bone problems often have osteoarthritis. But you may have osteoarthritis and no osteoporosis or vice versa. The term *osteoarthritis* defines a group of conditions that lead to painful joint symptoms that are associated with defective cartilage at the bone and changes in the underlying bone at the margins of the joints.[771] Risk factors of osteoarthritis are obesity, aging, joint injury, and prolonged occupational or sports stress causing cartilage damage.[37] Symptoms of osteoarthritis include restricted motion after you engage in mild to moderate activity and joint stiffness in the first thirty minutes after you awaken.[37, 798]

What you should know: Vitamin D helps. People with deficient levels of serum vitamin D had 3 times the risk of developing osteoarthritis at the knee, according to data from the Framingham study.[37] One recent study of 1,500 women over age 55 revealed that deficient serum vitamin D (less than 30 mg per ml) was found in more than half of the women.[356] So again, make a commitment to get your optimal vitamin D intake.

Do hormones help or hurt? The studies show both results! It is known that hormone therapy significantly reduces the severity and the loss of the subchondral (beneath the cartilage) bone thickness. For women who are obese or women who began using hormone therapy postmenopausally after age 50, however, the results are mixed. Some studies show that estrogen reduces osteoarthritis symptoms.[669, 806] One study showed that women with these problems were more likely to be using hormones.[809]

Timing is key. Studies that ask about the effects of taking estrogen before age 50 have unambiguously shown consistent benefits. Reviewers have agreed that hormonal therapy has limited benefits when administered *after* cartilage degradation has already occurred, but it may be protective for those who start hormones early.[771] For example, an Italian study of 43,000 women showed that "ever-users" of hormone therapies were at a decreased risk of developing osteoarthritis compared with "never-users."[771]

Osteoarthritis is clearly more common in women who are overweight. Women who were overweight at age 40 had about triple the risk of having osteoarthritis by the time they were postmenopausal.[806]

Bone-Saving Drugs

Table 8.2 shows the variety of treatment regimens that are currently approved and marketed for treating osteoporosis or osteopenia.[453]

Table 8.2 Agents That Reduce Fracture Risk

All Fractures

- Calcium and vitamin D_3
- Hormones: Estrogen and progesterone
- Bisphosphonates: Alendronate (Fosamax), Risedronate (Actonel), Ibandronate (Boniva), Zolendronic acid (Aclasta)

Vertebral Fractures

- Raloxifene (Evista, a SERM)
- Calcitonin-Salmon (Miacalcin)

The bone-specific therapies shown in the table—raloxifene and the bisphosphonates—do offer short-term bone benefits. Unlike hormones, however, these therapies fail to address the other issues (such as vaginal atrophy, blood vessel protection, aging skin and eyes) experienced by a woman who is progesterone- and estrogen-deficient. Prevention of fractures in the long term appears to require long-term therapy, regardless of treatment. I believe the persistent message for most women is: continue your sequential hormone regimen.

For women who should avoid hormonal therapies, bone-specific therapies may offer benefits.

Raloxifene

Raloxifene reduces vertebral fracture risk in osteoporotic postmenopausal women.[386] It is a SERM, a selective estrogen receptor modulator. This synthetic molecule, a patented drug, Evista, *selectively* reacts with some, but not all, estrogen receptors. Whether or not the women have already had vertebral fractures, the results showed that raloxifene worked to prevent future fractures.[386]

Women who began the experiment with a t-score of −3.1 (see the T-Score box on page 136) (very osteoporotic) were at the highest risk of developing new vertebral fractures over the next 3 years. At the end of 3 years, 5.5 percent of the placebo users who had such low t-scores experienced new vertebral fractures. In contrast, about 2.5 percent of the women who had been taking raloxifene (60 mg per day) at the end of 3 years had sustained fractures. A little over 5 percent was cut to a little over 2 percent.[385]

What you should know: Drugs alone may not be enough. Clearly, a drug can help. I would add that studies like this are not designed to simultaneously advise the women to exercise or change their nutrients to prevent fractures.

I say, make lifestyle changes first. Then decide on the drugs.

Bisphosphonates: Do They Help?

Drugs that work as antiresorptive agents appear to reduce the fracture risk by blocking (suppressing) bone resorption. Over-suppression, however, confers a potential risk because theoretically microdamage —micro cracks—would accumulate instead of being fixed.[453]

Bisphosphonates Work, but Long-Term Effects Are Unclear

Bisphosphonates definitely reduce the loss of bone mass and produce a significant 30 to 50 percent reduction in new vertebral fractures.[89] In studies examining bone mineral density in the lower spine, the bisphosphonate *alendronate* maintained or increased bone mineral density better than raloxifene did.[472] The molecules of alendronate attach themselves to the bone tissue, however, and accumulate in the bone.[818] Because these are "foreign particles" not naturally produced by the human body, the long-term effects cannot be determined until the drugs have been consumed for many years, and the adverse effects are recognized and reported. Osteonecrosis (the dying of bone) of the jaw is one such recently discovered adverse effect.[282]

Compared to hormone therapies, bisphosphonates have significant gastrointestinal side effects. And they are not adequate substitutes for estrogen with regard to organ systems other than the bones.[644]

Hormones Are Better

One study showed that taking estrogen with progestin, either sequentially, as NET 10 days per month, or continuously, as MPA at 5 milligrams per day, was superior to taking alendronate up to 5 milligrams per day.[358] After 1 and 2 years of treatment, alendronate did not prevent bone loss in the distal forearm, but doses of either hormone *did* prevent loss. (Since the time of that study, the recommended alendronate dose has doubled to 10 milligrams per day or 70 milligrams per week.) Adequate levels of bisphosphonates are generally effective to address bone loss, up to 10 years of use.[453]

For this reason, physicians who treat bone patients recommend keeping them on bisphosphonates for only up to 7 to 10 years, if they have osteoporosis and not the less severe osteopenia.[453]

These drugs are expensive, costing more than double the price of hormonal therapy. Because Fosamax went off patent in 2007, generic manufacturers will produce much cheaper substitutes for it. Issues of generic equivalence and quality control then warrant discussion. For now, I think bisphosphonates are worth considering only if you cannot take HRT.

Calcitonin

In the early 1980s, there were high hopes for the use of calcitonin hormone to help the bone-*building* component of the remodeling cycle. Unfortunately, for women who are osteoporotic, calcitonin has shown only a small (20 percent) reduction in the risk of new vertebral fractures and no effect on nonvertebral fractures (such as the hip).[89] For this reason, calcitonin is not currently in wide use.

The antiresorptive therapies that were previously described will effectively reduce bone turnover to maintain microarchitecture, improve mineralization, and increase the bone-mineral density. But they do not *reconstruct* bone.

Parathyroid Hormone (PTH)

PTH treatment works differently. It improves bone density by stimulating formation. The drug *teriparatide* is a fragment (a part of the molecule) of human PTH and is FDA-approved for the treatment of osteoporosis. Unfortunately, it has a black box warning on every package that is handed to the consumer, stating that there is an increased risk of osteosarcoma (cancer of the bone) in rats. So it's not a "magic" bone solution.

This PTH drug with the trade name Forteo increased bone mineral density and significantly reduced the risk of new fractures (65 percent reduction in the vertebral and 53 percent in the nonvertebral) in osteoporotic women who had had previous vertebral fractures.[74, 89] You would need to give yourself injections of PTH daily. This tricky regimen also requires careful medical monitoring. *But it does work* when an expert clinician switches the patient to other drugs after two years of use.[74]

What you should know: You may need PTH and then other drugs. Women who took this PTH drug experienced fewer fractures and also had substantial increases in bone mineral density. After stopping the PTH at two years, however, they experienced substantial bone *loss* unless they took antiresorptive drugs.[74] So, two-year use of PTH shows promise for postmenopausal osteoporotic women under careful medical management.

Conclusion

Here are some general recommendations for maintaining bone strength:

1. Exercise regularly. Maintain your balance and fitness through regular activity. Almost any local YMCA or the National Osteoporosis Foundation's Web site (www.nof.org/prevention/exercise .htm) would be a good resource. Every woman, and especially those who are at risk for fragility fractures, should also exercise daily by participating in regular weight-bearing exercises, such as walking. A daily 20- to 30-minute walk should be a *minimum* part of every woman's exercise regimen. Walk while you shop or do housework. Ideally, though, you should get out in the fresh air under that big sky, so that the walk will combine with UVB exposure and good respiration to enhance your overall health, along with your muscles. And practice good posture!

2. Stop smoking. Smokers should quit. There are many ways you can get help to break this bad habit. (See chapters 4 and 9.)

3. Control alcohol consumption. Enjoy alcohol in moderation but not in excess because inebriation can lead to falls. One or two drinks per day have not been shown to increase the risk of osteoporosis or fractures, are good for you, and will probably increase the joy in your life.

4. Practice good nutrition. A well-rounded diet of wholesome, unprocessed foods is part of a general healthy lifestyle. That includes getting enough calcium every day to at least compensate for what gets excreted (about 600 to 700 mg per day). Although many green vegetables do contain high levels of calcium, some, unfortunately, do not release their calcium for absorption, so it is then excreted. Assess your need for a calcium supplement if your diet isn't supplying enough. Take vitamin D_3, at least 1,000 IU per day.

5. Create safe surroundings. Do an environmental risk assessment of your living quarters and other spaces, as a wise precaution. Get rid of tripping hazards. Plug nightlights into sockets in areas you will navigate at night.

6. Consider hormone therapies first, drugs second. Pharmacological agents should be considered, if and when appropriate. Hormonal or bisphosphonate therapy can halt the excessive resorptive breakdown of bone. Progesterone use, preferably sequentially, with regular estrogen, can trigger new bone formation.

The behaviors you choose and the habits you set for yourself profoundly influence your bones, your muscles, and your very freedom to move about as you grow older. Your mother was right when she told you to stand up straight and drink your milk. Now we know more.

9

Keep Your Heart Strong and Your Blood Flowing through Unclogged Vessels

Your heart and blood vessels form a cardiovascular system: *cardio* means "heart" and *vascular* is the "blood vessels." If you are healthy, your blood vessels provide unclogged *pipelines* for your blood to flow throughout your body with each heartbeat.

Your cardiovascular system accomplishes profound tasks. First, the arteries transport red blood cells loaded with oxygen from your lungs to your cells as veins carry blue-colored waste gases from your cells back to the heart and on to the lungs for exhaling. Second, like a home heating-and-cooling system, the pipelines regulate body temperature. Third, these pipelines form an orderly network that delivers:

- Hormones
- Nutrients such as sugar to fire the nerves
- Building blocks such as calcium for the bones
- The cancer-fighting cells of your immune system
- Waste products for disposal to the liver, the kidneys, and the lungs

You want to keep this amazing system vibrant and healthy.

If your blood vessels are clogged with cholesterol or plaque, the pipelines shut down and your health deteriorates. If your veins have obstructions, you are at risk for developing a thromboembolism or having a stroke. Cardiovascular disease is silent for many years before it speaks with a big bang, like a heart attack and a stroke. Meanwhile, the natural onset of menopause starts the clock ticking for the onset of unwelcome cardiovascular changes.[481] Surgical menopause (removal of the uterus and the ovaries) produces an even higher risk of developing cardiovascular disease.[34] The earlier it happens, the earlier the changes start.

The Epidemic of Cardiovascular Disease (CVD) in Postmenopausal Women

- *It kills more women.* Cardiovascular disease (CVD) is the number-one killer of men *and* women in the United States. Worldwide, it accounts for 38 percent of all noncatastrophic deaths.[224, 639] If you look at the year 1950, you will see that for every 100,000 women, 485 died of heart disease, while only 32 died of breast cancer. Happily, death rates from both diseases have been declining since 1950. But 8 times as many women still die of heart disease as they do of breast cancer.

- *It puts more women in the hospital.* CVD accounts for more than one-third of the hospital stays in women over the age of 55.[520] Focus your attention on the actions you can take to feel good *and* prevent this deadly disease.

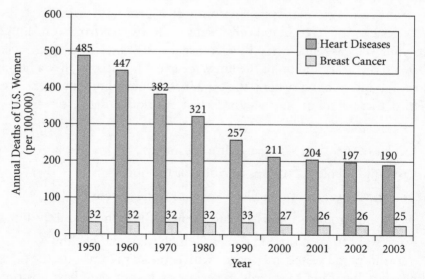

Figure 9.1. Deaths from heart disease and breast cancer in U.S. women, 1950–2003.[554]

Perspective: Start HRT Early

The published data convince me that most postmenopausal women who begin to take hormone-replacement therapy early enough show a favorable pattern that is similar to the cardiovascular condition of premenopausal women: a beneficial pattern that keeps the vessels unclogged and the heart pumping.

The Gender Difference

CVD in *post*menopausal women is silent and more deadly than in men.[770] Although men are worse off than intact *pre*menopausal women, with 4 times the incidence of cardiovascular disease and 40 times as many heart attacks, this ratio *reverses* after menopause, whether it is natural or induced by surgery. More women than men die after a heart attack.[459]

Fertility Cycles and Vessel Health

- *How hormones help:* Atherosclerotic disease (thickening of arteries) is rare in premenopausal women, rises in postmenopausal women who are not taking hormone-replacement therapy, but is reduced to premenopausal levels if women use HRT early enough. Why? The sex hormones directly affect the dilation of blood vessels and the coagulation of blood and act as antioxidants in fighting inflammation. (The sex hormones are the hormones of the reproductive system, secreted from the gonads or the ovaries, and include estrogen, progesterone, and testosterone.) Inflammation is bad. It accelerates the accumulations of fatty substances and blobs of clogging tissue, which are technically referred to as atherosclerotic plaques within the walls of the arteries.[224, 666] You want to prevent inflammation.

- *How sex helps hormones:* My initial research at Penn and then Stanford revealed that *weekly* sexual behavior improved women's sex hormone secretions.[169] At least one intimate sexual encounter per nonmenstruating week served as something like a "paycheck"; it promoted regular menstrual cycles and almost doubled the level of estrogen in both fertile-age and perimenopausal women. It resulted in better levels of progesterone, too. But half of the young women with sporadic (feast or famine) exposure to sex partners had *sub*fertile (irregular) cycles and estrogen levels that were characteristic of old women. For perimenopausal women, regular sex delayed their biological aging and kept their menstrual cycles regular much longer.

- *How regular cycles help:* Dr. Reijo Punnonen in Finland reported that 90 percent of the premenopausal women (ages 42 to 50) with *irregular* menstrual cycles had sclerotic arteries in their uteruses.[624] To me, this meant that a subfertile cycle (low progesterone, erratic estrogen) might be responsible for the arteriosclerosis.

How Fertility Protects You from Heart Disease

Dr. Punnonen examined the arterioles of these uteruses and saw arterial hardening (arteriosclerosis) when women's cycles were irregular. Confirmation in other studies followed, showing that the fertile sex hormone patterns (characteristic of regular cycles) promote the health of women's blood vessels.[147, 488, 730] Estrogen also contributes to long-term protection of the lining of the blood vessels, safeguarding them from injury.[155, 425, 513] The heart muscle itself has receptors for estrogen and progesterone.[64, 274] That is for a reason.

A stable love life is good for your hormones and your cardiovascular health. Likewise, if you start sequential hormonal replacement early in the perimenopausal transition, it should mimic this benefit.

Hormones and Clogging Vessels

Table 9.1, "The Effect of Aging on Blood Lipids," compares the blood levels of lipids (fats) in older versus younger women of the same weight. The postmenopausal women with low estradiol (no progesterone) show alarming increases in all four blood fats, even when they maintain a low weight.[304]

Any sex hormone—in moderation—can help. Women with *moderately high* levels of circulating testosterone had less atherosclerosis of their carotid arteries up to ten years after menopause.[72] But *high* blood

Table 9.1 The Effect of Aging on Blood Lipids

Substances Found in Blood	Reproductive-Aged Women	Postmenopausal Women
Estradiol	50–80 pg/ml[a]	Less than 15 pg/ml
Total cholesterol	178 mg/dl[b]	239 mg/dl
Triglycerides	71 mg/dl	136 mg/dl
Very-low-density lipoprotein cholesterol	15.3 mg/dl	232 mg/dl
Low-density lipoprotein cholesterol	109 mg/dl	154 mg/dl

Adapted from G. A. Berg, N. Siseles, A. I. Gonzalez, O. C. Ortiz, A. Tempone, and R. W. Wikinski (2001): Higher values of hepatic lipase activity in postmenopause: Relationship with atherogenic intermediate density and low density lipoproteins. *Menopause* 8:51–57.

[a]Picograms per milliliter.
[b]Milligrams per deciliter. (For clarity, standard deviation data are omitted.)

levels of testosterone are not so good. High testosterone coupled with low estrogen risks atherosclerosis and inflammation.[160, 324]

Inflammation of Your Blood Vessels

Inflammation is the protective response of tissues to irritation or injury. It can be acute or chronic. The process begins with the constriction of blood vessels and, if chronic, is followed by damaging arteriosclerotic changes to the vessel lining.

A simple blood test your doctor prescribes can check your lipids and other risk markers (such as C-reactive protein) for inflammation. It's easy to test. Lifestyle changes may be all you need to reduce your risk of cardiovascular disease! Table 9.2 lists some established risk factors for CVD.[770, 834]

Dyslipidemia (dysfunctional lipids) is unhealthy levels and ratios of blood fats. Examples include:

- LDL cholesterol level if greater than 100 mg/deciliter (dl)
- Triglyceride level if higher than 199 mg/dl
- Total cholesterol level if higher than 200 mg/dl
- Healthy HDL cholesterol level drops lower than 40 mg/dl

Table 9.2　Heart Disease Risk Factors: What You Can—And Can't—Change

Modifiable	Nonmodifiable
Cigarette smoking	Increasing age
Dyslipidemia (abnormal concentration of lipids in blood)	(male ≥ 45 yr; female ≥ 55 yr)
Hypertension (blood pressure ≥ 140/90 or on antihypertensive medication)	Family history of premature CHD (coronary heart disease)
	• Male first-degree relative < 55 yr
Diabetes mellitus	• Female first-degree relative < 65 yr
Obesity (BMI ≥ 29)	
Physical inactivity	

The National Cholesterol Education Program Expert Panel has concluded that if the "lousy" LDL cholesterol level is high, above 100, *and* lifestyle therapy fails to reduce it within three months, then drug therapy can be considered.[834] *Help your heart:* Save your blood-test printouts to compare the changes over time in your lipid numbers. Know what needs to change.

Hypertension, or blood pressure greater than 140/90, places women at four times the risk of developing coronary heart disease.[834] *Help your heart:* Track your blood pressure reading. If it's creeping higher, you can take action to lower it with a healthy diet and by reducing stress. (See chapter 4.) If these fail to improve your hypertension, you should strongly consider taking prescription drugs.

Diabetes mellitus. Cardiovascular disease is the main cause of death in diabetic people, with CVD death rates three to seven times higher than in nondiabetics. Hypertension and dyslipidemia commonly accompany diabetes mellitus.[834] *Help your heart:* If you have a family history of diabetes, ask for your blood-sugar numbers. If you are overweight, lose weight. If you are not overweight, maintain a healthy weight.

Obesity and physical inactivity. If your body mass index (BMI) is greater than or equal to 29, you are obese. If your BMI is between 25 and 28.9, you are seriously overweight and at risk for developing significant heart disease. *Help your heart:* You cannot change your genes, but you can change your diet and activity level. See chapter 4 to check your BMI.

Take Action to Improve Your Cardiovascular Health

You can't change getting older or your family history, but there is a lot you can do to modify and/or reduce your risk of getting cardiovascular disease.[606]

The American Heart Association has suggested eight lifestyle interventions. The American College of Obstetrics and Gynecology has endorsed them, after reviewing nearly 9,000 studies.[307]

- No cigarette smoking
- Regular physical activity
- A heart-healthy diet
- Cardiac rehabilitation
- Weight maintenance or reduction
- Checking for depression in women who have cardiovascular disease because it is an unwelcome "companion"
- Omega-3 fatty acid supplementation for high-risk women
- Folic acid supplementation or add it to your diet (avoid dangerous overdoses; ask your doctor before you do this one)

Save Your Own Life

Unfortunately, smokers inhale carbon monoxide, which tightly binds to the red blood cells and blocks the transport of needed oxygen. As a result, cells throughout the body (not only in the lungs) begin to die of asphyxiation and disease.

Help your heart: Smoking is an addiction; it is very difficult to stop, but effective help is available. Consider the Freedom from Smoking Online program from the American Lung Association (www.LungUSA .org) and QuitNet (www.quitnet.com), which operates in association with Boston University's School of Public Health. In chapter 4, I provided a breathing trick that works (and it's free!). The reward of quitting is immediate, a dramatic rush of energy.

Exercise: Aerobic exercises—those that cause you to breathe deeply and heavily—serve your cardiovascular system by increasing your oxygen consumption, thus bringing more oxygen into your bloodstream to nourish cells throughout your body, including your heart. Your cardiovascular system functions best when it receives plenty of oxygen.[581, 711]

The bonus of exercise: Deep-down relaxation. Remember, your heart is a muscle. After exercise, your muscles will automatically enter a state of relaxation. Muscle relaxation affects all of the muscles of the body, including those that form arterial vessels.

Biofeedback experiments show that you can lower your blood pressure by doing relaxation exercises.[157] Take a class or choose serenity-making activities, and log them on your calendar. Remind yourself that you deserve it.

Help your heart: To maximize your cardiovascular health, you need at least 180 minutes of athletic activity per week. Do whatever you like, and break it up any way you like into doable chunks of fifteen to sixty minutes each.

Walk as much as you can. Take the stairs instead of the elevator; park your car farther away. If you work at a desk, try to move around whenever you can. Keep in mind that during vigorous exercise, seemingly healthy older women who are *not* taking HRT are vulnerable to impaired leg vasodilation (muscle cramps).[532, 620, 833] This means that older vessels might not dilate enough to adequately supply the leg muscles with blood. As usual, age matters. Light exercise won't be a problem. But a study of older women has shown that at greater exertion, leg blood-flow responses were significantly weakened in the femoral artery that supplies the area. These losses in older women were not related to the total leg muscle mass, but rather to the declining capacity of the blood vessels to deliver oxygen where it was needed.[620]

Help your heart: Taking a daily walk and breathing deeply will keep you going as long as possible. Although life *is* terminal, walking will make it terminal later.

VO2: Your Maximal Volume of Oxygen

"Maximal oxygen consumption" measures the amount of oxygen consumed and delivered to the body when you are working as hard as possible. Measures of maximal oxygen consumption provide the most informative indicator of cardiovascular health.[531]

To Cope with Stress, Learn to Relax

Stress is your body's physical reaction to the threat of danger or sensory overload. The woman who overreacts puts an additional burden on her physiological system, and her prolonged stress generates higher cortisol levels in her blood. Cortisol is one of the stress-combating hormones that is secreted by the adrenal glands. But chronically *high* levels of cortisol increase your risk for developing coronary artery disease and are important predictors of significant clogging of the heart vessel.[409] Reduce stress, and your cortisol levels will drop. Here's how:

- Modify your philosophy or attitude.
- Seek out a religious orientation to help you find peace.
- Do regular, quiet meditation and/or biofeedback training.
- Get support, whether through a group, a psychotherapist, or courses of study.
- Get connected: revive friendships, make new ones.
- Seek a calm environment: go to a quiet beach, escape to the country, or contemplate something beautiful in nature. Write a poem. Start a journal.
- Exercise regularly. Exercise changes the way we *perceive*, as our brain chemistry is flooded with beta endorphins that produce feelings of well-being.
- Give love and not only romantic love. Find others to love, perhaps through community or social service volunteering, *and* maybe invite a dog to move in with you!

Eat Intelligently

A heart-healthy diet, like the Mediterranean diet described in chapter 4, combines at least three key components.[307] First, a variety of fresh produce, whole grains, low-fat and nonfat dairy products, fish, legumes, and sources of protein that are low in saturated fat. (If you can slice a fat when it is cool, such as butter or lard, it is "saturated" and this is bad!) Second, limit the saturated fat to less than 10 percent of the calories you consume. So for a typical 1,800-calorie diet, this would mean no more than 180 calories total of butter or other dairy or meat-related fats. Third, eliminate or reduce your intake of trans-fatty acids. These man-made fats are unambiguously dangerous and cause hardening of the arteries. Food labels will tell you where they are. Read them. Cherish your vessels by eating well.

Help your heart: The more whole grains a person eats, the less coronary artery disease she will suffer.[742] A croissant is a good example of a bad food. Refined white flour minus the nutritious wheat germ and bran, coupled with artery-clogging fat, is a really bad combination! (See chapter 4 for a table of whole grains and refined grain foods.)

Fruits and vegetables also promote good cardiovascular health.

Help your heart: The greater the consumption of a variety of fruits and vegetables, the lower the total death rate.[742]

Consider two key supplements: vitamin C and calcium:

- Vitamin C supplements will help your cardiovascular health. Vitamin C supplements reduced the incidence of stroke in the Women's Health Initiative study.[819] And intravenous vitamin C given to estrogen-deficient postmenopausal women improved the flow of blood in their vessels.[512]

  Help your heart: Take at least 500 milligrams of vitamin C per day. Possibly more might be even better when your air passages are stressed by pollutants, airplane travel, or pollen. Limit each dose to 500 mg because your body cannot absorb higher doses at one time. But you can take another 500 milligram capsule an hour later if you need it.[168]

- Dietary calcium also helps keep lipids in check. Women who consumed at least 1,000 milligrams per day had a healthier lipid profile than those who did not.[640]

  Help your heart: Particularly after a hysterectomy and/or menopause, it is important to make sure you get enough calcium—at least 1,000 milligrams per day. (See chapter 8 to review why you need vitamin D_3 with it.)

The Cardiovascular Argument for HRT

In 2005, researchers found that hormone-using women under 60 years of age had a significantly better likelihood of enjoying good cardiovascular health. The investigators reviewed 30 different studies, involving 27,000 postmenopausal women.[664]

The conclusions of this massive review are:

- It is reasonably clear that hormone therapy reduces cardiac events and total deaths in younger postmenopausal women;

- These benefits are not initially seen in older women who start hormone therapy after many postmenopausal years have elapsed. HRT increased the incidence of cardiac events in the first two years of late-onset use.

- Once older women have been using hormones for 2 years, there is no compelling CVD reason to stop because after 4 or 5 years of hormone use, the risk of developing cardiac problems declines.

Similar results were found for all of the studies, including the Women's Health Initiative, when the data were pooled and regrouped by age.[664] And in the Nurses Health Study, which used a cohort of 120,000 women younger than 55, who were followed for 20 years, a 40 percent reduction in coronary heart disease events and total death count was associated with the use of hormone therapy.[298, 664] This is fantastic!

A snapshot from the Nurses Health Study reveals:

- The best "scores" in cardiovascular health were in hormone-using women who had their uteruses and ovaries intact.

- The next-best performers were hormone users who had undergone ovariectomies.

- The worst record in cardiovascular health and longevity was in women who had never used hormones.[298]

- Once women stopped taking hormones, they lost that advantage over "never-users."

Animal studies show the same. If estrogen is administered in monkeys immediately after they have ovariectomies (even if they are then fed an atherogenic high-fat diet), the development of atherosclerotic disease is significantly reduced.[349]

Even More Proof of a Clear Advantage in Hormone Users

Lower triglycerides, lower LDL cholesterol, less obesity, and a lower incidence of diabetes mellitus were reported in hormone-using women in Sweden among 7,000 women enrolled in an observational women's health study.[690] These benefits were only for nonsmokers. Oral estrogens are *not* helpful to smokers.[63]

And less than half the amount of carotid atherosclerotic plaque formations were found in women who "had ever used hormonal-replacement therapy" compared to never-users (8.6 percent versus 19.1 percent) among 815 postmenopausal women ages 59 to 71.[438] Similarly, less thickening of the femoral arteries was found. Women who were also physically fit were even better off using HRT.[531]

In addition, current users of estrogen, in an upper-middle-class community of nonobese women, had a 60 percent lower risk of developing increasingly severe clogging of coronary arteries with calcium deposits.[53]

HT Users Have Decreased Coronary Heart Disease Risk

Overall, the many observational studies show a decreased risk of developing coronary heart disease in healthy postmenopausal women who used both estrogen-only therapies and estrogen plus synthetic progestin. HRT use slightly lowered blood pressure in women with higher levels and it slightly elevated low levels.[745]

Compared to women who were not taking hormones, coronary heart disease risk is about 30 percent lower in estrogen users and 40 percent lower in those who use estrogen and progesterone. These cardio-protective effects are associated with improvements in measures of blood lipids, hypertension, glucose tolerance, endothelial function, and inflammation.[80]

One Catch: You Have a Window of Time

Both advancing age and atherosclerotic injury to the vessel walls diminish the cardiovascular benefits of starting hormone therapy.[415] For women with documented coronary artery disease and also for women with high glucose (characteristic of diabetes), five recent studies have shown that the hormone therapy regimens that were tested did not produce any benefits.[144, 346, 347, 454, 578]

In the case of *coronary artery atherogenesis* (basically, the clogging of the artery that nourishes the heart), the benefits of HRT depend on how clogged the blood vessels are when you start HRT.[470, 480, 481]

Estrogens have major beneficial effects (70 percent inhibition of the progression) in the early stages of atherogenesis. But after plaque complications have already occurred, it's too late.[100, 146, 260, 349, 388, 479, 729]

The proof came from two randomized controlled experiments, EPAT, Estrogen in the Prevention of Atherosclerosis Trial,[745] and Well-Hart. Both used the same protocol to measure the same outcomes: the thickening of the carotid artery, which eventually leads to heart attacks. EPAT tested healthy women in early menopause. Well-Hart tested postmenopausal women taking lipid-lowering drugs who had already had at least one serious coronary artery mishap.[349]

EPAT showed that early in menopause, hormonal treatment was effective in *preventing* atherosclerotic thickening in women who had no preexisting disease. In contrast, Well-Hart showed that using the hormonal regimen later had no benefit. It was too late!

When to start HRT: If you are healthy, trim, exercise regularly, and have clear vessels, then with appropriate regimens of hormones you may be able to prevent CVD.[550, 745] If you have a regular sex partner as you approach menopause, you will have less need of taking estrogen during the transition because regular sex then delays the sex hormone decline. If you had a hysterectomy (whether or not you retained your ovaries) or are younger than fifty-six, starting a good hormone regimen will most likely be *very* helpful to you. If you don't have a regular sex life, I think you should consider beginning HT well before your last menstrual period.

But don't stop what is working. These findings lead thoughtful scholars to advise women with heart disease and also those who are overweight *not to start* hormone therapies in hopes of a cure, but *not to stop* if they have been enjoying the benefits of hormone therapies for more than a year. If hormones are serving the general health of the woman, they should be continued.

Another Catch: You Need to Choose Your Hormone Products Carefully

Some HRT products work better than others. Let's look at some of the research.

The continuous-combined regimen Prempro has been extensively studied. It has a lot of problems.

Prempro and Premarin Hormone Products

The first study: HERS (the Heart and Estrogen/Progestin Replacement Study) tested Prempro versus a placebo in 2,763 postmenopausal women.

The women: All of them already had cardiovascular disease when they began. Most of these women were seriously overweight, with an average body mass index equal to 29 and, not surprisingly, had many cardiovascular disease events during the 7 years of the study.

The result: Prempro caused an immediate increase in stroke, pulmonary embolism, and gall bladder disease. After 6.8 years of follow-up, the authors stated that Prempro "did not reduce [the] risk of cardiovascular events in women with coronary heart disease (CHD)."[286] They further concluded, "Based on the finding of no overall cardiovascular benefit and a pattern of early increase in risk of CHD events, we do not recommend starting this treatment for the secondary prevention of CHD events."[367]

The second study: The Women's Health Initiative (WHI) also tested Prempro versus a placebo in 16,000 intact postmenopausal women.

The women: Ninety-five percent had *no* history of cardiovascular disease, and most (74 percent) had *never* used hormones. At the start, they ranged in age from 50 to 79, and the majority were overweight.[819]

The result: As in the HERS study, the WHI also showed a significant increased risk of strokes, especially ischemic stroke and coronary heart disease, from taking Prempro.[166] By 2005, it was clear that this risk of Prempro on coronary heart disease was confined to the oldest group of women: those who started hormones more than 20 years after menopause.[729] Moreover, Prempro users who had high baseline levels of the "lousy" LDL cholesterol were in trouble. Prempro *increased* the coronary heart disease risk in these women . . . and "should not be prescribed for the prevention of cardiovascular disease."[494]

The conclusion of the final analysis was that the relative risk for strokes was (a little) worse for Prempro (in intact women) than for Premarin and both were worse than for a placebo.[166]

Blocked Blood Flow to the Brain: Risk of Dementia

The Women's Health Initiative Memory Study evaluated 5,000 of the 16,000 intact WHI participants and showed that Prempro caused a twofold increase in the risk of dementia in women over the age of 65.[778] Dementia was rare, however, so doubling a low rate was still very low and was primarily due to the higher rates of vascular-related dementia. The Prempro risk of dementia may have been due to the 50 percent higher incidence of strokes in the hormonal therapy groups.[778]

Animal studies of blood flow in the brains of mammals provide clear visual images of the effects of different hormone regimens on blood vessels. The results showed that synthetic progestins (both MPA, as in Prempro, and norethindrone) disrupt the endothelial tissue by forming clots.[778] In contrast, the natural progesterone combined with either conjugated equine estrogen or estradiol-17β did not produce this toxicity. Different synthetic progestins vary in toxicity and benefits.[716]

Other Continuous-Combined Hormone Products

Would a different continuous-combined regimen show cardiovascular benefits? Postmenopausal women with high cholesterol agreed to change their eating patterns to a lipid-lowering diet and tested 1 milligram per day of estradiol combined with 500 micrograms per day of another synthetic progestin, norethisterone. No benefits could be shown.[186]

MPA diminishes the benefit of estradiol in animal studies, too.[133, 378, 576] Stunning proof of the CVD dangers of the synthetic progestin MPA came from a 2005 study of large female mammals. (See figure 9.2.) Divided into 3 groups, all of the animals had hysterectomies and ovariectomies and were fed a high-fat diet for 18 months. One-third of them received placebos, one-third got ethinyl estradiol (EE) and norethisterone acetate (NETA), and one-third got EE and MPA. The question asked was which group had the most heart damage and, specifically, did NETA or MPA do more damage? Remember: all 3 groups had 18 months of a heart-damaging high-fat diet after being castrated.

When "the envelopes were opened," the EE/NETA group won, with only 4 percent of the animals' hearts sustaining damage. Note the

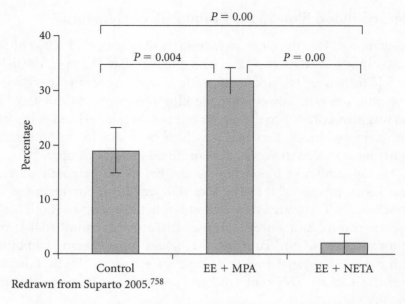

Redrawn from Suparto 2005.[758]

Figure 9.2. Heart damage in eighteen months of postovariectomy/high-fat diet.

bar on the right of the figure.[758] The EE/NETA provided some heart protection after the bodily insults of castration and a damaging diet, since the placebo-control group scored an average of close to 20 percent to the heart damage in each animal. The loser? MPA, because the third group showed more than 30 percent heart damage. Applying these animal studies to humans, I think these results show that postmenopausal women on a high-fat diet should not use MPA as the progestin that is needed to balance their daily estrogen.

Toxic versus Beneficial: Synthetic Progestins Compared to Progesterone

Two reports concluded that MPA applied in vitro (in a dish) may diminish estradiol's beneficial antisclerotic effects on the blood vessels. But a different synthetic progestin, NET, may be neutral.[539, 686] A third product, micronized progesterone (natural), produced much better effects. Unfortunately, the synthetic progestins may lessen or even reverse the beneficial lipid effects of the natural progesterones, according to research on monkeys.[242]

For older postmenopausal women in the huge WHI study, MPA was clearly dangerous because it increased the incidence of pulmonary embolism and venous thromboembolism.[602] Similarly, MPA appeared to be a bad progestin choice for its negative effect on lipids and atherosclerosis.[437, 539]

Choose Another Progestin

Although MPA *reduces* the beneficial effects of estrogens on the lipoprotein levels, the human-identical, micronized progesterone *does not.*[479] Sequential dydrogesterone (which is closely related to natural progesterone) balanced by estradiol also produced favorable long-term effects on lipids, according to a randomized, controlled trial of more than 550 women in the Netherlands.[746] And unlike certain synthetic progestins, micronized progesterone did not increase the risk of stroke.[112]

The Importance of the Delivery Route of Hormonal Therapy

Studies of cardiovascular responses to hormonal therapies have focused principally on comparing oral and transdermal routes. The results differ.

Oral Options to Swallow

For trim women who start hormone therapies *before* developing atherosclerotic changes, oral routes are convenient and unlikely to be harmful to cardiovascular physiology. But if HRT begins *after* atherosclerotic changes have occurred, these oral estrogen routes can cause undesired effects such as strokes.[425] Once the lining of your blood vessels has been damaged, your blood flow is compromised.[280] So, the timing, the route of delivery, and the current condition of the blood vessels determine the outcomes.

Stroke Sufferers Should Avoid Oral Estrogens

When estrogen pills are swallowed, the hormone concentrates in the liver, accumulating extremely high levels. This is not so for other delivery routes: transdermal as gels or patches on the skin, sublingually (pills absorbed under the tongue), or vaginally across the mucosa. This probably explains why oral (swallowed) Premarin increases the risk of stroke for a very small minority of women who take it.[476]

If you have had a stroke, avoid oral hormones. One study enrolled 684 women within 90 days of their stroke and tested oral estradiol or a placebo. After nearly 3 years, oral estrogen increased the incidence of having a fatal stroke.[807] A similar increase in risk for oral, but no problems for transdermal, estrogen was reported in 2007 in France.[112] Choose a different route to avoid the (admittedly low) risk of stroke.

Triglycerides—Dangerous Fats Found in the Blood

Premarin, but not an esterified estrogen, taken orally *raised* triglycerides about 18 percent.[320, 465] *Oral* estradiol offset by the synthetic progestin (norethisterone) taken sequentially produced a 21 percent increase in serum triglycerides in healthy women (age 53 with a body mass index of 25).[234] But transdermal estrogen therapy (a patch or a gel) *decreased* triglyceride levels in several studies.[341, 425, 667, 811] And in one experiment, the same estrogen taken *orally increased* the triglyceride levels by 12 percent within a year but applied *transdermally* to other women caused no change.[341]

Switching from Oral to Transdermal Estradiol Reduced Triglycerides

Simply switching 61 women to *transdermal* estradiol and having them continue on *oral* medroxyprogesterone acetate reduced elevated triglycerides that had been caused by oral Prempro.[668] Triglyceride elevations could potentially be dangerous. It is one reason to think about having blood tests done if you take oral estrogens.

You Should Know: Consider Inflammation

You probably know that high levels of LDL cholesterol and triglycerides in your blood each signal a risk for CVD. The Women's Health Initiative Observational Study discovered that inflammatory markers were even more predictive of CVD than was LDL cholesterol.[189]

Inflammatory Markers in Postmenopausal Women

- *C-reactive proteins (CRPs)* are proteins that are measured from blood samples. Think of them as footprints left by inflammation. A blood test showing CRP levels over 3 (micrograms/milliliter) places a woman at high risk for developing cardiovascular disease.[160] High CRP levels predicted CVD whether or not the women were using hormone therapy.[611] Oral Premarin elevates CRP levels.[476] And oral estradiol taken by itself increased CRP, but the same oral estradiol did not increase CRP when taken in combination with the testosterone derivative Gestodene.[610] Transdermal estrogen taken by itself did not increase CRP in the blood even when opposed by oral MPA.[432,610,867] Some other oral estrogen products combined with certain progestins also *elevated CRP*.[183, 433, 597, 612] This is not good. Most oral estrogens taken alone or with either MPA (the "pro" in Prempro) or NETA represent bad choices because they increased the CRP levels.[50,302]

- *White blood cell count* is measured by an inexpensive test. In the WHI, women with the highest levels had the highest likelihood both of dying and of incidence of stroke within the 6 years they were followed.[497]

- *Interleukin-6 (IL-6).* About 5 percent of postmenopausal 46- to 63-year-old women are at risk of developing an early inflammatory reaction shortly after they begin taking oral hormone therapy.[808]

- *Homocysteine (HCY)* causes spontaneous blood vessel constriction.[723] Estradiol reverses this bad effect.[868] Both oral (2 mg) and transdermal (50 micrograms/day) estradiol routes combined with norethisterone (NET) lowered HCY from baseline.[110, 139] Lower levels of HCY were reported from a variety of hormone regimens compared to nonusers.[302] This is good news! But Prempro produced variable effects: no change[50] or decline.[789] And Premarin or placebo alone caused an elevation of HCY, while Premarin supplemented with folate lowered HCY.[781] Folic acid supplements (1 mg) with vitamin B_{12} (400 mg) and vitamin B_6 were therefore suggested for women who were going to use Premarin.[464]

To protect yourself from inflammation, the most rational choice seems to be estrogen through a nonswallowed route and a bioidentical progesterone capsule swallowed, if formulated in oil, or sublingual, if compounded.

You should know: Check your triglycerides and CRP if you start any oral estrogens. If you want to begin oral estrogen, it seems prudent to me to get a blood test three and/or six months after you start, and switch regimens if your CRP or triglycerides rise.[667] As always, do this in consultation with your doctor.

Sequential Progestin: Three HRT Regimens Compared

A study of healthy postmenopausal women compared a placebo to three different hormone regimens of estrogen every day with synthetic progestin used variably against two cardiovascular disease risk factors that can be measured in the blood.[80]

- The best results were from the sequential regimen of progestin half of each month.
- The next best used progestin every third month.
- The worst used no progestin.

Estrogen and Sequential Progesterone Can Be a Winning Combination

Progesterone elevates your body temperature by raising the metabolic rate. (This is why fertile women can monitor their daily basal body temperature to predict ovulation. Ovulation is the event that starts the progesterone-secreting half of the monthly cycle.) Since progesterone increases the metabolic rate, it also helps women stay trim.[584]

Nature's Design for Women: A Good Model for HRT

Fertile women (who rarely experience cardiovascular disease) have a normal estrogen-progesterone cycle, in which progesterone is absent the first half of each month, but estrogen circulates *every* day (at least 50 pg/ml): what I call nature's design. Very few research studies have considered mimicking nature in testing regimens of hormones, but the few that have done so provide compelling evidence for the wisdom of nature's design.

I favor estrogen therapy taken daily through a *nonswallowed route* and natural progesterone taken sequentially the second half of each month instead of any of the synthetic progestins. Progesterone can be prescribed for oral use or as a lozenge that is absorbed across the cheek or sublingually and possibly vaginally. Both the Big Pharma product Prometrium and a compounding pharmacy can supply progesterone when your doctor writes the prescription. Such regimens produce very good physiological results.[109, 795]

What about the Estrogen?

All oral regimens are not the same. Like progesterone versus progestins, different oral regimens of estrogen should not be viewed as a single "class." In 1997, the Group Health Cooperative (GHC) pharmacies switched postmenopausal estrogen therapy pills: from esterified estrogen to conjugated equine estrogens, for example, like Premarin.[720] Until that time, these two formulations had been thought to be therapeutically interchangeable. They aren't.

This large health maintenance organization in Washington state evaluated 2,000 postmenopausal members, looking for hormonal patterns that would reveal the risk of having a first deep venous thromboembolism (VT) or a pulmonary embolism (PE). The results revealed that current users of oral esterified estrogen had *no* increased risk of VT (stroke) compared with nonusers, but that current users of conjugated equine estrogens had 165 percent the risk. Similar results were obtained for myocardial infarctions and for ischemic stroke.[444] (This increased hazard is about the same magnitude as that shown in the Prempro data of HERS and WHI.)

Avoid These Estrogens

The GHC study made it clear that conjugated equine estrogen (for example, like Premarin) was significantly more hazardous than esterified estrogen.[720] When the researchers restricted their analysis to current users of *combined* conjugated equine estrogen and synthetic progestin, the Prempro-type regimen was even worse—it had double the increase in VT risk, compared with combined esterified estrogen and synthetic progestin. Compared with a placebo, a different synthetic estrogen, the SERM (selective estrogen receptor modulator) raloxifene, also doubled the risk of VT events: vein thrombosis, PE, and retinal embolism.[285] Again, this was double a low risk.

Another synthetic estrogen is ethinyl estradiol. It appears to be a poor choice for postmenopausal women. By 1998, an early warning signal was sounded after the testing of triphasic oral contraceptives and cardiovascular events because studies in monkeys showed that the long-term use elevated cortisol levels, a known stress response that promotes inflammation.[342, 701]

The fact that outcomes vary from taking estrogen should prompt you and your doctor to choose carefully.[707]

Choose Estrogens Wisely

A good choice is estradiol-17β, which is a powerful antioxidant.[26] This estrogen, concomitantly taken with norethisterone acetate (NETA) as the balancing progesterone, whether the two are combined in a swallowed pill or an intranasal spray, produced beneficial lipid changes. In the study, the women's triglycerides and LDL cholesterol levels both declined.[340] But oral estradiol-17β taken without any progestin increased triglycerides.[341] Transdermal estradiol does not alter triglycerides and has other benefits: enhanced heart rate variability, which reduces the risk of acute myocardial infarction in postmenopausal intact and hysterectomized women.[131]

There have been no studies of oral estriol (a weaker human estrogen) lessening a cardiovascular disease risk. Therefore, no benefits should be claimed as a class effect.[167]

Conclusion

This chapter has covered a lot of ground. It was quite a workout, but for a very good cause. The two key take-home messages for you are:

- Consider taking hormones: the right kind.
- Live a healthy life, too.

I think one could reasonably conclude that oral Premarin has been shown to increase the risk of strokes, myocardial infarction, and deep venous thrombosis in a small proportion of users, but that certain other forms of estrogen may not be implicated. Prempro has been shown to have many adverse cardiovascular effects as well. Taking a hormonal regimen that most closely mimics nature's design appears to benefit the cardiovascular system. Bioidentical Estrace and bioidentical Prometrium or a compounding pharmacy filling a prescription for estradiol-17β and progesterone tablets to be taken sublingually, are some good options.

Nothing works in isolation. All of the hormones in the world, even a regimen that mimics nature's design and that you begin before menopausal changes occur in your vessels, cannot overcome unhealthy lifestyle habits and behaviors. As outlined in this chapter, you can help your cardiovascular system by

- *Exercising regularly.* Pick an activity that you enjoy. This is supposed to be a pleasure, not a punishment!
- *Eating intelligently.* Choose fresh foods that are as close as possible to the natural product, with little processing and packaging.
- *De-stressing daily* (or more!), using whatever technique works for you.
- *Consider getting a puppy* if you need more love in your life.
- *Living free of smoke.*

Help your heart!

10

Protecting the Breasts: The Hidden Truth about Mammography, Radiation, Hormones, and Cancer

Breast cancer is the subject of a perpetual barrage of fear-inducing headlines. And as of April 2006, the U.S. Department of Health and Human Services advises: "Women 40 years and older should get a mammogram every one to two years" (www.4women .gov/mammography.htm).

Symbolic pink ribbons are everywhere. Famous personalities urge us to have mammograms to detect our cancer early. And an emerging "breast-terror industry" alarms women with marketing methods that are ostensibly designed to generate money for research but that also coincidentally increase product sales and support an army of people who do not do any research. I find that these messages subtly misinterpret data. The excessive search for disease can stress and traumatize a woman. Stress is unhealthy. It damages our immune systems and reduces our natural capacity to fight cancer and other diseases. We should focus our energies on what to do to be healthy. First, let's take the fangs out of the fearmongering.

Here's what the current science has to say—and it's not as frightening a picture as the breast-terror industry would have you believe:

- The actual incidence of breast cancer is much lower than that of cardiovascular or bone disease.

- Breast cancer is highly unlikely to kill you.
- You can cut your risk dramatically by making wise food choices, cultivating good exercise habits, getting exposure to fresh air and sunshine, and taking steps to promote mental health.
- Mammograms are not "treatment"; they are stressful detection techniques.
- Users of some types of HRT have less cancer than nonusers do. And 99 percent of women will not be at *increased* risk of developing breast cancer, regardless of which hormones they take.

What You Should Know

You do have choices. This chapter outlines your options by reviewing the real facts behind the scientific research. My goal is to expose how the misunderstanding of statistical jargon distorts results. I'll show you the actual studies and the good news that a correct interpretation can offer. Let's start with death rates.

Figure 10.1 clearly shows that in 53 years of "public awareness campaigns," the breast cancer death rate of about 25 deaths per 100,000

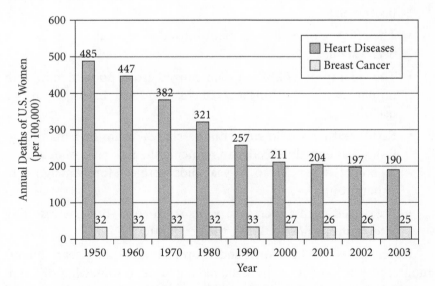

Figure 10.1. What disease is most likely to claim your life? Death from heart disease and breast cancer in U.S. women, 1950–2003.[554]

women in the United States is low and has barely changed. The data from the National Center for Health Statistics for 2005 reveal how different the media messages are from the reality.

Does Mammography Reduce Mortality Rates? Maybe Not.

We hear that more breast cancers are occurring, but what this really means is that more breast cancer is being "discovered" when mammograms are used to search for it. Breast cancer screening seems to explain recent increases in breast cancer *detection*.[219] If you're looking for something (such as cancer) and you look regularly, chances are, you're more likely to find it.

Does mammography reduce the devastating experiences of developing incurable metastatic breast cancer or having a mastectomy or does it lower mortality rates? The science behind such claims has not proved that it has.

In 2002, the U.S. Preventive Services Task Force commissioned a review of everything published up until that time, in order to update its recommendations. The task force findings were sobering to me:[368]

- There were no randomized, controlled treatment-outcome trials. In other words, no current breast cancer treatment had been proven effective.

- The efficacy of early treatment on reducing death rates has *not* been established.

- The quality of published data ranged from poor to fair, with numerous flaws limiting any conclusions about mammography's usefulness.

- Early treatment following either a clinical exam or a mammography was equally effective in reducing the risk ratio of death (by 3 percent) when 50- to 59-year-olds were randomly assigned to either group.

- Breast self-exams increased visits to doctors, but the resulting interventions did not affect the death rates.[368]

Nevertheless, the task force ended up recommending yearly mammograms. But looking at the same data, I come to somewhat different conclusions. In my opinion, the public information is unbalanced and falsely marketed when it suggests that mammographic screening is always good, leads to early detection, and implies that early intervention thereby improves lifespan. This message contradicts the data.[869, 870]

Can a Mammography Hurt You? Yes.

- *Stress effects.* Adverse effects include anxiety, discomfort, loss of work, and increased stress if one is called back for additional tests that reveal no disease. Stress itself is now recognized to generate a cascade of endocrine responses (such as a reduced ability to fight infection) that increase a person's vulnerability to many diseases, including cancer.[846]

- *Radiation exposure.* Recent estimates from the U.S. Preventive Services Task Force state that radiation from 10 annual mammograms will cause up to 8 deaths from breast cancer for every 100,000 women.[368] Since 25 deaths per 100,000 women per year occur from breast cancer, 8 fewer would be substantial.

   Although infrared imaging is painless and has been touted as a useful noninvasive new method of detecting pathology, unfortunately it is not very specific.[590] Neither is ultrasound useful as a screening tool.

- *The "costs" of biopsies.* More than one million breast biopsies are performed each year in the United States and 80 percent of these yield a benign outcome.[590] Biopsy costs vary from under $1,000 to several thousand dollars. *What does the stress "cost" the woman?* I think the economic waste is stunning for the individual, and the economic gain is substantial to those who profit from these tests.

- *The costs of incompetence.* Women who choose screening by mammography should select a competent evaluating center.[399] In the United States, radiology physicians are required to read *only* 480 mammograms per year in order to fulfill the Mammography Quality Standards Act. In the United Kingdom, physicians must read more than 5,000 mammograms a year to maintain certification. This tenfold lower certification standard required of U.S. physicians may well explain the excess false positives that U.S. women suffer. Although the open surgical biopsy rate is two to three times higher in the United States than in the United Kingdom, the cancer detection rate is similar.[722] Lots of unnecessary biopsy procedures may be profitable for some people but not for you; they are bad for your health.

Mammograms are stressful. The WHI analysis reported that 36 percent of Premarin and 28 percent of placebo users had been called back to evaluate "abnormal" mammograms in the first 7 years.[741] That is surely stressful. And worse yet, scheduling and then undergoing a biopsy has been recently shown to hurt the immune system for several months afterward.[846] This means that a biopsy itself inhibits a part of the cancer-fighting machinery of an intact, healthy woman.

Is There a Benefit to Finding Smaller Tumors Earlier?

* In Norway, investigators concluded that the increased detection from screening led to a dramatic overdiagnosis, not to an improvement in life circumstance.[869, 870] There was some good news about HRT regarding mammograms that show calcifications. Taking hormones did not affect the malignancy rate for women who showed calcifications that were "indeterminate" when diagnosed at a routine screening.[466]

    By 2004, in the *Journal of the American Medical Association*, Dr. Lisa M. Schwartz commented that finally, there is a growing awareness among physicians that cancer screening is a double-edged sword. If early detection of breast cancer and the resulting treatment fail to lengthen life and do harm its quality, is it useful to detect it?[684]

* In California, among the 13-million-member HealthNet HMO, mammograms were reported to detect small tumors at earlier stages than would otherwise be found without frequent mammographic screening. The discovery of smaller tumors, however, did not increase the number of surgeries that conserve breasts, as had been expected from "early detection."[441]

* In a Swedish study, a slight reduction in the death rate was attributed to earlier treatment.[569] The study did not test whether teaching women self-examination would have been just as good. Yet exactly this finding was reported when the Canadian National Breast Cancer screening study compared mammography to self-examination.[519]

What you should know: The data suggest to me that for reducing the future death rate from breast cancer, having one clinical exam by a competent clinician, followed by regular self-examination, is just as protective as four or five annual mammograms without any self-examination. Some women will prefer a mammogram; others, a self-exam. And there is no radiation in a self-exam. But women should not believe it is unanimously accepted that annual mammograms are required. Discuss this with your physician. Remember, it is effective prevention and treatment, not detection, of breast cancer that decreases the death rate.

Hormones and Breast Cancer

Hormones are biologically active substances that are clearly designed to have an effect on target tissues. If you take hormones (to arrest hot flashes and other hormone-deficiency symptoms), you can expect some changes in your breasts. Let's look at two major changes: cell proliferation and breast density.

Cell Proliferation

Both estrogen and progestin therapies can stimulate mitogenic growth in your breasts. The term *mitogenic* refers to the capacity of a substance to induce cells to divide and multiply, that is, proliferate.

Knowing that "cancer" is basically cells that exhibit uncontrolled growth can lead you to mistake proliferation as an inevitable sign of breast cancer risk. It's not. Breast tissue's normal "lifespan" can involve cell growth without cancer issues.

Breast Density

Twelve studies revealed that women with very dense breasts are at a significantly increased risk for developing breast cancer, compared to women who have the very lowest level of density.[318] Although one study reported it, the others found there was no trend to show that medium-density breasts were at higher risk than low-density breasts.[90] Likewise, an increase in density does not clearly increase the risk of breast cancer.[318]

Effect of Hormonal Therapies on Breast Density

Some hormonal therapies increase breast density; others do not. But whatever change the hormones generate tends to occur immediately, with no further changes after the first few weeks.[319]

What you should know: Different HRTs produce different effects:

- Increased mammographic density is most likely with oral continuous-combined estrogen and certain synthetic progestins. Up to 50 percent of women who start such combined regimens experience this phenomenon.[153, 319, 474, 687] In comparison, several different *sequential regimens* that more closely mimicked a fertile menstrual cycle produced no significant increase in the density of the breasts.[687]

- An increase of more than 25 percent in the breast-density score was experienced by 16 percent of those whose estrogens were *oral* but by only 4 percent of those whose estrogen was taken *transdermally* in HRT regimens that used continuous-combined synthetic progestin that was available in Europe (NETA).[319]

- An oral estrogen used in Finland (*estradiol valerate*) that was combined with a low dose of the progestin *levonorgestrel,* which an *intrauterine device* released slowly, produced minimal effects on breast density.[474] This was considered a promising new regimen.

- Oral conjugated equine estrogen such as Premarin appears to substantially increase cell proliferation and breast density for most women.[793]

- Fibrocystic breasts have also been tested for their response to hormone therapies in postmenopause. Experiments in Turkey showed that some regimens (Prempro) increased the size of the cysts, whereas two regimens (transdermal estrogen alone or with oral medroxyprogesterone acetate) were neutral.[865]

Hormones and Breast Cancer: Do Circulating Levels Disclose Cancer Risk?

Hormones secreted from the ovaries and the adrenal glands in normal ranges appear to protect against breast cancer, if you consider the facts.

- The incidence of breast cancer is age-related, starting to rise as hormones diminish. At age 50, 1 in 50 women reveal breast cancer; at 70, 1 in 20; and at 90, 1 in 10 women.[853]

- Pregnancy at a young age elevates sex hormone levels and reduces risk.[181]

- Oral contraceptives in medium and low doses of synthetic estrogens and progestin are not associated with increased risk.[496]

- Measurement of estrogen levels in the specialized fat cells immediately adjacent to breast cancer reveals 20 to 30 times the concentration as found in the general circulation. This implies local, rather than systemic, sources of hormone manufacture associated with breast cancer.[853]

Because the incidence of breast cancer increases as women approach their menopausal years and continues to increase with age after menopause, it seems likely that diminishing sex hormone levels might be involved. That's the general overview; now let's get specific.

The Nurses Health Study has provided a great deal of data. Among women not using HRT when their blood was collected, these researchers find:

- *DHEA: Timing counts.* High baseline levels of DHEA increase the risk that *post*menopausal women subsequently develop breast cancer.[583] But high baseline levels in the *pre*menopausal nurses were *not* a predictor of risk.[524] So the pre- and the postmenopausal women's breasts were apparently responding differently to the same hormone.[217]

- *Estrogens.* Postmenopausal women with highest circulating levels of estrogen had an increased risk for developing breast cancer, but HRT reduced that risk.

- *Progesterone.* Postmenopausal women who circulated the highest levels of progesterone (10 times as much as those with the lowest levels) had no increased risk for developing breast cancer.

- *Take away.* The authors suggested that synthetic progestins in many hormonal regimens might be harmful—in fact, *the* harmful agent—while natural progesterone would likely be benign.[524]

How Various Hormone Prescriptions Affect Normal and Cancerous Tissue

Clearly, all hormone therapies are *not* alike. Experimental evidence reveals profound differences among different synthetic progestins on breast tissue.[143, 192] Most studies also show that postmenopausal women who develop breast cancer when they are on hormones *are less likely to die from it* than are postmenopausal women who have breast cancer and are *not* on hormonal therapy.[207]

Hormone Therapies Slightly Increased Detection but Not the Risk of Death from Breast Cancer

In 2006, a 5-year observational study of all Finnish women over the age of 50 who had been on unopposed estrogen therapy in pills swallowed (no progestins) after their hysterectomies reported an increased incidence of breast cancer detection—by about $\frac{3}{10}$ of 1 percent per year of continued use, compared to women who did not take hormones.[478] In contrast, no increased risk was found in the first 5 years of use among 84,729 transdermal and 18,314 vaginal estrogen users.

The Nurses Health Study followed 70,000 apparently healthy women who were older than age 44 at enrollment in 1976; by 1995, 972 of them (1.4 percent) had discovered that they had breast cancer. In 20 years, only 1.4 percent—are you surprised? Less terrified? Hormone use for more than 5 years increased the risk ratio of cancer detection among 60- to 64-year-olds. But hormone users had *no* increased risk in deaths from breast cancer. Oral conjugated equine estrogen (e.g., Premarin) was the predominant estrogen used; the synthetic MPA was the main progestin.[151]

In healthy breast tissue, natural progesterone, but none of the synthetic progestins, appears to protect normal human breast epithelial cells. (*Epithelial* describes tissue that forms a thin protective layer on exposed bodily surfaces and forms the lining of internal cavities, ducts, and organs.) Estradiol creams applied to healthy breast tissue of postmenopausal women stimulated the proliferation of epithelial cells.[143] Progesterone dramatically limited the estrogen-induced proliferation of normal human breast epithelial cells when applied as a cream directly on the breast.[244] Since progesterone can counteract the estrogen-induced proliferation, the natural form of the hormone "progesterone," rather than a "synthetic progestin," may protect against hyperplasia (excess cell proliferation).[219, 353, 540]

Apoptosis is a biological term for a major "natural death" mechanism whereby old or damaged cells are removed from the breast. It has been shown that natural progesterone and certain progestins stimulate cell-death apoptosis in normal cells, as well as in hormone-dependent breast cancer cells. The removal of progestins for a short period, as in a sequential regimen, triggers the maximum apoptotic mechanisms. That's good. But continuous administration, as in a continuous-combined regimen, alters the normal cell cycle. A fertile woman's half month without progesterone secretion and half month with seems to direct the mammary cells correctly. Scholars have proposed that progesterone supplementation should be given sequentially in order to inhibit proliferation and to restore apoptosis.[219] I agree.

It makes sense biologically that sequential regimens should be preferred over continuous-combined ones, in order to optimize the protective mechanisms of apoptosis. Apoptosis helps prevent the runaway proliferation of cells that is so commonly seen in the growth of tumors. Table 10.1 shows which progestins to avoid: those with significant glucocorticoid effects (positively correlated with breast cancer). It also shows those that have estrogenic or androgenic effects. Bioidentical progesterone does not have these potential negative effects.

Experimentally, conjugated equine estrogen stimulated the proliferation of human breast cancer cells. None of the synthetic progestins was able to inhibit this. Only natural progesterone, when given in high doses, could inhibit cell proliferation.[540] The scientists concluded that (human bioidentical synthesized) progesterone has no deleterious breast effects, even when given at very high dosages.

Human breast cancer cells can be studied in experimental dishes. They proliferate when they are given estrogen alone. Adding either MPA or certain proteins slows their growth. That's good. But norethisterone (NET), a synthetic progestin used widely in Europe, did the opposite; it had proliferative effects. This is bad because it would cause an increase in the growth of breast cancer cells. Bioidentical progesterone had no significant effect on cancer cell proliferation in the presence of estrogen.[418] But even progesterone had some dangerous effects on cancer cells, increasing their metastasis-inducing chemicals.[2] This suggests that all progestins and progesterone can stimulate breast cancer cells in dishes.

Healthy human breast cells do not respond the same way that cancer cells in experimental dishes do. Progesterone inhibits the tendency of estrogen and other growth factors to stimulate growth in healthy breast cells.[417, 418] This is a very good effect.

Table 10.1 Partial Effects of Progesterone and Synthetic Progestins[219]

	Estrogenic	Androgenic	HDL-Ch[a] vs. estrogen monotherapy	LDL-Ch[a] vs. estrogen monotherapy	Gluco-corticoid	Glucose tolerance	Anti-androgenic	Anti-mineralo corticoid
Bioidentical to Human								
Progesterone	—	—	—	—	(+)	—	(+)	+
Synthesized Progestin Derivatives								
Dydrogesterone	—	—	—	—	—	—	—	(+)
Medrogestone	—	—	—	—	+	—	(+)	—
MPA[b]	—	(+)	→	—	+	⇊	—	—
Synthesized Nortestosterone Derivatives								
Norethisterone acetate (NETA)	+	+	→	↑	—	⇊	—	—
Lynestrenol	+	+	→	↑	—	⇊	—	—
Levonogestrel	—	+	→	↑	—	⇊	—	—

Key:

— No partial effect;
(+) Weak partial effect;
+ Significant partial effect;
→ Decrease;
⇊ Marked decrease;
↑ Increase

Modified from Druckmann (2003), "Progestins and Their Effects on the Breast," *Maturitas* 46:59–69.
[a]Ch—Cholesterol. The progestins vary in their effects. Each synthetic reveals some less desirable effects; for example, 19-Nortestosterone derivatives increase the bad LDL-Ch.
[b]Medrodyprogesteroneacetate.

Are some hormone-replacement therapies safe or safer than others? Yes, but you have to look closely to see it.

A closer look provides me—and you—with a clearer picture. The randomized, controlled trial evaluates outcomes in women who are willing to submit blindly to either a placebo or a drug and be followed for a certain number of years. But huge dropout rates (close to half on Premarin or Prempro) tend to limit the conclusions because the FDA-mandated statistical methodology scores the dropouts as if they had continued taking the drug. A woman who stopped taking the drug after six months because she did not like the way she felt and five years later developed breast cancer becomes one of the statistics for hormones causing breast cancer. Some researchers believe this "loads the dice" in favor of misleading conclusions.[489] I find these objections sensible and think that such trials should be considered in context with the observational studies.

Observational studies test whether women who have breast cancer are more or less likely to have used hormones, compared to their contemporaries who are cancer free.[739] Some studies ask whether particular regimens might be safer. More than 65 observational studies provided data by 2007. In 1997, 51 of these studies were reanalyzed into one large "meta-analysis," pooling the previously published data of 53,000 women with breast cancer, compared to 108,000 without.[68] A meta-analysis attempts to provide a global overview of a great deal of data and a large number of individual studies.

Overall, this first broad-brush approach judged a slight increased risk of developing breast cancer for women who have ever used hormone-replacement therapy.[68]

In 2001, a different group of authors reviewed all 65 studies and published their findings. The second meta-analysis showed:[107]

- Hormone users were less likely to die from breast cancer than nonusers were.

- There was a lack of agreement among studies. Some found increased risk; others found decreased risk of breast cancer. This disparity persisted throughout the entire 25 years of investigation.

- The overall risk of breast cancer with hormone use compared to nonuse has hovered around 1; that is, not higher or lower than no hormone use.

In 2005, a third meta-analysis reported its conclusions.

- Of 2,474 published studies, only 204 met the investigators' criteria that would allow comparisons of hormone therapy influence on breast cancer risk.[688]

- Of these, 8 studies totaling 655,559 women provided sufficient data to suggest that current use of combined hormone therapy *did* increase the risk compared to nonusers by about 40 percent. (But this does not mean that 40 percent of women taking hormones *got* breast cancer, as some media reports suggested, only that their risk was 40 percent higher but still low.)

- The main discriminating risk factor appeared to be the type of progestin chosen.

Observational studies have to take what they get. By their very nature, they rely on what women chose to do after consulting with their clinicians. And when women die, we are not told the causes of their deaths; in other words, was it a heart attack, an automobile accident, or breast cancer? In the United States, more than 80 percent of the progestin prescribed has been oral MPA (medroxyprogesterone acetate). The very composition that appears to be least beneficial forms the basis of most of the published research. Oral estradiol with MPA appears to increase the risk of lobular and ductal breast cancer when women who are not menstruating are tested.[134] Sequential regimens usually score better for women.

One study (detailed in the box) evaluated 3,534 women for the risks of sequentially taking synthetic progestins added to estrogen and reported a worse outcome.[654] But another study of 7,545 women found that sequential regimens were better.[485]

Figuring Your Odds: "Odds Ratios" as Scientific Jargon

The study that reported an increased risk lacked the normal rigorous requirement of "blinding."[654] Researchers *knew* which subjects had breast cancer when they asked them to *recall* their HRT usage. A closer look at the data shows that 97 percent of the 3,534 women studied were not taking any hormone therapies. Here is what the researchers actually found:

- 2.6 percent of the 1,897 women with breast cancer had been using a sequential regimen for 10 years or more.
- 2.1 percent of the 1,637 women without breast cancer had also done so.[654]

"Odds ratios" compare the odds of one group to the odds of the other by dividing their ratios: 2.6 percent divided by 2.1 percent = 1.5. So a published "OR" equal to 1.5 can produce misleading headlines that imply a 50 percent increased risk in cancer for women using hormones.

To my mind, the odds ratio message distorts reality since 97 percent of the breast cancer patients and 98 percent of the non–breast cancer patients had *not* been using hormone-replacement therapy. I believe it is illogical to conclude that hormone therapies are a major cause of breast cancer; doing so would fail to explain the 97 percent who did not use hormones and had breast cancer anyway.

Another investigator, the late R. Don Gambrell, MD, had a 35-year history of prescribing sequential regimens for women after they had undergone hysterectomies. His training and perception told him that the most rational regimens are those that most closely resemble the fertile time of life. He also followed this pattern for intact women, titrating the dose in response to the feedback each patient provided about her unique response to her regimen. In 2006, he reported on the 1,200 patients, who had been followed on average for 22 years. The women used 18 different progestins (oral, vaginal), but never continuous-combined, and 16 different estrogen types (implants, oral, transdermal, injectible), and the data were clear in showing an extremely low incidence of breast cancer: 16 cases, 1 metastasis out of 1,200 patients over 35 years.[258] This work is significant because it evaluated women individually, making sure that each one had a regimen that produced a healthy quality of life. When the qualified clinician worked respectfully with each patient, listening to the feedback she provided, he was able to titrate the dose based on her body's reactions, which she reported to him. This is the practice of medicine at its noblest level.

Recent International Studies

A close look at the international studies allows a useful perspective into the variation in prescribing practices in these different countries. If you want to know whether hormone therapies increase or decrease the incidence of breast cancer, focusing by country adds some important information.

Study #1: A Big Study: Incendiary Conclusions

Where: England.

What: The Million Women Study (MWS).[47, 67, 522]

Who: One million postmenopausal women, 50 to 64, from a pool of women who were eligible for free mammographic screening who permitted their medical records to be reviewed for this study. Any woman who had begun HRT while perimenopausal was excluded, so no information was available about these women who would have been ideal HRT users.

What the study found: Overall, breast cancer was detected in less than 1 percent (9,364) of women who underwent mammographies. (That part is reassuring.) Comparing these 9,364 women by hormone usage revealed that cancer was detected in

- 1.35 percent of the MWS women who had used estrogen-progestin regimens,
- 0.85 percent of those who had used estrogen without progestins, and
- 0.7 percent of those who had never used hormones.

Those are the main findings. A major strength of this study was the double-blind examination of the hormone regimens from prescription records.

So women whose mammograms detected cancer were more likely to be using hormone-replacement therapy.

But put the results in perspective: Remember that 99 percent of the one million women had no breast cancer and more than 98 percent of the 1 percent with breast cancer were not using any hormone therapies. There were not enough women on sequential regimens, natural progesterone, or progestins other than MPA, NET, and norgestrel/

levonorgestrel to allow an analysis of specific progestins or regimens. The study's table showed 2 estrogen products in use: conjugated equine estrogen and the powerful synthetic ethinyl estradiol.[47, 67, 522]

The two most substantial criticisms were:

1. Conflict of interest. The governmental body that was charged with evaluating the study and setting governmental health policy consisted in some cases of the same people who had authored the study.[235]

2. Choice of subjects. "Detection bias" raises the issue that women who are hormone users tend to use health services more, so they have more frequent physical exams and more frequent breast screening. This combination of events increases the chance of detecting a cancer that is present in this short-term study, increasing the risk of bias.[797] Many other detailed criticisms followed.[93, 245, 256, 557, 585, 796, 797]

The bottom line: So, 99 percent of the one million women did *not* have breast cancer. Of the 1 percent who *did* have cancer, the difference was 0.7 percent for nonusers and 1.35 percent for users of combined estrogen and progestin. Given the modest elevation in risk ratio that was actually observed, the criticism concluded, "It remains impossible to distinguish between bias and causation as alternative explanations for the observed associations."[691] In my opinion, these criticisms of the MWS are compelling and suggest that the risks if real are limited, and the hysteria that the study (and the media) generated was irrational.

Study #2: Hormone Regimen Is Key

Where: Denmark.

What: The Danish Nurses Study, published in 2 reports, 2004 and 2005.[735, 736]

Who: Starting in 1993, there were 10,874 intact women older than age 44 who enrolled; some were postmenopausal and others were using hormonal therapy and still menstruating (so they were still perimenopausal, unlike women in the MWS). Most of the women had never used hormonal therapy (60 percent), but 25 percent were current users.

What the study found: By 1999, 2.2 percent of the women had been diagnosed with breast cancer; that is, 244 emerging breast cancer cases had been detected in the 10,874 intact women.

What you should know: Hormonal therapies increased the risk of breast cancer, but not all regimens were equal.

- The continuous-combined regimen produced double the rate of cancer that the sequential regimens did. The longer the duration, the higher the risk.
- Sequentially applied MPA was more likely to increase the risk of breast cancer than were the sequentially applied androgen-type progestins such as NET.
- There was no significant increased risk for past users of hormones, nor was there any increased risk for women hormone users of longer duration on sequential regimens.
- Unopposed estrogen also increased the risk of breast cancer in the intact women.

The key statistics: From the many measures reported, a few are most telling. Compared to "never-users" of any type of hormone therapy:

- The MPA-type of sequential HRT produced a *risk ratio (RR)* = 3.02;
- The NET-type of sequential HRT that is available in Europe yielded a lower RR = 1.94;
- The MPA-type of continuous-combined regimen was the most hazardous: RR = 4.16;
- For unopposed estrogen, the RR = 1.84.[736]

By 2004, of the 71 women with breast cancer who had died (of any cause): 37 had never used hormones, 12 were past users, and 22 were current users.[735]

Study #3: Hormone Therapy May Result in Less Lethal Tumors

Where: Australia.

What: The 2006 Melbourne (Australia) Collaborative Cohort Study.[268]

Who: Of the 24,479 women who enrolled, 99 percent were ages 40 to 69. At enrollment, 13,444 were postmenopausal and 16 percent of these were using hormone therapy.

What the study found: Twelve years later, of these 13,444 women, 336 (or 2.5 percent) had developed invasive breast cancer. The authors reported a 50 percent increased risk ratio for recent use of hormonal therapy on invasive breast cancer, which was consistent with other international studies. No information was provided on which hormones were used.

The bottom line: Compared to women who were not using HRT, the prognosis for women who developed tumors while on hormonal therapy was better. The tumors were more differentiated, rendering them less dangerous and more treatable.

Study #4: Hormone Delivery Route Is Key

Where: Finland.

What: National registry data.

Who: The study consisted of all 110,371 Finnish women over the age of 50 who had undergone hysterectomies and had filled a first prescription for unopposed estrogen therapy between 1994 and 2001. (None of these prescriptions was for a conjugated equine estrogen, such as Premarin.)

What the study found: By 2002, there had been 2,171 breast cancers (1.967 percent) detected in this group. Again, take note of how few cancers were found in a group where doctors were searching for them! Comparing these cancer rates to those of the general population, there was no increased risk for detecting breast cancer in the first 5 years of unopposed estrogen use. Women on transdermal or vaginal routes of estrogens did *not* have an increased risk. The authors calculated that 5 to 10 years of continued *oral* estradiol use would result in 2 or 3 extra cases of breast cancer per 1,000 women over a 10-year period.[478]

The bottom line: The increase in breast cancer if you take hormones is real, but it's tiny and it's avoidable if you use non-swallow, such as transdermal or vaginal, delivery routes.

Study #5: The Type of Hormone Is Vital

Where: France.

What: The French Cohort Study.

Who: 3,175 postmenopausal women who were studied for an average of 9 years in an observational study.[193]

What the study found: HRT users had no worse of a prognosis than untreated women did. There were 105 cases of breast cancer in 3,175 women (3.3 percent of the group during the 9 years they were followed).

The bottom line: A major difference in the hormone-prescribing pattern in France was described by the authors. Eighty-three percent were using mostly transdermal estrogen, while the progesterone tended to be an oral micronized version (a human bioidentical form) with less than 3 percent of the population using medroxyprogesterone acetate. The use of natural progesterone appears, consistently, whenever it is reported, to be the optimal choice for women on the issue of breast health and progesterone use.

The Protective Power of Testosterone in Hormone Therapies

Androgens such as testosterone also may limit the estrogenic stimulation of breast cell proliferation.[469] Using monkeys' mammary biopsy material because of their close biological similarity to humans, scientists discovered that androgens serve to reduce mammary epithelial proliferation and help maintain the integrity of breast tissue and health.[214]

In 2004, the beneficial role of testosterone in human breast cancer (when added to estrogen and progestin regimens) was suggested by authors who analyzed data collected over 25 years. They had acted as a referral center for physicians, who sent them hundreds of women with testosterone-deficiency symptoms such as loss of libido, fatigue, impaired concentration, sleep disturbance, muscle weakness, and osteoporosis. The authors supplemented testosterone with the conventional hormone therapy that each patient was using, titrating the dose to increase symptom relief and minimize common side effects, notably acne and hirsutism (the abnormal growth of hair).[213]

Thus, as in Dr. Gambrell's 1,200 patients, the HRT doses were individualized to the woman and her reactions. Medical treatment doesn't get much better than this. Only 1.4 percent of the 500 postmenopausal patients (7 women) during the 25-year period developed detectable invasive breast cancer. The women had baseline mammograms when they started and every 2 years thereafter. Consistent with international studies, the data revealed that compared to no progestins, continued-combined progestin-estrogen regimens increased the risk of developing breast cancer. In all cases, adding testosterone to the women's hormone therapy lowered the cancer incidence to levels that were much lower than would be expected, using either England's MWS or the U.S. WHI rates. The authors suggest that testosterone is protective when added to estrogen and progestin and is certainly not a risk factor for developing breast cancer.[213]

By 2007, more studies had been published. The 2006 Nurses Health Study found that either oral methyl testosterone or synthetic progestin, in addition to estrogen, were equally likely to modestly increase the odds of developing breast cancer, much as the other cited studies have found for synthetic progestins when they were added continuously in combination with estrogen.[764]

It remains unclear whether testosterone transdermally absorbed and added to various HT regimens will turn out to be safe, because no study has yet been randomized and controlled for more than a brief six-month trial.[352] The issue is promising, but unresolved.[103] Transdermal bioidentical testosterone did seem to be a safer choice than oral methyl testosterone was.

A Randomized, Controlled Trial of Hormone Therapy and Breast Cancer

The WHI enrolled 161,809 postmenopausal women who were 50 to 79 years old to test whether hormone therapies would affect breast cancer. The randomized, controlled parts of the trial were divided into two arms: first, estrogen (Premarin) or a placebo was to be tested on women who had had hysterectomies; and second, conjugated equine estrogen with medroxyprogesterone acetate (Prempro) was tested on women who were still intact.

After 5.2 years, the Prempro arm of the study was stopped because of excess cases of invasive breast cancer, compared to the placebo group. In the 8,506 women assigned to Prempro, 166 cases of invasive breast cancer had occurred; in the 8,102 women assigned to a placebo, 124 cases of breast cancer had occurred, that is, 1.95 percent versus 1.53 percent. These differences, 1.95 percent divided by 1.53 percent, produced the

1.26 risk ratio (also defined as 126 percent) or a 26 percent increase in risk above the 1.53 percent expected in women who did not use hormones. The WHI also revealed that 98 percent of the women assigned to continuous-combined hormones and 98.4 percent of the women assigned to a placebo did *not* get invasive breast cancer.[856]

Premarin did better. With its use being studied for 7.1 years, it did not increase the risk of developing invasive breast cancer. The most common form of ductal cancer showed a significantly lower incidence for Premarin users than for placebo users.[741]

Unfortunately, in 2006, a new analysis of the Nurses Health Study revealed that hysterectomized postmenopausal women who were currently using conjugated equine estrogens (such as Premarin) had an increase in breast cancer risk that kept increasing the longer the women stayed on the hormone. But that risk did not become statistically significant until their use had exceeded 20 years.[136]

By 2006, a plethora of comments had been published about the WHI randomized, controlled trial.[231] Perhaps the issue was best articulated by the editors of the *International Menopause Society Journal*: "The risks of estrogen therapy have been overstated and are now mainly those of the venous and arterial thromboembolisms."[604]

Weighing Your Risk

According to epidemiologist Dr. Janet Daling, although epidemiologists have used the term *attributable risk* for more than thirty years it has only recently appeared in gynecology journals. *Attributable risk* refers to the incidence (in this case, of breast cancer) in women with a behavior (in this case, using hormone therapy) minus the incidence without the behavior. To calculate the attributable risk of hormone therapy on cancer, first one would have to know the incidence of cancer. For the WHI data, that incidence was 30 cases per 10,000 per year for "no-hormone" users at baseline.[391] Since there were 8 extra cases in the hormone users, 38 per 10,000, the attributable risk for those who used Prempro was 8 per 10,000 women per year.

Another way of describing the attributable risk is: the proportion of the disease due to a particular factor. Using data from the Million Women Study, this was calculated to be a 3.27 percent additional risk

Table 10.2 Behaviors That Influence Breast Cancer—Attributable Risks

Risk Factors over 20 Years for Women 50–70 Years Old	Breast Cancer Cases (out of 10,000)	Extra Cases (out of 10,000)
Never Used HRT	45	—
> 5 yrs. HRT	47	2
> 10 yrs. HRT	51	6
>15 yrs. HRT	57	12
Menopause after age 60	59	14
Alcohol (2 drinks/day)	72	27
No daily exercise	72	27
Weight gain (>20 kg)	90	45

with combination therapy after 15 years of use.[154] You should note that it is not 3.27 percent of the women who will get this cancer, but rather an additional 3.27 percent of the 2 percent who will get cancer.

3.27 percent × 2 percent = .06 percent

Translation: This is 6 one-hundredths of 1 percent, extremely tiny numbers. Table 10.2 compares some factors that are now known to increase a woman's risk of developing breast cancer, showing their relative influence.[23] Intemperate use of alcohol, a lack of exercise, and excessive weight gain have a much greater influence on a woman's potential to get breast cancer.

Different HRT Regimens Have Different Attributable Risks

I don't think you can throw all "hormone use" into the same pot. We should differentiate between the various regimens in discussing attributable risk and breast cancer. Here's why.

Beginning in 2002, there were studies being conducted on which hormone regimens are the most risky. The National Institutes of Health Contraceptive and Reproductive Experience (CARE) study was one of the few efforts to examine breast cancer risk in relation to *specific* hormone regimens. This was a multicentered, population-based, case-control study conducted in five U.S. metropolitan areas (Atlanta, Detroit, Los Angeles, Seattle, and Philadelphia) from 1994 to 1998.

The study followed 3,823 cases of women with breast cancer, compared to 1,953 local women contemporaries who didn't have cancer.[832] It collected detailed information on the lifetime use of hormones from a large number of women residing in 5 geographical areas of the United States.

What the study found: The association between the risk of developing breast cancer and undergoing hormone-replacement therapies varies by regimen.

The U.S. multicentered study reported that only continuous-combined HRT for 5 years or more (the Prempro type) increased the risk of developing breast cancer, which worsens the longer the duration of its use. The risk appeared to evaporate when the regimen was discontinued. Former users had no elevation in their risk of developing breast cancer. Nor did the women who used sequential progestins opposed to their estrogens. Only current users of continuous-combined regimens were at risk. Apparently, this risk was confined to the rarer lobular type of breast cancer.[181, 182]

The outcomes in CARE observational studies were roughly similar to the outcomes of the Women's Health Initiative and observational studies that found an increased risk of breast cancer detection in Prempro users.[181, 182, 561, 736]

Confirming data on the deleterious effects of continuous-combined regimens were reported in another study of older women, ages 65 to 79, in the Seattle metropolitan area.

What the study found: Unopposed estrogen-replacement therapy did not increase the risk of developing breast cancer, even with up to 25 years or more of use. But continuous-combined hormone therapy (with MPA as the predominant progestin) of more than 5 years *did* increase the risk of both ductal and lobular breast cancer.[449] Further studies determined that if women had previously used oral contraceptives, this appeared to be protective in reducing the likelihood of breast cancer for postmenopausal women using hormone therapy.[561]

Another Attributable Risk: Absence of Sunlight UVB-Radiation

Sunlight, the principal source of vitamin D (see chapter 8), has long been recognized to be a risk factor for developing skin cancer. As a consequence, many dermatologists and the media urge women to avoid the sun or to block it with sunscreens. One investigator noticed a large geographic variance in the United States in mortality rates for many cancers. In fact, except for skin cancers, he noted that rates of breast, colon, ovary and prostate, non-Hodgkin's lymphoma, bladder, esophageal, kidney, lung, pancreatic, rectal, stomach, and uterine cancers varied by geography. The rates were approximately twice as high in the Northeast versus the Southwest.[291] He concluded that many lives could be extended with solar exposure or vitamin D_3 supplementation. *I agree.*

What you should know: In addition, the scientists reviewed breast cancer mortality rates from 1989 to 1996, along with dietary supplement data and latitude (which is an index of solar UVB) from 35 countries.[290] They calculated that 80 percent of the variance of breast cancer mortality rates was explained in this order:

- Fraction of calories derived from animal products (more risk)
- Fraction of calories derived from vegetable products (reduction in risk)
- Exposure to sufficient solar UVB (reduction in risk)
- Alcohol use (increased risk)
- Fish intake (reduction in risk)

HT after Breast Cancer: Is It Safe?

After patients undergo breast cancer treatment, estrogen-deficiency symptoms are a major problem for many women. Some women will take hormonal therapy when alternative treatments fail. For example, for debilitating hot flashes, no benefit from high-dose phytoestrogens (herbals) was recently shown scientifically.[559] Although synthetic progestins are an effective hot-flash treatment for up to one-third of breast cancer patients,[546] they can increase the risk of developing breast cancer. It appears that various progestins act differently, depending on when they are given and for how long. They seem to transiently increase the rate of progression of actively cycling breast cells but do not accelerate quiescent cells into activity.[546]

What you should know: Since many physicians are justifiably worried about recommending hormone therapy to a woman who has survived breast cancer, it is unfortunate that only one 2-year randomized, controlled trial appears to have been published. Overall, the findings are not very informative. Of 434 women enrolled, only 345 showed up in at least one follow-up to supply data. Altogether, 26 women in the HRT group versus 7 in the non-HRT group had new breast cancers within 2.1 years after enrollment. So, overall, "hormone treatment" was apparently worse in causing a recurrence of cancer.[140, 357] I could not evaluate which hormones might be safer or riskier because the regimens were not systematically controlled but were instead left up to each local physician's prescribing preference in Europe and Scandinavia.

But at least 6 recent studies have reported that for women who made a decision to take hormones to cope with debilitating symptoms such as hot flashes and vaginal atrophy, the outcomes were good.[196, 197, 207, 223, 300, 571] In 2004, a study of 524 women who had menopausal problems and prior breast cancer revealed that those who had taken hormones for up to 27 years (average 6.3 years) had no more recurrences than did those who had chosen not to use HT. As figure 10.2 shows, the survival rate of hormone-takers was certainly not worse and even looks a bit better (but not enough to be statistically significant).[222]

Give women a choice. Other investigators analyzed 2,755 women in an Oregon HMO who were first diagnosed with invasive breast cancer between the ages of 35 and 74. Using medical records, a comparison

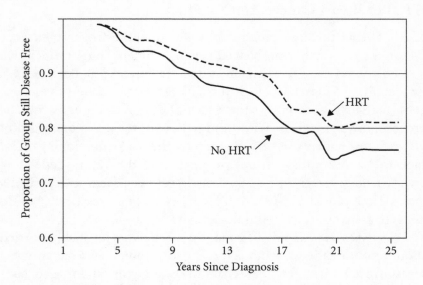

Figure 10.2. Adjusted survival curve for disease-free interval.

was made between women who had chosen hormonal therapy after their cancer and HMO cancer patients who had not.[571] Hormone users had half the recurrence rate of cancer as nonusers.

Conclusion

There is little doubt that the general practice of hormonal therapy, by prescribing it with concomitant mammography, has caused a slight overall increased incidence in breast cancer detection. But you have to put that risk in perspective. We increase our chances of having an automobile accident by getting into cars, but we also know that we can choose safer vehicles, safer routes, and safer times for road travel. Similarly, hormonal therapy can take you to good, healthy places—provided that you choose hormone products wisely.

The *route* of estrogen should also be carefully selected, based on weighing the overall benefits of each. (See the chapters on your cardiovascular health, bones, and cognition.)

Among women who were diagnosed with breast cancer, most, but not all, of the evidence suggests lower death rates and a better cure rate in women who had menopausal symptoms that reflected estrogen deprivation and who chose to use hormone-replacement therapy. Many women who undergo hysterectomies and who want to begin hormone therapies will opt for unopposed continuous estrogen therapies. These appear to be without increased breast cancer risk for the first five years. After five years, however, the unopposed estrogen starts to show an increased (but small) risk of inducing breast cancer in women in some, but not all, of the published studies. Most women who have undergone hysterectomies will be considering twenty to fifty years of hormonal support, not five. So I think it makes sense to weigh the benefits of a sequential regimen of human bioidentical hormones, with perhaps a sporadic dash of testosterone. Long-term use of these may actually reduce the risks of developing cancer.

Women should recognize that all hormone-replacement therapies are not alike. Their fear about the risks of developing cancer should not necessarily mandate against the marvelous health benefits that a well-managed hormone-replacement regimen can provide. Breast self-exams, assisted by a competent clinician, may be as effective as a mammogram and without the adverse effects. Women should not believe that annual mammograms are "required."

The healthy body's natural anti-cancer defense mechanisms have recently been in the news. Prostate cancer is no longer immediately treated aggressively in its earliest stages because of the recognition that an otherwise generally healthy body's internal defenses can produce "spontaneous remissions." It may be the same for the natural history of early stage breast cancer, according to a large November 2008 study by the Norwegian researchers discussed earlier. They concluded: "It appears that some breast cancers detected by repeated mammogramic screening would not persist to be detectable by a single mammogram at the end of 6 years." [871b]

Finally, when alarming media headlines trumpet "risks doubled" or "27 percent increases shown," you should ask, "Double what? Or 27 percent of what?" Is this from 1 in 10,000 to 2 in 10,000? Is this 27 percent of 2.2 percent? Remember, breast cancer deaths in 1950 were 32 per 100,000 women; in 2003, they were 25 per 100,000 women; this is one-eighth the cardiovascular disease death rate. We sorely need to keep this perspective when bombarded by seemingly terrifying advertisements and headlines.

11

Hormones and the Brain: Preserving Memory, Alertness, and Optimism

For many years I worked closely with two California colleagues. Both were brilliant scientists. Both were intensely focused on our shared efforts through the Stanford Menopause Study to contribute to knowledge about aging, sex hormones, and sexuality. One was skinny and wiry with high triglyceride blood levels; the other was full-bodied and gaining fat with age. They both showed evidence of clogged blood vessels. And I watched sadly as they began to lose their capacity for intellectual thought, eventually becoming two more "cases" of dementia.

Our thoughts, emotions, dreams, and memories are fundamental to our identity. Mild cognitive impairments can be the transitional state that catapults you from independence to utter dependence and loss of freedom. If you can't find your keys and don't remember where you parked the car—or whether you turned off the oven—you will need a full-time caretaker, as both my former colleagues eventually did.

Memory

Dementia describes severe symptoms of memory loss that occur without compromising the normal arousal of emotion, such as anger or joy. Strokes and Parkinson's disease are common dementia-inducing illnesses.[408] Alzheimer's disease accounts for 60 to 80 percent of the cases of dementia.

Take action now, through the habits you form, to keep your blood vessels healthy, your mind sharp, and your memory fluent. Add to the vibrancy of your own optimal mental energy by adhering to healthful patterns of eating, exercising, cultivating a rich spiritual life, and undertaking correctly timed hormonal therapies.

Memory and Age

Cognition includes perception, memory, and judgment.[830] Tests of 800 upper-middle socioeconomic California women (older than 64 years in 1972) on 12 cognitive skills showed real vulnerability to aging. Ten of the 12 test scores had clearly declined 15 years following the original tests.[52]

Memory and Menopause

Before menopause, mental capacity tends to be stable.[345] The greatest predictors of a 53-year-old woman's IQ, verbal memory, and concentration at early menopause are the combined effects of childhood cognitive ability (tested at age 8) and lifetime socioeconomic circumstances.[49, 410, 424] But after age 60, for most women, memory gets worse.[553]

Since a clear decline in mental function seems to begin about 10 years after menopause, researchers began to ask whether declining sex hormone levels might be responsible. If so, would adding HRT help? In 2005, some researchers said no.[471] But the first researchers asked the question the wrong way and drew an invalid conclusion.

Just because it's "research" doesn't make it right. The mistake they made? They relied on the women's memories at age 70 when they were asked for their ages at ending—and starting—menstruation and compared that data with their mental ability scores. If their memories were declining, their data were unreliable and the findings would be flawed.

By 2007, there were enough published valid data to prove exactly the opposite conclusion. Yes, naturally secreted estrogen, progesterone, and testosterone, before menopause, all serve to keep the intellect functioning optimally. Timely initiation of hormone therapy—an early start—seems best for reducing the likelihood of intellectual and hearing deficits 10 to 30 years later.[117, 343, 486, 643] And a healthy cardiovascular system that provides freely flowing blood to nourish the brain and the central nervous system seems crucial.

Memory and Cardiovascular Disease

People with cardiovascular disease are more at risk for developing memory problems. People (ages 53 to 84) with hypertension or poorly controlled blood pressure show an "exaggerated neuroendocrine reactivity"—extreme sensitivity—to stress.[8] They tend to perform worse on cognitive tests, even when they have not had a stroke and are still free of dementia.[812] And treatment for hypertension improves cognitive test scores. That makes sense: the brain needs blood to supply nutrients, and any impairment in the cardiovascular system would necessarily weaken mental abilities. Check your blood pressure and take action to keep it within reasonable bounds.

Current users of estrogen therapies showed a better aging cognitive profile than "never-users" in one large study, except for a subgroup of women with a genetic blood-fat abnormality.[861] That lipoprotein abnormality (APOE ε4 allele) increased the risk of women developing Alzheimer's disease if the subgroup had a longer span of reproductive life. For the main group, a later menopause did not increase the risk.[262] A likely explanation: cardiovascular diseases block the benefit that sex hormones provide. So estrogens are helpful, provided that the blood vessels—and their contents—are in good shape.

Poor sleep is also a serious health concern that is associated with an increased risk for coronary artery disease, as well as for death from heart disease.[249] Women who had nightmares more than once per week also tended to have spasmodic chest pains, as was shown in a study that collected data from 6,000 women, ages 40 to 64. Since these symptoms may reflect coronary artery disease, women with sleep disturbances should have their cardiac symptoms evaluated.[30] We need good circulation, and we need to sleep restfully.

Memory and Attitude

Your outlook on life, what I call your cognitive style, has an impact on your memory. People who become easily distressed are at an increased risk of experiencing cognitive decline in old age.[389, 845]

Norman Vincent Peale had it right when he wrote *The Power of Positive Thinking*, one of the best-selling books of all time.[595] In large measure, we decide how we will view our world. We can decide to find the best in others; to see the beauty of the flower, rather than the weeds surrounding it; to be an optimist and choose compassion. Such habits pay rich physiological dividends: lower levels of stress hormones, lower blood pressure, and increased lung function. We become what we do, and we can decide to make wise choices. Why else read a book like this one? There are many ways to develop a more positive focus; here are six.

Exercise Regularly to Increase Vitality

Consistent exercise promotes good feelings and optimism. Unsurprisingly, a poorer sense of well-being and a high body mass index (BMI) consistently occur among sedentary women.[65] Whatever your weight, walking for thirty minutes a day, three days a week, will increase your *vital capacity* (the amount of oxygen you can bring to your lungs per minute). And as vital capacity increases, so does your optimism.[227]

In other words, the healthier your lungs are, the greater your optimism. Vital capacity does decline with age, but the severity or steepness of the slope determines how soon your capacity is too low to sustain your life. (A nonsmoking athlete who gives up exercise, moves to a smog-laden city, and takes up cigarettes will have a steep downhill slope!) For some people, this occurs before age 60. For others, age 98. An optimistic cognitive style—your optimism—slows the decline, and you age more slowly.[422] Exercise, optimism, and love are intertwined.

Get a Pet to Love

Imagine receiving an enthusiastic greeting whenever you return home, a being who expresses joy when you approach. A pet will bless you with improved physical and mental health. For the last 25 years, Dr. Erika Friedmann and her colleagues at the University of Pennsylvania, Brooklyn College, and the University of Maryland have published findings that demonstrate the profound benefits of pet ownership on the cardiovascular system and, therefore, I suggest, on memory. Studying patients who recently had healed from their myocardial infarctions (heart attacks), she discovered that pet owners scored better on heart rate variability (HRV). And stroke victims who came home from the hospital to a dog were most likely to survive the next year. HRV measures the heart's flexibility in changing the rate of beats per minute. A better HRV predicted a better prognosis: in other words, a longer life. Dogs were the most effective pets, providing the best long-term outcomes.[252] I think their unconditional love, loyalty, and optimism can teach us what matters.

Develop a Compassionate Attitude

According to recent research, people who have a compassionate attitude tend to have greater psychological health.[743] A *compassionate attitude* is an elemental teaching of all major religions.

- Christianity (2 billion members): Teaches that people should love others as themselves and give to others in need; should promote justice, love kindness, and walk humbly with their God.
- Islam (1.3 billion members): Preaches the sharing of wealth, which helps the needy, as well as the spiritual well-being of the giver.
- Hinduism (900 million members): *Karma* is the law of cause and effect, and one can improve the outcome of one's life by caring for the poor and seeking the good for others. *Dharma* means living one's life according to what is right; it emphasizes doing good to oneself, one's family, and others.
- Buddhism (360 million members): Three elements of the eight-fold path are right action, right speech, and right thought. Buddhist teachings emphasize compassionate conduct toward others and the alleviation of suffering.
- Judaism (15 million members) and the Bahá'í faith (7.5 million) emphasize compassion as central tenets.

Cultivate an Inner Spirituality by Your Compassionate Practice

Religion can enhance your compassion, or it can increase your bigotry and exclusion of others. (The "evil twin" of pride in belonging to a group is disdain for nonmembers.) Disdain and arrogance are self-destructive.

Recent scientific studies separating "intrinsic" from "extrinsic" religious attitudes confirm the benefit of compassionate practices.[502] *Intrinsic* religion, practicing as an end unto itself for spiritual development and growth, leads to better self-reported health. The *extrinsic* approach involves being a member for social affiliation or social gain. This form of religious practice is related to depression and anxiety.

Research using the Duke University religion index on both college students (ages 18 to 22) and adults (average age 72) showed that people who have a compassionate attitude experience less stress and lower blood pressures.[502, 743] If you are nonreligious, consider the next two options as an alternative pathway to practicing compassion.

Whatever path you choose, I hope you will add the regular practice of compassion to your own health habit disciplines.

Consider Mindfulness-Based Stress Reduction

One scientifically tested method is the *mindfulness-based stress reduction* (MBSR) program developed by Dr. John Kabat-Zinn.[382] MBSR programs are rooted in the contemplative spiritual traditions that actively cultivate conscious awareness. Within a mind-set of nonjudging, acceptance, and patience, these meditative practices guide you to focus your awareness on your breathing, a process that typically leads to a combined state of relaxation and alert "observant detachment."[114]

The two hormones of the adrenal gland, cortisol and DHEA, provide reciprocal actions. Cortisol rises and DHEA falls when we are stressed. Practitioners of MBSR have lower levels of cortisol and higher levels of DHEA than nonpractitioners do.

Although undergoing psychotherapy to cure metastatic cancer has *not* withstood claims of improved longevity,[158] breast cancer survivors who were tested after 8 weeks of comprehensive, disciplined training in the MBSR program showed dramatically decreased symptoms of stress and an improved quality of life.[114]

Investigate Cognitive Behavioral Stress-Management Training

Other university-based programs achieved similar results.[310] They all involved cognitive restructuring; in other words, being less judgmental and more compassionate. They employ self-instruction and progressive muscle-relaxation programs, each of which helps lower the rise in cortisol that would otherwise occur in stressful situations.[310]

Hormones Affect Memory and Learning

Your way of being—your spiritual and physical disciplines—profoundly influence your cognitive functioning. Your hormones are intimately involved in the process.

Verbal Memory

Memory is studied in various ways. One test assesses *verbal work-ing memory*, which counts how many words you can study, then remember. Both estrogen and progesterone contribute to this capacity. Verbal working memory shows a cyclic variation that is aligned with the menstrual cycle. You can remember more when your estrogen levels are high.[653] The same principles apply for monkeys, who, after having ovariectomies, must have cyclic estrogen therapy to "rescue" the loss of their cognitive skills.[628]

The cyclic rise in progesterone on the few days immediately after ovulation also promotes peak cognitive performance. Progesterone enhances your performance on tasks that demand concentration and memory.[725]

Testosterone and Memory

The main male sex hormone, testosterone, enhances memory in men but not in women. Sex differences in the hormone testosterone are shown in figure 11.1.[777]

These 2006 testosterone graphs comprise data of 2,400 men and women who enrolled and retested every 5 years over a 20-year span.

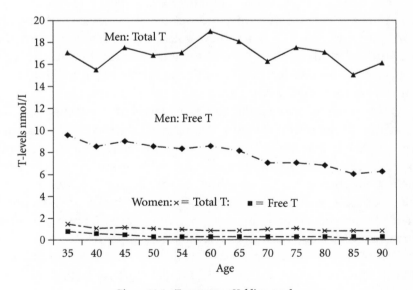

Figure 11.1. Testosterone: Holding steady.

They provide the first substantial records to reveal the changing patterns of cognitive ability, along with testosterone levels, as people aged.

Blood tests for testosterone measure *total testosterone per mg of blood*. Then, using complex formulas, calculations are made of how much of that testosterone is traveling "*free*."

Only the free testosterone (which is not bound to blood proteins such as sex hormone binding globulin [SHBG] and thereby inactivated) is "bioavailable." Only bioavailable testosterone can act as a neurosteroid to affect cognition.

The graph shows that men who are 35 and men who are 90 had about the same amount of *total* testosterone. Until this study was published, with one exception, studies in men *did* report an age-related decline in total testosterone. The earlier studies were cross sectional, "snapshots" of small numbers of men, and took only one blood sample per person without following anyone across time.[169] The 1980 Baltimore Longitudinal Study, which followed a group of healthy, non-obese, 25- to 89-year-old men who did not consume excess alcohol, was the first to report that total testosterone of *healthy* men did not decline with age.[315] This newer 2006 graph of 2,400 people shows a rather gentle downhill slope with advancing age in the group's average level of *free* testosterone for men.

Compared to men, women circulate dramatically lower levels of *both* total and free testosterone, and women also showed little change across their lifespans.[777] These new data were collected as part of a longitudinal study in Sweden, and the analysis was done at the well-respected Karolinska Institute. Healthy people seem to maintain their *free* testosterone levels as they age.

Until a man reaches ages 60 to 65, the levels of free testosterone he circulates do *not* affect his mental performance, but after age 65, men with higher free testosterone levels perform better than those with lower levels of free testosterone.[777] So, testosterone protected men's mental function after 65, much as estrogen does for women after menopause. A testosterone-deficient group of men who were more than 50 years old showed improvements in their spatial reasoning performance when they were given testosterone supplements.[138]

For women, it works the opposite way. *Lower* levels of free and total testosterone were "significantly linked to *better* performance on verbal fluency."[777]

What you should know: Our sex hormones affect our memory, mental agility, mood, and cognition. But our cognitive *style* helps determine how we respond to the stress we experience or even whether what we experience is processed as stress at all.

Stress

Webster's New World College Dictionary, 3rd edition (1991) defines the noun *stress* as (1) mental or physical tension or strain; (2) urgency, pressure, etc., causing this. Hormones don't merely influence a target organ such as your blood vessels; they are actively involved in your nervous system.[266, 660] Progesterone, estradiol, testosterone, and cortisol are each "neuroactive steroids." Like the traffic cop directing the flow of cars, they help direct the transmission of nerve communications. And just as electricity moves down a wire, once fired by an "on" switch, these hormones switch the nervous system on and off. Your hormones affect your nervous system, mood, and energy levels.

Hormones Fuel Moods: Progesterone Affects How Alert You Are

High levels of progesterone that are characteristic of pregnancy can anesthetize a woman, making her restful and sleepy, or can even, under certain metabolic circumstances, cause a persistent fatigue.[596] But in the normal fertile cycle as a woman's progesterone levels rise each month, so does her metabolic rate, increasing her energy. A week later, the progesterone levels start to fall. Progesterone can be metabolized into seven different hormonal variants. One of these, allopregnanolone, apparently causes fatigue. Most women taking a sequential HRT regimen showed no difference in negative mood over those thirty days.[22] But a few of the women developed high levels of allopregnanolone, and they experienced a deterioration in positive mood.

A single injection of a high dose (100 mg) of progesterone to fertile-age women, or much smaller doses to postmenopausal women, raised their allopregnanolone. The high dose tested on young women acted like a sedative. It reduced their sense of vigor and arousal when the levels of allopregnanolone rose.[194] But in postmenopausal women, these brief elevations in blood did not disturb their mood or energy.

You probably know that hormone cycles among intact fertile women can trigger monthly negative mood changes (i.e., PMS) in the last (premenstrual) week of the cycle ("late luteal phase").[842] This is the last week before menstruation, when the corpus luteum in the ovary (which manufactures the progesterone) is shrinking, and progesterone and estrogen levels are falling.

Mood alterations in the late luteal phase may be a consequence of the declining levels of progesterone before menses.[642] If the rollercoaster downhill slide of progesterone is steep, you might feel moodier than if the changing levels vary more subtly. If you take sequential hormonal therapy regimens, you may notice mood and physical energy cycles, too.[842]

Either the synthetic progestin medroxyprogesterone acetate or human bioidentical micronized progesterone taken *sequentially* improves sleep quality.[527]

Stress Hormones: Cortisol and Synthetic Sex Hormones (E&P)

The adrenal glands produce cortisol and DHEA. Endocrinologists think of cortisol as the main stress hormone because it rises during stressful experiences. Elevations of cortisol can trigger memory loss. Certain synthetic HRT regimens cause elevations in this stress hormone. Although biologically identical estrogen is good for your mood, the synthetic estrogen-type drugs such as tamoxifen are not. Tamoxifen is prescribed to prevent breast cancer. Unfortunately, it also causes dramatic negative mood changes.[528]

In a test on monkeys, another synthetic, ethinyl estradiol, combined with the synthetic progestin levonorgestrel, caused large elevations in cortisol, as well as great increases in their heart rates.[342, 701] This is the hormone that's used in some triphasic oral contraceptives, raising questions about the impact of that synthetic hormone on a woman's cognitive function and memory. I recommend that women avoid ethinyl estradiol after age forty-five because it also increases their risk of having a stroke.

What you should know: "Estrogen-like" is not the same as estrogen. Estrogen and progesterone can trigger different cognitive effects than their synthetic versions do. Synthetic hormones can change the way you feel, but if this is an unwelcome change, you can change your prescription!

DHEA: The Feel-Good Hormone

The two most abundant hormones of the adrenal glands, DHEA and cortisol, are reciprocal. As one rises, the other falls. Unfortunately, senile dementia patients show elevated cortisol levels and reduced DHEA levels and shrinkage of their brains. This is not good! Their cortisol-DHEA ratio is double that of normal people.[500] Higher DHEA and lower cortisol are better.

- *DHEA improves performance.* When vigorous men underwent physical training for paramilitary survival, high ratios of DHEA to cortisol were found in their bodies. Their objective performance scores (i.e., their ability to *survive* extreme stress) were directly related to how high their ratio of DHEA to cortisol went. As the DHEA levels rose, their performance got better. As their performance levels dipped, the cortisol rose, while the DHEA fell, and symptoms of dissociation occurred: sounds disappearing, feeling "spaced out," and colors fading.[533]

- *DHEA declines in the presence of pain.* DHEA levels decline with age in women, as well as in men. But in women, levels drop more sharply in those who have either musculoskeletal pain or psychological stress.[241]

- *Lower levels of DHEA are associated with depression.* A comparison of depressed and nondepressed women in postmenopause showed that the depressed women had significantly lower levels of DHEA.[679] But a small group of patients with major depression showed a hormonal anomaly: significantly higher levels of DHEA, testosterone, and androstenedione, as well as significantly higher levels of cortisol.[829] It is not clear whether these high levels of DHEA and cortisol reflect abnormalities or a lab anomaly; high DHEA is almost universally associated with a better sense of well-being.[65]

- In fact, therapy with high daily doses of DHEA (starting at 90 mg per day and moving up to 450 mg per day) helped 48 patients with midlife onset of major and minor depression. It worked.[678]

Because these doses are dangerously high and may cause liver damage, however, you should not use DHEA to self-medicate. Excess DHEA poses serious risks to your cardiovascular health.[304] A simple blood test can measure yours.

What you should know: DHEA supplementation is not advisable unless your doctor confirms that your levels are very low. Only then, under careful medical monitoring, you may find that supplementation offers benefits.

Stress Alters Your Hormones

Chronic stress elevates cortisol. This is not good. And several hormone patterns change when we are stressed. Therefore, stress can affect memory. A simple but crucial message is: *try to avoid chronic stress.* The hormone cortisol is manufactured in the adrenal gland, is secreted into the bloodstream, and tends to rise in response to stress.[843, 858]

Unfortunately, people who suffer from persistent diseases (cardiovascular, psychiatric, and autoimmune) have chronically high levels of cortisol circulating in their blood.[423] Healthy people show a different cortisol pattern, with a daily cyclical variation throughout the day, rapidly rising within a few minutes after they get up, then declining over the next 12 hours.[365, 423]

In the short term, sudden elevations of cortisol energize a person to cope with stress or to get started and address the day. But for a woman who continually feels overwhelmed, excessive cortisol can cause real bodily damage. The higher the level of cortisol, the slower the wound healing after a surgical biopsy.[225] Chronic increased elevations of stress hormones cause both memory impairment and a shrinking of the brain, according to the work of Sonia Lupien, PhD, the director of aging and Alzheimer's disease research and the codirector of the McGill Center for Studies in Aging in Canada. Over a ten-year period, she and her colleagues demonstrated that chronic high levels of stress and the resulting hormonal secretions are very bad for cognition.[475]

Stress and Gender

Other experiments illustrate relationships among cortisol, estrogen, and progesterone. In one experiment, young men and women were given a math test in front of others, an experiment that is known to induce stress for most people, followed by a memory test.

In the men, the examination caused an increased secretion of cortisol. The higher their cortisol increased, the worse their memory performance.

In the women (tested during the postovulatory phase of their cycles), the combined estrogen and progesterone secreted at that time protected them from showing this stress result and the memory impairment that ordinarily goes along with it.[848] Nature seems to have endowed fertile progesterone-estrogen rich women with a natural "stress-management system."

In another experiment, 76 healthy women between ages 65 and 80 were tested on cognitive performance, blood pressure, and cortisol measures, as well as heart rate. Those whose cortisol shot upward had impaired memories. It was difficult for them to remember pairs of words they had just seen, such as "dog-cat"; however, their reasoning skill was preserved.[855] This implies that short-term memory impairment is vulnerable to elevations in cortisol as women age, but that reasoning is less vulnerable.

The Yin and Yang of Hormones and Emotion. The complex connection between your mind and your body is also present with other "emotion" hormones. Psychological stress generates the release of a hormone called vasopressin, which elevates blood pressure. Think of "red in the face" anger. But pleasurable intimate contact, massage, breast stimulation, and breast suckling stimulate the release of the opposing hormone, oxytocin. These two hormones, vasopressin and oxytocin, have been likened to a kind of yin-yang relationship because of their reciprocal roles of stimulating or decreasing the levels of cortisol.[442]

Positive emotions also alter hormones. "Falling in love" can elevate the levels of cortisol and simultaneously (and counterintuitively) *reduce* levels of testosterone in men. "Falling in *lust*" is different and acutely *elevates* testosterone levels in men. When reproductive-age women "fall in love" both their cortisol and their testosterone levels rise.[495] This implies that women become less rational then. (No comment.)

Estrogen and the Central Nervous System

When we consider estrogen's effects on the brain and the nerves, we hit the mother lode! Estrogen promotes the growth of neurons, prevents atrophy of neuronal (nerve) cells, regulates the plasticity of the synapses—those connecting sites from one nerve to the next—and increases a key enzyme that is needed for learning and memory, choline-acetyl-transferase.[21]

Estrogens also act as neuroprotectants because, unlike the other steroids, they are antioxidants. (Oxidative stress and free radical damage also contribute to Alzheimer's disease pathology.) This antioxidant activity of estrogen protects our nervous systems.[521] So, although a number of hormones are integrally involved in stress, cognition, and well-being, estrogen appears to be particularly beneficial. Let's look at specific areas of the brain and the corresponding mental functions affected by the remarkable female sex hormones.

Prefrontal Cortex

Executive functioning describes a cognitive skill of learning and subsequent memory that involves formulating successful plans and prioritizing one's actions. Brain-imaging studies have shown that the front, or *prefrontal cortex* of the brain, is actively "on fire" during executive-functioning activities.[380] This area (near your forehead) is crucial for higher cognitive functions such as working memory, mental imagery, and willed action.

In one study, when ovariectomies (which eliminate the main source of female sex hormones) were performed on monkeys, it reduced the density of the nerves in the prefrontal cortex, *creating a "dumbed-down" animal.* Estrogen and progesterone restored the diminished nerves' density.[395] There is a close parallel in humans, as the following study of 40 healthy women shows.

In 2006, using high-resolution MRI brain imaging, researchers in Italy reported significantly more "gray matter" in castrated women who were using estrogen versus those who used no hormones. Gray matter is the part of the brain that is composed of nerve fibers: the electrical circuitry required for thinking. Former and current estrogen users showed significantly better cognitive ability than did those who had never undergone hormone-replacement therapy. The anatomical findings matched the cognitive test results. Former estrogen users also had more gray matter than did those who had never used estrogen.[85]

What you should know: Sex hormones protect against the age-related loss of brain tissues.

More Beneficial Estrogen Effects

- Estrogen increased the electrical activity in the frontal cortical regions of the brain when women took tests of verbal and spatial working memory.[380] This occurred in monkeys, too, after they had ovariectomies but only if they were given estrogen promptly.[708, 767]

- Elderly people show reductions in the firing patterns of their prefrontal cortex nerves on MRI.[21]

- Hormone users performed better in tests of executive functioning in one study that used estradiol valerate and Dienogest,[395] but not on another that tested estrogen with the synthetic progestin MPA.[296] MPA was not a helpful hormone.

When women who had ovariectomies (i.e., were castrated) viewed three different films that excited the brains of intact women, this produced quiescent (quiet, unexcited) brain-firing patterns in their brains.

After the ovariectomized women had used a transdermal estradiol patch for 6 weeks, the firing in their brains was more active, similar to that of intact women.[24] Adding testosterone further enhanced the excitability of the brain but specifically to sexually oriented films.[767]

The hippocampus, located at the base of the brain, is a "way station" for impulses that are heading toward the prefrontal cortex. Its blood flow increases when a woman is involved in tasks that involve verbal memory, figures, images, and shapes. The hippocampus is also rich in estrogen receptors.[421]

Even old monkeys that were ovariectomized while they were still fertile can show dramatic responses in their hippocampal firing when they are given estrogen,[314] provided that the estrogen is a bioidentical form such as estradiol-17β.

You should know: Not all estrogen is alike. Researchers have argued that the conjugated equine estrogens (such as Premarin, Prempro, and generic equivalents) do not produce these active results in the brain that bioidentical estradiol produces.[314] This might explain why Prempro and Premarin were both associated with increased risks of cognitive declines in older postmenopausal women who started taking hormones 17 years after menopause (see page 227). The WHI study reported an increased incidence in dementia in its Prempro users,[629] which was attributed to cardiovascular clogging that caused strokes. (See the box on page 227, "Both Premarin and Prempro Were Not So Great for Brain Power.")

"Nutritional" Sources of Estrogen Products and Cognitive Function

Soy. Although there is a large army of marketers selling soy and soy derivatives as natural sources of estrogen, the experimental evidence is not as supportive. A 2004 study concluded that *cognitive function* was unlikely to be affected by soy proteins that contain *isoflavones.*[390] Other researchers have found some effects, but they are slight.[120] And very high levels of tofu consumption were linked to dementia in a study described in chapter 4.

Red clover. The isoflavone contained in red clover did not show any substantial cognitive benefit in a study of 30 postmenopausal women older than 60.[369]

Other supplements. Healthy Woman Soy Menopause Supplement (McNeil PPC, Inc.) showed some clear cognitive benefits in postmenopausal women who were not using hormone-replacement therapy but only with the very youngest postmenopausal women.[421]

What you should know about supplements: If supplements have any benefit at all, it is likely to be limited to the very early stages of menopausal decline. Moreover, since there is no federal regulation of supplement sales, many products will not be as effective as claimed. Let the buyer beware!

Hormone Prescriptions and Cognitive Function

According to Dr. Uriel Halbreich, a psychoneuroendocrinology scholar, hormonal therapies may be able to slow age-related declines in cognition just as they can for cardiovascular health.[306] I agree! Both structural and functional changes in the brain precede cognitive decline by many years.[152] For hormonal therapy to be effective in preventing cognitive deficits, the evidence shows that it's best when started early. Irreversible changes in brain microanatomy (decreased cerebral blood flow, glucose metabolism, and neurotransmitters) and shrinkage of brain matter occur after prolonged estrogen deficiency.[152] If clogged arteries impede blood flow to the brain, how can your cognition not be impaired?

You should know: It's not necessarily age-related. Life *stage* appears to be more important than *age*; when hot flashes begin is the time when *estrogens* are diminishing. Your body sends you important signals to let you know that your level of estrogen is plummeting.

There are convincing arguments for starting hormone-replacement therapy earlier. Women with the *longest* lifetime estrogen exposure had the *least degree of cognitive impairment*, when exposure was calculated by adding up the number of years of hormonal therapy, plus the number of years of reproductive fertility.[630]

Cognitive tests showed that the sooner a woman started wearing an estradiol patch, the greater the cognitive benefit.[220]

Both Premarin and Prempro Were Not So Great for Brain Power

Premarin was also tested in the Women's Health Initiative Memory Study on hysterectomized women ages 65 to 79 who were free of dementia at enrollment. Those who took a placebo did better than those who took Premarin in delaying dementia. More stroke incidents (6.5 percent versus 4.5 percent) in the Premarin compared to the placebo group appears to explain this, since no difference between the placebo and the Premarin groups was found when women who had suffered strokes were excluded from the analysis.[228]

In another study of 800 older menopausal women, Premarin did not slow memory loss in old age either.[52] But for 60 postmenopausal women (33 to 51 years old), their everyday activities such as reading showed better scores in Premarin than in placebo users.[693] Another study of 120 women who had undergone hysterectomies found that Premarin did not slow the disease progression in a group that already had mild to moderate Alzheimer's disease.[541]

The two randomized, controlled trials that compared Premarin to Prempro both concluded that Prempro was even worse.[704, 708, 721]

An eminent neuroendocrinologist explained the neutral to negative results of human studies of Premarin, concluding that the higher levels of estrone in the blood worsened cognition in healthy women and that conjugated equine estrogens, which contain mainly estrone sulfate, may have worsened dementia (see tables 3.1 and 3.2 in chapter 3).[354]

Can Estrogen Therapy Reduce Alzheimer's Disease (AD)?

In distinct contrast to the neutral to negative findings reviewed in the box on page 227, that focused solely on Premarin and Prempro, other estrogen studies showed positive results.[354]

What: An analysis of 14 studies.

Who: 1,565 women who used HRT, compared to 4,425 non–hormone users.

The result: Among the hormone users, 215 developed Alzheimer's disease, or slightly under 14 percent of elderly women. Among non–users, 941 out of 4,425 developed Alzheimer's disease, or 21 percent. HRT users had one-third less risk.[354, 375, 648, 766] This is not trivial.

Three observational studies, in the United States, Denmark, and Australia, all found that the earlier the hormonal therapy began, the lower the incidence of cognitive impairment up to 15 years later.[42, 392, 482]

Five other studies provide powerful support for the benefits of *estrogen* on cognition. But there are insufficient data to determine whether it matters *which form* you take and whether you need to start early enough.

- Among 81 women, ages 50 to 65, of equal educational level living in a Melbourne, Australia, community, those who had never used hormonal therapy had (nonsignificantly) lower verbal memory scores than the people who had used hormones or were currently using them.[538]

- In Manhattan, among 1,300 elderly women with no dementia, estrogen users experienced a significantly reduced risk of developing dementia within 5 years. Most of these estrogen users were taking Premarin.[766]

- In London, tests of post-hysterectomized, ovariectomized women ages 55 to 70 showed that estrogen users had significantly better cognitive function.[159]

- In London, once postmenopausal women started taking estrogens, the longer they continued, the stronger their cognitive test responses were.[794]

- In a Missouri study of 1,900 women after at least 10 years of hormone use, those in their mid-70s who had been using hormones had less than half (41 percent) the incidence of impairment.[871]

Overall, the brain works faster and better when it is estradiol-rich, provided that it has not been deprived of estrogen for many years.[676] A Swedish study of identical twins, which was described earlier, tested their cognitive functions against their hormone history.

What: This is the only published population-based study to examine both the glandular and the therapeutic (HT) estrogen exposure and cognitive decline. (That is why it is such an important study.)

Who: Of close to 6,000 individuals between 65 and 84 years of age who had cognitive evaluations, the scientists studied the 325 twin pairs in which only one sister had dementia. They were searching for the effects of long exposure to an estrogen-rich environment.

The results: Women with the longest lifetime exposure to estrogen had the least degree of cognitive impairment.[630]

In Sweden, women generally start HRT early, when they start having hot flashes, rather than years after they have already transitioned *past* that stage, the way that the WHI tested U.S. women. The Swedes use the bioidentical versions of human hormones, too. Only 2.2 percent of their HRT prescriptions are Prempro-type products, which the WHI found caused an increased risk of dementia when they were started late in life. The authors explained that the prescribing patterns favor using estradiol-17β (human bioidentical) 1 or 2 mg per day and progesterone that is *not* medroxyprogesterone acetate. That is because MPA is known to block the intracellular calcium rise: a rise that is considered to be the way estrogen works to benefit cognition.[630] Swedish clinicians routinely avoid both conjugated equine estrogens and medroxyprogesterone acetate (MPA) because of their belief that those products are not appropriate for the best clinical practice. I agree with them, not only for cognitive effects, but for cardiovascular and other body-wide systems.

Mood and Estrogen Therapy

Since estrogen is recognized to improve mood and cognition if taken in the right dosages, forms, and timing, a series of experiments in macaque monkeys tested *how* this occurs. Researchers took away a monkey's estrogen by removing her ovaries, recorded the expected decline in mood and cognitive function, and then added back estradiol or tamoxifen or raloxifene. Some products worked. Others did not. Tamoxifen was ineffective, but the other two (estradiol-17β forms) were effective in influencing the central nervous system through alterations in a neurotransmitter that was being tested (serotonin).[73]

You should know: Not all estrogens are alike. Estrogen therapies that provide a 17β form (such as Estrace or estradiol-17β) are the ones that seem to help cognitive function the best.[847] Conjugated equine estrogen (such as Premarin) contains a little 17β, but it is diluted by many other ineffective variants (as shown in table 3.2, "What Are You Swallowing?" in chapter 3), thereby diluting its cognitive benefit.

Why is there so much confusion about hormone therapy? Because of inconsistent reporting on which "estrogen" was tested and researchers not recognizing the relevance. Dr. John Studd, an eminent British researcher, clinician, and academician, has lamented the misunderstanding in the field: "In spite of the clear clinical history of a woman who will probably respond to estrogens, most psychiatrists believe that such patients are ideal for the use of antidepressants when they are depressed."

Dr. Studd said that psychiatrists often fail to recognize the individual life history of the woman whose relapsing depression often coincided with the lifetime troughs in her own estrogen: the postnatal, premenstrual, and perimenopausal transitions.[753] I agree, and I would also add that after a woman has had a hysterectomy, her estrogen is likely to plummet, and this may cause depression.

If you take estrogen therapy, request a prescription for estradiol-17β, rather than conjugated equine estrogen.

Be picky about progesterone product prescriptions, too. Brain-imaging studies in postmenopausal women who took cognitive tests have shown that some progesterone added to estrogen therapy improved memory, more than estrogen alone did.[553]

Postmenopausal women who were moderately depressed also experienced a significantly reduced severity of depression when taking a progestin product called Dienogest.[658] This European progestin comes very close to being identical to the natural human progesterone form. (See table 3.3 in chapter 3.) Prometrium is available in the United States and is an excellent bioidentical progesterone.

Continuous-Combined versus Sequential Therapy

While the studies just reviewed showed benefits from continuous combinations of estrogen and progestins, none have yet tested sequential regimens.[521] My view is that sequential regimens provide a better choice for women overall. At puberty, a girl's brain diverges neuroanatomically from the male pattern. From then on, her physiology is designed for the hormonal symphony of progesterone's presence half of the month, while estrogen is always there until our aging decreases both hormones. A sequential regimen most closely supplies the amounts that bone and brain tissues have developed molecular receptors to receive. The most rational regimen would mimic the design of nature that occurs when a woman's mental capacity is powerful.

What you should know: Rhythm is central to our mental health. Depressed premenopausal women showed a loss of the natural, rhythmic, pulsed release of brain hormones (luteinizing hormone) that is normally found in nondepressed women.[288] I conclude that mental health flourishes with normal rhythmicity.

Sequential progesterone and synthetic progestin regimens were tested in a group of 56-year-old women for 15 months. A clear improvement of mental functioning that was independent of mood was shown during the P time of each woman's cycle, when the progesterone or the synthetic progestin was taken sequentially.[11, 553]

Women probably recognize that during their menstruating years, the premenstrual (progesterone) half of the month tends to be the moodier time. In fact, there has even been a suggestion that women's irritability comes from the sharpness in their thinking process, their increased perception, and their ability to see everything that is "wrong" in great clarity.[580] This makes sense to me.

You should know: You have options. Experiments on another newer, more natural progesterone, dydrogesterone, given sequentially and opposed to 17β estradiol that was prescribed every day, showed that this sequential regimen improved blood flow to the brain.[795]

Bioidentical versus Synthetic

Synthetic progestins can be toxic. Added to estrogen, either of two synthetic progestins (MPA or norethindrone) injected in an animal model were tested in both the cerebral and the peripheral blood vessels for cognitive or cardiovascular effects. Both estrogens were benign. Both synthetic progestins were toxic to blood vessels.[778] This is very bad.

Since cognitive declines may be a consequence of the atherosclerotic disruption of blood flow to the brain, I believe that women over 40 would be wise to avoid these synthetic progestins. They are commonly found in birth control pills and some hormone regimens.

What you should know: Insist on knowing the name of the hormone. Consult with a knowledgeable physician who will respect your knowledge and work with you.

Conclusion

Consider the benefits of a lifelong use of hormone therapies to keep your mind as sharp as possible, unless this is contraindicated by your personal condition. The brain is receptive to estradiol-17β, so be sure your prescriber knows that this is the form of estrogen that makes sense—not other forms. And mimic the design of nature, taking estradiol every day and progesterone (not synthetic progestin) for the last fourteen days of each month to optimize your brain's cognitive abilities. At the same time, cultivate a disciplined lifestyle of right thinking, right eating, and regular exercise, while you make daily contributions to the well-being of others. This should improve the quality of your own life and the lives of those you love.

12

Your Changing Sexual Life and What You Can Do about It

SEXUAL WELL-BEING WAS CORRELATED with overall happiness in both men and women of every culture and every location around the globe, according to a 2006 global study of more than 27,000 women and men who were 40 to 80 years of age.[436]

And sexual well-being inevitably changes. Sexual difficulties were some of the more frequently reported health concerns of menopausal women.[202] The problems begin well before the last menstrual period. A decline in sexual responsiveness, frequency, and libido, with a significant increase in painful intercourse and partners' performance problems are common.[82, 200] These changes are most drastic for women who have pelvic surgery, but every woman can expect menopause-related changes.

Factor In Our Culture

Clearly, culture plays a role in our attitudes toward aging and sexuality.[83] Consider the U.S. movie industry's preoccupation with youthful women paired to older men. Is this the mind-set of male Hollywood producers who—living in a movie star culture—are focused on short-term "arm candy" relationships that they glamorize in movies? Does it consign such young wives to become nursemaids and "first wives" to living out their mature years devoid of intimacy? Or consider polyga-mous cultures that replace old wives with secondary young wives: cul-tures that teach the older ones not to be sexual.[490]

Much of Western culture highly values long-term commitment to a partner who ages as you do. But keeping a rich intimate life may collide with the physiological realities of thinning vaginal tissue in menopause that can be vulnerable to abrasions, ulceration, and infection.

What's a woman to do if she has, or wants to search for, a partner? Good studies offer useful insights to help you make some critical deci-sions.

Studying Sex

Studying sexual behavior research is not as simple as checking a wom-an's blood pressure. What's normal? There's no easy answer to this question.[221, 510] Instead, the complexities include *both* partners' physi-ology, attitudes, and skills. Even when one partner has a "dysfunction," it is the couple's sex life that is impaired.

For functional men, it's straightforward and linear: they experience a stimulus, get erect, engage, move to the rhythm that "scratches their itch," climax, and relax. Women are more complex, and their pattern is anything but linear; it's almost circular, with on- and off-ramps at every stage. At every level, a woman's heart and head are inextricably linked with her physical response.[287]

Getting in the Mood

When women watched erotic films, their blood flowed to their vagi-nas much as blood would flow in men to produce erections. But in women, the blood flowed whether or not they *perceived* arousal.[430] The increased blood to the genitals provides a natural lubricant that permits smooth massage by a dry penis during sexual intercourse. If women engage in exercise, like dancing or bicycling, just before watch-ing such a film, this increases the amount of blood that flows to their genitals during an erotic, but not a neutral, film.[517] Having a hysterec-tomy reduces this sexual reflex.[516]

For intact women, when sex is on the brain, the act of exercise increases blood flow, which diverts blood to the vaginal tissue, intensifying local pressure. As in men whose blood flow to the penis generates a pressure that triggers erection, blood flow to the vagina generates pressure. Intact women respond vaginally to "erotic" films whether they are created by men (women-as-object-type film) or by women (generally, a more gentle and loving display).[430] And women learn fast. After a woman has seen both types of film, her lubrication response is much greater to the female film and is more inhibited as she watches the male film. Although women report aversion to the male-produced abusive films, their blood still flows to the vagina as they watch. My interpretation of these facts? Nature's design attempts to provide lubrication as protection from injury whenever intercourse is imminent, whether the woman's potential partner is welcome or not—if there is adequate circulating estrogen and she is intact.

Our Sexual Perceptions Count, Too

Researchers can also measure *perceptions* if they are able to overcome the tendency to label women's sexuality using male terminology.[70, 76, 491, 649] When women are asked, they explain that sexual intercourse is rarely the main goal of their sexuality.

What you should know: Women's sexual pleasure commonly stems from a need for intimacy, not from a male-type need for sexual arousal and orgasm.[55] For a couple to have a good sexual relationship, they must first understand the simplicity of his needs,[750] then the complexity of hers.

Sexual Desire

For many men, this sexual appetite or libido can easily dominate their experience.[750] But women are more complex: desire covers a spectrum that ranges from aversion to disinclination, to indifference, to interest, to need, and, finally, to passion, wrote psychiatrist Steve Levine.[448]

His observations match other research. About 30 percent of women do not generally experience sexual desire. And unlike in men, in women desire follows genital arousal as often as the other way around.[55, 57, 58] And for some postmenopausal women, sexuality has become irrelevant.

Desire Decreases with Time, Too

One study of young men and women in steady relationships found that for women, sexual desire decreases but the desire for tenderness increases as time passes. For men, sexual desire remained steady but the desire for tenderness decreased.[405]

A national social life survey of 3,200 U.S. residents, from 18 to 59 years old, likewise reported that the quality of marital sex declined with time for both men and women.[458] Men seemed less sensitive to the problem. Women were less satisfied with sex in their marriages, maybe due to having fewer orgasms than their men had.

These disparities in long-term relationships create imbalances,[148] but since sexual behavior is a partnership issue, these differences need to be negotiated.

An increase in sexual desire and sexual interest is consistently reported with a new relationship, even in women who are many years postmenopausal and with very low levels of sex hormones.[58]

The 2005 U.S. Study of Women's Health Across the Nation confirmed that starting a new relationship is related to greater emotional satisfaction, sexual arousal, frequency of sexual intercourse, and desire.[38] But whenever women began their perimenopausal changes, they were vulnerable to having an increase in painful intercourse because of hormonal changes. Even very young women, with plenty of estrogen, are vulnerable to sexual difficulties.[518] For a more mature woman, her feeling for her partner is the key to sexual response.[55, 58, 202]

Painful Intercourse (Dyspareunia) and Related Problems

Vaginal stimulation will lead to tension (i.e., arousal) and then a spasmodic release of tension (orgasm) as long as the nerve endings have not atrophied and the rhythm of the stroking creates "harmonious," rather than "discordant," music. Two people involved in romantic attraction create a kind of dance. But lubrication is needed to avoid abrasions and the tearing of tissue.[799]

A University of Pennsylvania study followed 300 healthy women who were 35 to 47 years old. Over 4 years, the best predictors of a decline in libido were vaginal dryness, depression, their children still living at home, and highly variable testosterone levels from one month to the next. Women who had stable testosterone hormone levels during the 4 years did not show these declines.[284] Investigators could not tell which came first, the hormone fluctuations or the change in libido. Or maybe the behavior of their partners.

Exercise and Sexuality

Exercise affects sexuality in other ways:

- Only the frequency of exercise, not testosterone or age, was significantly associated with having better sexual satisfaction.[267]

- Women who exercise at least once or more a week were more likely to continue participating in studies of sexual behavior in women as they aged.[203]

- Women who were not sexually active had a significantly higher body mass index than did those who were sexually active.[827, 828]

- Obesity (a BMI greater than 30) was a significant predictor of being sexually inactive.[5]

- And in the short term, rigorous exercise enhances the blood flow to the vagina when exercise precedes sex.[517]

Does keeping physically fit promote interest in sexual behavior? Or is it the other way around? These studies did not, and perhaps could not, address those questions. But the media in developed nations unanimously proclaim that a fit and trim woman is more sexually attractive than a grossly obese woman. So exercise is a good thing in itself and helps maintain a warm romantic life, which is also good for you.

The Effect of Age and Estrogen

In 2005, the first investigation that attempted to standardize an evaluation of how the vagina's inner walls age was published by researchers at the Cleveland Clinic. Both age and lowered estrogen predicted declining tissue vigor; the tissues become thinner, flatter, less spongy, and less able to withstand the pummeling of vigorous intercourse.[840]

As I see it, nature's design includes some time for learning about one's own best rhythm, after puberty has ripened into the fertile years and estrogen levels have risen to those shown in table 3.1 in chapter 3. Young people rarely start their sexual lives understanding their own best rhythms. Most of them learn as they go. Fortunately, nature provides an estrogen-rich young woman with lubricant to spare. So an estrogen-low older woman in a long-term relationship is likely to need much more loving and petting before her lubrication response is activated, especially if she is involved with an aging man whose best erection occurs as he awakens in the morning—when she may be the opposite of "aroused."

As a woman ages, if she is not aroused, she is more likely to suffer painful intercourse (dyspareunia), which can lead to tearing, bleeding, and infection. Although over-the-counter lubricants are helpful in alleviating such dyspareunia, they do not restore the elasticity of a healthy vagina.

The Brain-Cervix Connection

In 1992, Drs. Beverly Whipple and Barry Komisaruk and their colleagues studied the physiological components of orgasm in women that were induced either by imagination or by a vibrator in a private hospital room. The main finding of their study was that pain-tolerance thresholds increased during genital stimulation that included both vaginal-cervical vibration and self-guided imagery.[838] Vaginal-cervical stimulation worked to reduce pain, whether or not the woman perceived that she was sexually aroused. In other words, an intact woman could tolerate more pain when she was sexually aroused. Resting and relaxation worked the opposite way; they lowered the pain tolerance threshold.[412, 414, 837]

So, a woman has a capacity to respond to sexual relations that triggers widespread analgesic effects, assuming her nerves are in place.[232, 413] This capacity has not previously been recognized; the nerves that are responsible have not been studied to determine the impact of a hysterectomy or other pelvic surgeries on them. Nature's design for an intact sexual system has barely been probed by scientific research, for understandable reasons of privacy and delicacy. But disruptions in the system have some now-recognized sexual consequences. First came the myths, however, which compounded medical confusion.

Surgery and Sexuality

Hysterectomy myth #1: The procedure improves your sex life. Researchers of several studies have provided data about women before and after they underwent hysterectomies that they claim show that hysterectomies improve the measured sexual behaviors.[39, 113, 317, 826] Or that cervical removal or retention was irrelevant to postoperative sexuality.[427] I think their conclusions are invalid because the researchers did not choose the proper baseline.

For example, in November 1999, researchers published the Maryland Women's Health Study.[641] Updates followed in 2005.[427] The study reported that 2 years after having hysterectomies, more women were sexually active (from a baseline of 71 percent before the hysterectomy to 77 percent after the hysterectomy), more women were orgasmic, and more women were frequently sexually active (greater than 5 times per month). This sounded like an endorsement for having a hysterectomy, until we took a closer look.

Notice what the researchers chose to measure from: For the baseline, women were asked about their prior-30-days' sexual functioning after they had been diagnosed with disease in their genital areas, heard and accepted their physicians' prescription for surgery, and scheduled the surgeries. In the hospital, just before surgery, each woman was asked how much intercourse she had in the 30 days before surgery.

What woman, during that presurgical time when she is awaiting surgery and experiencing and fearing pain, would have her normal interest in sexual activity? I think a scheduled hysterectomy would turn off most sexual interest.

With a low baseline, any post-hysterectomy increase leads to a misleading conclusion of "improvement." Unless you stop and think, "Compared with 'what' will her sex life be improved?"

Hysterectomy myth #2: It's a cure. A panel of professors of gynecology from the Agency for Health Care Policy Planning reported that by

2007, no data have yet shown that a hysterectomy has a better efficacy than more conservative treatments for benign conditions such as fibroids.[487] Therefore, it behooves the clinician and you, the consumer, to recognize the erroneous logic of well-meaning assumptions that lead to false conclusions.

After reviewing these pro-hysterectomy studies, my colleagues and I concluded that this defective baseline renders the information not useful and even harmful.[175]

In 2000, my colleagues and I presented our findings on sexual response in women at the American College of Obstetrics and Gynecology meeting. Tables 12.1 and 12.2 show the proportion of women who reported that they were sexually active (at all), as well as the proportion of women who reported frequent (at least once a week) sexual activity. In both cases, women who were scheduled to have hysterectomies were less likely to be either sexually active or frequently sexually active, just as logic would predict. They were "turned off" just before surgery. After having hysterectomies, two years later or much later, as shown in both tables, more women engaged in sexual behavior. But women who had retained their uteruses had the highest likelihood of being sexually active, as well as sexually active at least once a week.[177, 178]

We concluded that a hysterectomy can be expected to negatively impact a woman's sexuality. Our data contradict the conclusion that having a hysterectomy enhances the sexuality of women.

Table 12.1 The Proportion of Women Reporting Frequent Sexual Activity

Group	Total Number	Sexual Activity ≥ 5 Times/Month
1. Intact uterus (*Athena*)	81	58%
2. Intact uterus with fibroids (*Smith*)	30	57%
3. Post-hysterectomy .5–20 yrs. (*Athena*)	22	45%
4. Post-hysterectomy at 2 yrs. (*Rhodes et al.*)	1,101	41%
5. Scheduled for hysterectomy (*Rhodes et al.*)	1,101	31%

Table 12.2 The Proportion of Women Reporting Frequent Orgasms

Group	Total Number	Frequent Orgasm
1. Intact uterus (*Athena*)	118	61%
2. Intact uterus with fibroids (*Smith*)	34	58%
3. Post-hysterectomy .5–20 years (*Athena*)	21	61%
4. Post-hysterectomy at 2 years (*Rhodes et al.*)	1,095	55%
5. Scheduled for hysterectomy (*Rhodes et al.*)	1,095	46%

What you should know: A hysterectomy is not an innocuous procedure. It removes a significant part of your sexual anatomy. Be clear that "the research" may not always be in your best interest. Don't make a decision based on a headline or a conclusion; ask how the researchers arrived at that conclusion.

A hysterectomy can impair your sex life. Although a group of studies purported to show that hysterectomies improved the sex lives of women, other researchers began to search for the influence of testosterone therapy to help "fix" this problem.[108]

First, they asserted that post-hysterectomized women had sex problems by using common sense to gather data. Dr. Rosemary Basson and colleagues found that 30 percent of the hysterectomized women they studied had experienced little sexual desire and that woman often engage in sexual behavior before they feel, or independent of, any desire. For some women, their partners' behavior triggers their arousal and then desire.[57]

Dr. Jan Shifren, at Harvard, surveyed post-hysterectomy patients and learned that close to 30 percent of these women might want to enter a study of their own sexual dysfunction after having hysterectomies.[697]

In 2000, other researchers published their "Brief Index of Sexual Functioning," a validated questionnaire for surgically menopausal women who would be complaining of impaired sexual function compared to their pre-surgical experience.[505]

Among 104 surgically menopausal women in monogamous relationships who had sexual dysfunction complaints, they reported significantly worse scores in 7 domains of sexual response than did intact women of comparable ages who were in relationships without complaints. The women who had undergone hysterectomies experienced less arousal, less frequency of sexual activity, less receptivity and initiation, less pleasure/orgasm, and less satisfaction with their sexual relationships, as well as more problems and fewer thoughts and desires about sexual activity.

In 2006, three more studies were published that supported this finding.

Study #1: Dysfunction and dissatisfaction. In the Kaiser Permanente Study, 2,109 participants in a survey of sexual function and incontinence in women ages 40 to 69 found that 32 percent who had had hysterectomies had some sexual dysfunction, and 28 percent had no sexual activity in their lives.

What they found: The authors concluded that a hysterectomy is a significant predictor of having no sexual activity thereafter, as is having a body mass index greater than 30 or being incontinent.[5]

Study #2: A higher rate of divorce and low desire. This was a study by the Women's International Study of Health and Sexuality of 952 U.S. women.

What they found: Surgically postmenopausal women were more likely to be divorced (19 percent of those who had had hysterectomies or ovariectomies versus 7 percent of those who were intact).[443] The surgical group was 3 times more likely to be in a state of distress over their sexual lives than were intact women, despite the fact that 80 percent of them were presently using hormonal therapy. They reported feelings of frustration, hopelessness, anger, and a loss of femininity or self-esteem.[443]

Study #3: Loss of ovaries = loss of desire. Also in 2006, Dr. Susan Davis and her colleagues reported that after undergoing ovariectomies, 30 to 50 percent of women reported diminished sexual desire, which was twice the rate for women who had had hysterectomies but *retained* their ovaries. If the woman answered "yes" to the 5 following questions, she was advised to see a specialist to evaluate

Table 12.3 Female Sexual Dysfunction and Drug Management[56]

	Generalized Female Sexual Arousal Disorder	Genital Arousal Disorder	Missed Arousal	Dysphoric Arousal
Mental excitement	Absent	Present	Absent	Absent
Genital congestion	Absent	Absent	Present	Present
Vasoactive medication logical?	No	Yes	No	No

treatment for "hypoactive sexual desire disorder." (You can check yourself, too.)

1. Before the ovariectomy, was your sex life good and satisfying?
2. Since the ovariectomy, have you experienced a meaningful loss in your level of desire for sex?
3. Since the ovariectomy, have you experienced a significant decrease in sexual activity?
4. Are you concerned or bothered by your current level of desire or interest in sex?
5. Would you like to see an increase in 4?

These data look pretty grim. Fortunately, there is good news because regimens and treatments are available to offer help. But drugs that are used for erectile difficulties in men are rarely effective in women.[59] Vasoactive medication, such as Viagra, would be logical only in a small subset of women who experience mental excitement but don't have genital congestion when they engage in sexual encounters. (See table 12.3.)

The Impact of Prolapse, Incontinence, and Corrective Surgery

The study: Gynecologist and scholar Anne Weber evaluated the sexual functions of 81 women who were undergoing surgery for uterine prolapse and incontinence. Before surgery, these women were comparable to 30 women without those problems in the measures of sexual frequency, dyspareunia, masturbation, and sexual satisfaction.[827]

What happened after surgery: After 3 years, painful intercourse had developed in 26 percent of women who had a "posterior colporrhaphy" procedure and in 38 percent who had a "Burch" procedure.[825] These classic procedures in common surgical use had never been evaluated this way before.

What you should know: The surgery has side effects. Dr. Weber and colleagues discovered previously unrecognized adverse outcomes of these surgical procedures. A different investigator evaluated 343 women older than 45 who were randomized to different treatments.[48] In the short term, comparing outcomes up to 6 months after treatment, no improvement or adverse outcome could be identified. Overall sexual satisfaction did not change and appeared to be independent of either diagnosis of or therapy for urinary incontinence or prolapse.

Hidden Sexual Problems

In a reverse type of "Don't ask, don't tell," researchers evaluated the incidence of sexual problems even in women who did *not* ask their doctors to be evaluated for sexual dysfunction. In 1997, Drs. Julia Heiman and Cindy Meston reported on data of more than 1,600 women who had not approached their doctors.

What you should know: Women have lots of sex problems. Most common were a lack of interest in sex among 30 percent of women (ages 18 to 59); insufficient lubrication and painful intercourse in 21 percent of women over age 45; and an inability to have an orgasm in from 20 to 30 percent—this problem was more prevalent for inexperienced younger women and in older women with declining hormones. Lack of pleasure in sex was most common in the very young groups and in the oldest groups.[334] (The women's hysterectomy status was not reported.) Remember, the *partner* might be "the problem."

Unfortunately, sex was not pleasurable for 15 to 27 percent of each age group from 18 to 59. Those percentages are a shame; sex should feel good.

The dysfunctions were low desire, low arousal, orgasmic disorder, and sexual pain disorders.[69] The causes included surgery, inadequate blood flow, nerve damage, declining hormone levels, and prescribed drugs, such as mood-altering SSRIs (selective serotonin reuptake inhibitors). But the body is one interconnected system.

Seeking Help for Sexual Complaints

By age 57, more than two-thirds of women experience vaginal dryness, which will cause pain during both a gynecological exam and sexual intercourse.[671] Estrogen alone will often help resolve this dryness, provided that blood levels of estradiol reach the levels that reproductive-age women have. (See table 3.1 in chapter 3.)

A Web-based survey of more than 3,800 women reported that 1,900 (half) had sought medical help for sexual dysfunction. Most of them

Table 12.4 Sex 911: Whom Should You Call?[293]

Professional Specialists for Different Sexual Problems

If:	You Should See This Specialist:
You're menopausal and want to consider hormone therapy	Gynecologist
You have sexual dysfunction that requires specialized evaluation and/or treatment	Gynecologist with a special interest in sexual dysfunction
Your partner has erectile or ejaculatory dysfunction that may require medical treatment	Urologist
Either of you has sexual dysfunctions	Internist/family practitioner with an interest in sexual medicine
You're a cancer survivor and want to consider hormone therapy for sexual symptoms	Oncologist or gynecology specialist
You're menopausal and experiencing depression and anxiety	Psychiatrist
Your altered hormonal status or his situational erectile dysfunction is creating orgasmic difficulties or dampening sexual motivation in either of you	Sex therapist
You have relationship issues that are contributing to your sexual dysfunction	Couples therapist
You have personal psychodynamic issues that may be inhibiting sexual function	Individual psychotherapist
Hyper- and hypo-tonicity of your pelvic floor is contributory	Physical therapist

said that their doctors did not want to hear about their problem, did not appreciate its significance to them, and made no attempt to reduce their nervousness or to thoroughly examine their complaint; 76 percent of the women received no diagnosis and 88 percent had doctors who did not develop a specific treatment plan.[71] Although discussing a female patient's sex life with her is an essential part of good medical care, physicians often feel very uncomfortable doing so.[59, 671] This is understandable.

If you need expert sexual counseling, take charge and locate the appropriate specialist. (See table 12.4.) And involve your partner.

Hormone Therapies and Sexuality

Both estrogen and testosterone therapies have been studied to investigate their influence on sexual life. But these studies have been funded by competing Big Pharma manufacturers with disparate interests. For this reason, I have tried to tease apart what was shown from what was missing from the experimental design, in order to determine what I think you need to know.

Estrogen Fuels Your Sex Life

For women, the capacity to respond genitally requires adequate estrogen that is equivalent to that of a menstruating fertile woman just before she is ovulating, to nourish the vaginal tissue as well as to enable the blood flow to that area.[490]

Why a low dose might not get you going: Dr. Lorraine Dennerstein and her colleagues concluded that the low doses of estrogen that are promoted by some medical "authorities" would not be effective in sustaining a woman's sexual function. I agree. For adequate sexual function, a woman needs levels of estrogen that are relatively high, or at least as high as when she was sexually active and comfortably so.[203]

What you should know: It was the circulating level of estrogen, not testosterone, that declined concomitantly with both the sexual interest and the sexual responsiveness in a cohort of healthy women who had not sought help for sexual dysfunction.[203] Although a vital part of the sexual function equation is the behavior and skill of your male partner, there is no substitute for adequate circulating estrogen to preserve vaginal tissue from atrophying.

How estrogen helps: Dr. Norma McCoy focused a comprehensive review of the scientific research to show the relationships between estrogen therapy and sexuality, as listed below.[507] Here is what she found:

- *Vaginal dryness.* Researchers reported that in 7 of 8 studies that examined vaginal dryness or vaginal cytologic (cell swabs) evidence, there were significant improvements with estrogen-replacement therapy, whether oral, transdermal, human, or conjugated equine estrogens.

- *Dyspareunia (painful intercourse).* Only 1 of 6 reports was able to show improvement on hormone-replacement therapy; this one positive study used a structurally human estradiol-17β transdermally.

- *Orgasm.* Of 5 placebo-controlled studies, only 1 found a significant increase. That one used ethinyl estradiol at .05 milligrams, which is a very powerful synthetic estrogen that is not recommended because of its association with an increased risk of developing breast cancer and cardiovascular problems. (See chapters 9 and 10.) The other estrogens that were tested provided no help.

- *Sexual interest (libido).* Overall, 7 studies have allowed some tentative conclusions. In naturally menopausal women, structurally human estrogens can sometimes increase the women's sexual interest, but conjugated equine estrogens like Premarin are not effective. Since the human forebrain has no receptors for most of the Premarin components (see table 3.2 in chapter 3), this makes sense.

Androgens and Your Sexuality

Although women circulate dramatically lower levels of testosterone than men do, as shown in figure 11.1 in chapter 11, the testosterone they do produce and circulate is essential to their well-being, vigor, and sexual function. Testosterone therapy shows some modest effects in increasing women's interest in sex for about 40 percent of women who have experienced surgical menopause (a hysterectomy and an ovariectomy), with its consequent loss of the ovarian contributions to their supply of androgens.

In 1996, Dr. Susan Rako, a highly intelligent and articulate psychiatrist, published *The Hormone of Desire: The Truth about Sexuality,*

Menopause, and Testosterone, chronicling her own embarrassing and infuriating experience as a woman seeking help for her postmenopausal loss of sexual sensation. She found an endocrinologist who, after reviewing the data she had presented, prescribed testosterone. The testosterone worked, and Dr. Rako wrote of the restoration she experienced.[627]

What you should know: You can get testosterone if you need it. By 1998, the pharmaceutical industry was focusing its attention on the possibilities of developing a testosterone drug for postmenopausal women who had sexual complaints. In mid-2008, FDA approval of testosterone for female sexual complaints had not been achieved, but physicians could legally prescribe it.

Is Low Testosterone Your Problem?

In 2002, a "female androgen insufficiency syndrome" was defined as a pattern of clinical symptoms: low libido, low responsiveness, and low sexual pleasure in the presence of very low levels of bioavailable testosterone.[41] (In some cases, I suspect the "insufficiency" might be in the sexual skills of a male partner.)

Testosterone is hard to assess. Adequate blood tests of bioavailable testosterone are difficult to obtain because the "T" (testosterone) quantities are so tiny that test results are often inaccurate. But another androgen—DHEAS (dehydroepiandrosterone sulfate)—is different. Produced in the adrenal glands, this hormone can be accurately and reliably measured in women. It is a "master hormone," in that our bodies can use it to convert into other androgens, such as androstenedione and testosterone. If DHEAS levels are high enough, you will not experience testosterone-deficiency symptoms. Of 311 women from the Penn Ovarian Aging Study, higher levels of DHEAS appear to be protective against sexual dysfunction. Among women with sexual dysfunction, significantly lower levels of DHEAS were circulating in their bodies.[283] In the Penn study, no other significant relationships with sexual dysfunction occurred: it was not related to testosterone, age, education, or a smoking habit. Circulating DHEAS has been consistently identified for its beneficial role in good health. *Don't self-medicate, however!*

Typically, men circulate 20 to 40 times the concentration of testosterone that women do. In men, testosterone has been long recognized to have profound influences on sexuality. As testosterone levels begin rising at puberty, so does the sexuality of boys, in a sort of lock-step hormone-behavior relationship.[309]

Women are not like men! Testosterone levels in women across their lifespan seem to remain relatively low but do not decrease with age. In 1995, one small study of 33 women reported that by age 35, almost none had high levels of testosterone.[879] But the 2006 data of more than 1,200 women, shown in figure 11.1 in chapter 11, reported no overall age-related change in testosterone across the lifespan of a very large group of healthy women.

The Melbourne Women's Study of more than 500 intact women (ages 45 to 55), from 4 years before to 3 years after the last menstrual period, reported stable unchanging DHEAS and testosterone levels, compared to dramatically declining *estrogen* levels, in these women who had not been seeking help for a sexual dysfunction![203, 267]

What you should know: You are unique. Women as a group cannot be demonstrated to show a trend for age-related changes in testosterone as they do for estrogen.[777]

What you should know: It may not be hormonal. In 2007, given the "news impact" that testosterone may help women with their low sexual desire, a report from Dr. Dennerstein's group provided clear perspective.[322] Close to 2,000 European women from 5 countries and 1,600 women from the United States (ages 20 to 70) completed the same validated questionnaires that were used in the testosterone patch studies. The incidence of "hypoactive sexual desire disorder" occurred in less than 13 percent of the population, regardless of age. Although there was an age-related decline in sexual interest, there was a simultaneous age-related decrease in concern about the situation.

Dissatisfaction can occur for other reasons; for example, dissatisfaction that the football captain Adonis she married has gained 80 pounds, mostly in his middle, and is a couch potato. In short, the cause of a woman's "hypoactive sexual desire" may not be "chemical"—it might be "spousal."

Which Hormones to Consider for HRT

Estrogen-replacement therapy is essential for estrogen-deficient women who want to have good sex lives.[203, 671] The recommendation for androgen-replacement therapy in women is much less certain.[269, 305] Consider the following key points:

- The blood levels of androgens may not be relevant to the target tissue action because local enzyme and hormone production would not be observable at the blood levels tested.[111] This means you can't get a blood test to reliably identify a problem with your androgen production.

- An androgen-insufficiency syndrome caused by an abrupt loss of the ovaries (an ovariectomy) may trigger an abrupt loss of libido. The symptoms of an androgen-insufficiency syndrome include:

  Low libido with persistent unexplained fatigue, decreased sense of well-being

  Blunted motivation, depressed mood

  Thinning pubic hair, body mass with more fat, less muscle, osteopenia and osteoporosis

If you're swallowing estrogen to replenish your sexual function, ask for a different prescription. Oral estrogen increases the liver production of SHBG (sex hormone binding globulin), which attaches or binds to the testosterone, thereby *reducing* the amount of bioavailable testosterone. The result: androgen insufficiency. Switch from oral to a sublingual, transdermal, or vaginal route for the estrogen.

If you've had a hysterectomy, will testosterone work? It might.[16]

Will testosterone restore your declining sexual interest during the menopausal transition? Maybe. One 2007 study of 441 "sexually active" women, 45 to 54 years old, showed that the 156 women who "wanted sex more often" had much higher testosterone blood levels than did the 237 women who were "satisfied" and the 27 who "wanted sex less often."[255] I believe these data show a direct relationship: either high testosterone does stimulate sexual appetite, or unsatisfied sexual hunger elevates testosterone.

Researched Regimens

Different hormone products are available with differing benefit and risk outcomes.

Methyl Testosterone with Estrogen versus Estrogen Alone

Several studies have evaluated a product known as Estratest, which is an oral pill that combines esterified estradiol with methyltestosterone. The Big Pharma manufacturer Solvay has achieved FDA approval for this drug for hot flashes but not for sex problems, "as of 2008."

Study #1: Effective, but bad for cardiovascular health. In 1993, the first well-controlled trial tested this regimen in 26 women (average age 52) who were more than one year postmenopausal. They found that the two regimens, Estratest versus Estratab (estrogen by itself without any testosterone), were both equally effective in reducing menopausal symptoms and were well tolerated. But they noted a potentially adverse impact on blood lipids from the added testosterone in Estratest. Although there was no change in triglycerides, there was a decrease in the beneficial HDL cholesterol.[348]

Study #2: Estrogen alone is better for cholesterol. In 2003, 218 healthy estrogen-using postmenopausal women (naturally or surgically) complaining of low sexual interest were tested to compare pills: Estratab versus Estratest.[465] About half who took the added testosterone reported an increased sexual interest and responsiveness, but the added testosterone was not effective for the other half of Estratest users. *Lipid changes:* There was a beneficial reduction in triglycerides but an adverse reduction in the good HDL cholesterol levels in women who took both estrogen and testosterone. Estrogen without testosterone, however, increased the good HDL cholesterol.

Study #3: The impact of higher doses. A 2005 study enrolled 102 women in stable, monogamous relationships who were bothered by hypoactive sexual desire after surgical menopause (i.e., after having hysterectomies and ovariectomies).

The study showed an improved outcome in the Estratest group compared to the Estratab (just estrogen) group in the sexual interest scores. The improved outcome did not occur for everyone, but was more likely for women using these higher doses of Estratest than for women taking Estratab. Unfortunately, there were adverse effects: the Estratest users had an average 26 percent decline in their good HDL cholesterol levels in their blood. *Other adverse events:* more weight gain, nervousness, and vaginitis (in 6 percent of the Estratest versus 0 percent of the Estratab users).[817] Two editorials about this study appeared at the same time. Dr. Susan Davis suggested that concerns should be raised about the substantial decline in the good HDL cholesterol in women taking the Estratest.[185] Dr. Jan Shifren commented in the medical journal *Menopause* that methyltestosterone (which is used in Estratest) does not "aromatize" (change its molecular form into estrogen, as other types of testosterone do); this indicated that the sexual effects obtained were true testosterone effects, not estrogen results. At the same time, both scientists were conducting studies on a competing testosterone product.

Other Oral Testosterone Regimens

In Sweden's Karolinska Hospital, surgically menopausal women who had not complained of hypoactive sexual desire were tested on either testosterone undecanoate or a full 2-milligram dose of estradiol valerate. (Neither is sold in the United States.) The results fit what we are learning about oral estrogens and testosterone products. The testosterone addition to the estrogen produced a stronger sexual benefit than estrogen alone did. The strongest effect noted was for enjoyment of sex and sexual thoughts and fantasies, which were much more marked when testosterone was added. No serious adverse effects were found in women using either of these regimens.[243] For a woman to obtain such a regimen in the United States, she would need a prescription for a generic equivalent from her doctor to be obtained through a compounding pharmacy.

Testing a Testosterone Patch

In 2000, a randomized, controlled trial of 75 women who believed their sex lives had deteriorated after surgical menopause and who continued to use their oral conjugated equine estrogens (at least .625 mg/day) tested 3 different doses of transdermal (patch) testosterone for 3 consecutive 12-week treatment periods.[696]

Study #1: Benefit, but not for everyone. Overall, the study showed a dose-dependent benefit of testosterone in 41 percent of the women who had impaired sexual function. Not everyone received this benefit, but for those who did, testosterone clearly improved their sexual lives. On a numerical scale, the improvement was modest.

Study # 2: Individual improvement. A 2005 confirmation followed from a 24-week study of surgically menopausal women who had hypoactive sexual desire disorder. The testosterone patch produced an average change of one additional satisfying episode of sexual activity per 4 weeks.[108] Do you consider these modest results? If you think results like these will improve your life, the decision belongs to you.

Study #3: Estrogen plus testosterone patch. Adding a testosterone patch to an estradiol patch *did* increase the women's scores on sexual desire, improved sexual function, and overall well-being. And it reduced the distress among surgically menopausal women in stable monogamous relationships who had hypoactive sexual desire disorder. Adverse effects were minimal and not different from a placebo.[188] Again, the results were modest in the 77 women.

Study #4: The patch in premenopausal women. The first test of the use of transdermal testosterone in healthy premenopausal women experiencing low libido also reported a clinically meaningful improvement in psychological and sexual well-being.[272] Half of these women were taking oral contraceptives, a choice that was previously shown to frequently inhibit libido if the regimen was a continuous-combined one, rather than sequentially changing to mimic the natural female cycle.[508]

Study #5: The patch in postmenopausal women. In 2006, 433 women who had concerns about their low sexual desire completed a randomized, controlled trial of the 300 µg/d (microgram) testosterone patch. These women, with an average age of 54, were using various estrogen therapies and adding either a placebo or a testosterone patch for 24 weeks, changed twice a week. Results showed some clear, but again modest, benefits of testosterone added to estrogen regimens.[695] Dr. Dennerstein previously concluded that estrogen therapy that fails to elevate the blood levels of estrogen to those of young women will probably be too low for sexual adequacy. So these results make sense. The women all had lower levels of estrogen than fertile women do, at any time of the cycle. The testosterone in this circumstance was helpful.

What you should know: What none of the testosterone studies was designed to ask was whether merely elevating the estrogen levels would have achieved the same results.

This question is important because there are some serious unresolved issues about the long-term safety and risks of testosterone use.[694, 872] The testosterone patch studies do show dose-dependent effects, but their testosterone levels were *supra*physiological (above normal levels). No long-term studies have yet tested whether this will be harmful to women, and I would suggest extreme caution.

Keep your perspective. Chemical tests of the women ignore the sexual skills and behavior of the partnership.

What a High-Quality Sexual Life Requires: Knowing Yourselves Respectfully

Aging undoubtedly influences sexuality. So does surgery. But researchers have found that mutual respect for the other person's needs and wishes is key to a satisfying sexual life in every age group and becomes even more important as women age.[317]

A sensuous sex life requires self-knowledge and the unabashed ability to communicate your needs. For example, if a man moves to the rhythm of his own approach to orgasm and does not know that yours is different or changing, he may be well intended but may fail to engage you in the dance that leads to your orgasmic approach and release of tension.

The two key predictors of sexual satisfaction, according to research studies,[599] in the age group 40 to 60 are

- Whether a woman always experienced orgasm when she had intercourse
- Whether she enjoyed embracing her partner

If the answers to those two questions are "yes," the women were sexually satisfied. Unfortunately, according to other research of more than 400 presumably healthy women between 35 and 59 years of age, less than 20 percent experienced orgasm on all occasions of sexual intercourse. The incidence of experiencing an orgasm during every intercourse begins to decline from a peak of 38 percent of women in their late 30 (if their pelvic organs are intact) and drops to about 21 percent of women by ages 55 to 60.[321] I think it matters that women tell their partners what they need to experience orgasm. If you can experience orgasm every time he does, then you will be nourishing your intimate bond, securing its stability.

As estrogen levels decline with menopause or with surgical changes, both anatomy and physiology change. Some of these issues can be addressed with hormones, but not all. Sexual functioning in a woman is directly influenced by her feelings for the partner and by the partner's sexual problems.[204] Even so, by midlife, 40 percent of women have acknowledged that there had been a change in their sexual response in the last year.[492] Many of the changes are normal, not dysfunctional. But both Big Pharma and certain physician specialists have an economic incentive to apply the "dysfunctional" label to that change. As a discerning consumer, you need unbiased facts to choose what's best for you.

There are huge differences in findings between women who seek professional help for low sexual desire and those who answer "no problem" to questions about their sexuality. Women who have satisfying sex lives tend to report that their intimate lives improve with age; their satisfaction increases as they grow older in their relationships with partners they love. And their sexual satisfaction is dependent on their partners.[317] This is not surprising since it takes cooperation from, and communication with, your partner in order to recognize and fulfill each other's needs. There are two dancers, but just one dance.

Conclusion

Sex hormones are important for a good sex life. If your natural supply has "gone south," buy some if you want your sex life back. Obtain a prescription from a doctor with whom you establish a mutually respectful communication.

I believe that testosterone therapy added to estrogen could be helpful, but the need for titrating the dose of each hormone and checking the individual's reaction necessitates a reliable doctor-patient relationship.

Estradiol, rather than conjugated equine estrogen, used on a daily basis by a non-oral route, and testosterone taken sporadically as relevant, combined with sequential progesterone taken 10 to 14 days per month (described elsewhere) seem to me, hands down, the best way to optimize an individually titrated regimen.

A loving sexual dance has two performers. Warm sexual relations require trust, intimacy, comfort with each other's vulnerabilities, respect, communication, affection, and pleasure from sensual touching. A sense of humor too. And the needs of both people must be met.

Work at communicating your needs. Learn your partner's, if you are blessed to have one whom you love.

A Note to the Reader

I understand the enormous undertaking of your reading this book. This one is not for dummies. I hope that this book will provide you with an ongoing resource as you make key decisions about your life.

As you have seen, every system in which your mind and your body functions is critically influenced by the decisions you make: about health habits, hormonal therapies, surgical options, and your choice of medical professionals with whom to consult. Congratulations on engaging in this important work with me. I end, as I began, with the motto we have established at the Athena Institute for Women's Wellness:

> When a woman refuses to be treated with disrespect and conde-
> scension, she becomes empowered to evaluate options and make
> intelligent choices. By doing the work of learning about her body
> and improving her health habits, she is in a position to assert her
> power. Power begets dignity. Dignity is essential to well-being.

References

1. Abbott J, Hawe J, Hunter D, Holmes M, Finn P, Garry R (2004): Laparoscopic excision of endometriosis: A randomized, placebo-controlled trial. *Fertil Steril* 82:878–884.
2. Abdallah MA, Abdallah HI, Kang S, Taylor DD, Nakajima ST, Gercel-Taylor C (2007): Effects of the components of hormone therapy on matrix metalloproteinases in breast-cancer cells: An in vitro study. *Fertil Steril* 87:978–981.
3. Abramov Y, Borik S, Yahalom C, Fatum M, Avgil G, Brzezinski A, Banin E (2004): The effect of hormone therapy on the risk for age-related maculopathy in postmenopausal women. *Menopause* 11(1): 62–68.
4. ACOG Committee Opinion (2004): Uterine artery embolization. *Obstet Gynecol* 103(2):403–404.
5. Addis HB, Van Den Eeden SK, Wassel-Fyr CL, Vittinghoff E, Brown JS, Thom DH (2006): Sexual activity and function in middle-aged and older women. *Obstet Gynecol* 107:755–763.
6. Affinito P, Di Speiezio Sardo A, Di Carlo C, Sammartino A, Tommaselli GA, Bifulco G, Loffredo A, Loffredo M, Nappi C (2003): Effects of hormone replacement therapy on ocular function in postmenopause. *Menopause* 10(5): 482–487.
7. Aiello EJ, Yasui Y, Tworoger SS, Ulrich CM, Irwin ML, Bowen D, Schwartz RS, Kumai C, Potter JD, McTiernan A (2004): Effect of a yearlong, moderate-intensity exercise intervention on the occurrence and severity of menopause symptoms in postmenopausal women. *Menopause* 11:382–388.
8. al'Absi M, Wittmers LE (2003): Enhanced adrenocortical responses to stress in hypertension-prone men and women. *Ann Behav Med* 25(1):25–33.
9. Al-Fozan H, Tulandi T (2003): Left lateral predisposition of endometriosis and endometrioma. *Obstet Gyn* 101:164–166.
10. Al-Sunaidi M, Tulandi T (2006): Adhesion-related bowel obstruction after hysterectomy for benign conditions. *Obstet Gynecol* 108:1162–1166.
11. Albertazzi P (2003?): Letters to the editors: Effects of progestins on olfactory sensitivity and cognition. *Climacteric* 302–304.
12. Albertazzi P, Sharma S (2005): Urogenital effects of selective estrogen receptor modulators: A systematic review. *Climacteric* 8:214–220.
13. Albertazzi P, Steel SA, Howarth EM, Purdie DW (2005): Comparison of the effects of two different types of calcium supplementation on markers of bone metabolism in a postmenopausal osteopenic population with low calcium intake: A double-blind placebo-controlled trial. *Climacteric* 7:1:33–40.

14. Albright F, Smith PH, Richardson AM (1941): Postmenopausal osteoporosis–its clinical features. *JAMA* 116:2465–2473.
15. Albright TS, Garlich CL, Iglesia CB (2006): Complications after laparoscopic Burch with hernia mesh and surgical tacks. *Obstet Gynecol* 108:718–720.
16. Alexander JL, Kotz K, Dennerstein L, Kutner SJ, Wallen K, Notelovitz M (2004): The effects of postmenopausal hormone therapies on female sexual functioning: A review of double-blind, randomized controlled trials. *Menopause* 11(6):749–765.
17. Alexander NJ, Baker E, Kaptein M, Karck U, Miller L, Zampaglione E (2004): Why consider vaginal drug administration? *Fertil Steril* 82(1):1–12.
18. Allison M, Manson J (2006): Observational studies and clinical trials of menopausal hormone therapy: Can they both be right? *Menopause* 13:1–3.
19. Altgassen C, Michels W, Schneider A (2004): Learning laparoscopic-assisted hysterectomy. *Obstet & G* 104:308–313.
20. Amato P, Marcus DM (2003): Review of alternative therapies for treatment of menopausal symptoms. *Climacteric* 6:278–284.
21. Anderer P, Semlitsch HV, Saletu B, Saletu-Zyhlarz G, Gruber D, Metka M, Huber J, Graser T, Oettel M (2003): Effects of hormone replacement therapy on perceptual and cognitive event-related potentials in menopausal women. *Psychneuroendocrinology* 28:419–445.
22. Andreen L, Sundstrom-Poromaa I, Bixo M, Andersson A, Nyberg S, Backstrom T (2005): Relationship between allopregnanolone and negative mood in postmenopausal women taking sequential hormone replacement therapy with vaginal progesterone. *Psychneuroendocrinology* 30(2):212–224.
23. Archer DF (2006): Hormone therapy and breast cancer issues in counseling women. *Menopausal Medicine* 13:5–12.
24. Archer JS, Love-Geffen TE, Herbst-Damm KL, Swinney DA, Chang J (2006): NAMS Fellowship Findings: Effect of estradiol versus estradiol and testosterone on brain-activation patterns in postmenopausal women. *Menopause* 13(3): 528–537.
25. Armas LAG, Hollis BW, Heaney RP (2004): Vitamin D2 is much less effective than vitamin D3 in humans. *JCEM* 89:11:5387–5391.
26. Arteaga E, Rojas A, Villaseca P, Bianchi M (2000): The effect of 17b-estradiol and a-tocopherol on the oxidation of LDL cholesterol from postmenopausal women and the minor effect of g-tocopherol and melatonin. *Menopause* 7:112–116.
27. Arteaga E, Villaseca P, Rojas A, Marshall G, Bianchi M (2004): Phytoestrogens possess a weak antioxidant activity on low density lipoprotein in contrast to the flavonoid quercetin in vitro in postmenopausal women. *Climacteric* 7: 397–403.
28. Asbury E, Chandrruangphen P, Collins P (2006): The importance of continued exercise participation in quality of life and psychological well-being in previously inactive postmenopausal women: A pilot study. *Menopause* 13:561–567.
29. Asikainen T, Miilunpalo P, Oja M, Pasanen M, Vuori I (2002): Walking trials in postmenopausal women: Effect of one vs two daily bouts on aerobic fitness. *JCEMSc and J Med Sci Sports* 12:99–105.
30. Asplund R, Aberg HE (2003): Nightmares, cardiac symptoms and the menopause. *Climacteric* 6:314–320.
31. Asplund R, Aberg HE (2004): Nocturia in relationship to body mass index, smoking and some other life-style factors in women. *Climacteric* 7:267–273.

32. Atkinson C, Compston JE, Day NE, Dowsett M, Bingham SA (2004): The effects of phytoestrogen isoflavones on bone density in women: A double-blind, randomized, placebo-controlled trial. *Am J Clin* 79:326–333.

33. Atkinson C, Warren RML, Sala E, Dowsett M, Dunning AM, Healey CS, Runswick S, Day NE, Bingham SA (2004): Red clover-derived isoflavones and mammographic breast density: A double-blind, randomized, placebo-controlled trial. *Breast Can* 6:R170–R179.

34. Atsma F, Bartelink M-L EL, Grobbee DE, van der Schouw YT (2006): Postmenopausal status and early menopause as independent risk factors for cardiovascular disease: A meta-analysis. *Menopause* 13:265–279.

35. Attar E, Bulun SE (2006): Aromatase inhibitors: The next generation of therapeutics for endometriosis? *Fertil Steril* 85:1307–1318.

36. Aungst M, Wilson M, Vournas K, McCarthy S (2004): Necrotic leiomyoma and gram-negative sepsis eight weeks after uterine artery embolization. *Obstet Gynecol* 104 (5):1161–1164.

37. Avci D, Bachmann GA (2004): Osteoarthritis and osteoporosis in postmenopausal women: Clinical similarities and differences. *Menopause* 11:615–621.

38. Avis NE, Zhao X, Johannes CB, Ory M, Brockwell S, Greendale GA (2005): Correlates of sexual function among multi-ethnic middle-aged women: Results from the Study of Women's Health Across the Nation (SWAN). *Menopause* 12:385–398.

39. Aziz A, Brannstrom M, Bergquist C, Silfverstolpe G (2005): Perimenopausal androgen decline after oophorectomy does not influence sexuality or psychological well-being. *Fertil Steril* 83:1021–1028.

40. Bachmann, G (2006): Expanding treatment options for women with symptomatic uterine leiomyomas: Timely medical breakthroughs. *Fertil Steril* 85: 46–47.

41. Bachmann G, Bancroft J, Braunstein G, Burger H, Davis S, Dennerstein L, Goldstein I, Guay A, Leiblum S, Lobo R, Notelovitz M, Rosen R, Sarrel P, Sherwin B, Simon J, Simpson E, Shifren J, Spark R, Traish A (2002): Female androgen insufficiency: The Princeton consensus statement on definition, classification, and assessment. *Fertil Steril* 77:660–665.

42. Bagger YZ, Tanko LB, Alexandersen P, Qin G, Christiansen C (2005): Early postmenopausal hormone therapy may prevent cognitive impairment later in life. *Menopause* 12:12–17.

43. Bain C, Cooper KG, Parkin DE (2002): Microwave endometrial ablation versus endometrial resection: A randomized controlled trial. *Obstet Gynecol* 99 (6):983–992.

44. Bair YA, Gold EB, Azari RA, Greendale G, Sternfeld B, Harkey MR, Kravitz RL (2005): Use of conventional and complementary health care during the transition to menopause: Longitudinal results from the Study of Women's Health Across the Nation (SWAN). *Menopause* 12:31–39.

45. Ballard K, Lowton K, Wright J (2006): Balancing the risks and benefits of different diagnostic interventions for chronic pelvic pain. *Fertil Steril* 86:1317.

46. Ballard K, Lowton K, Wright J (2006): What's the delay? A qualitative study of women's experiences of reaching a diagnosis of endometriosis. *Fertil Steril* 86:1296–1301.

47. Banks E, Beral V, Cameron R, Hogg A, Langley N, Barnes I, Bull D, Reeves G, English R, Taylor S, Elliman J, Harris CL (2001): Comparison of various characteristics of

women who do and do not attend for breast cancer screening. *Breast Cancer Res* 4:R1.1–1.6.

48. Barber MD, Visco AG, Wyman JF, Fantl JA, Bump RC (2002): Sexual function in women with urinary incontinence and pelvic organ prolapse. *Obstet Gynecol* 99(2):281–289.

49. Barlow DH (2006): Editorial: What do we think about cognition and menopause? *Menopause* 13:4–5.

50. Barnes JF, Farish E, Rankin M, Hart DM (2005): Effects of two continuous hormone therapy regimens on C-reactive protein and homocysteine. *Menopause* 12:92–98.

51. Barr SI, Prior JC (1994): The menstrual cycle: Effects on bone in premenopausal women. *Advances in Nutritional Research* 287–310.

52. Barrett-Connor E, Kritz-Silverstein D (1993): Estrogen replacement therapy and cognitive function in older women. *JAMA* 269:2637–2641.

53. Barrett-Connor E, Laughlin GA (2005): Hormone therapy and coronary artery calcification in asymptomatic postmenopausal women: The Rancho Bernardo Study. *Menopause* 12(1):40–48.

54. Barrett-Connor E, Wehren LE, Siris ES, Miller P, Chen Y, Abbott TA, Berger ML, Santora AC, Sherwood LM (2003): Recency and duration of postmenopausal hormone therapy: Effects on bone mineral density and fracture risk in the National Osteoporosis Risk Assessment (NORA): Study. *Menopause* 10: 412–419.

55. Basson R (2000): The female sexual response: A different model. *J Sex & Marital Therapy* 26:51–65.

56. Basson R (2001): Female sexual response: The role of drugs in the management of sexual dysfunction. *Obstet Gynecol* 98:350–353.

57. Basson R (2004): Introduction to special issue on women's sexuality and outline of assessment of sexual problems. *Menopause* 11(6):709–713.

58. Basson R (2004): Recent advances in women's sexual function and dysfunction. *Menopause* 11:714–725.

59. Basson R, Nachtigall LE, Leiblum SR, Heiman JR (2005): Clinicians' Forum. *Menopause* 14:25–27.

60. Baumann L (2005): A dermatologist's opinion on hormone therapy and skin aging. *Fertil Steril* 84:289–290.

61. Bazi T, Abi Nader K, Seoud MA, Charafeddine M, Rechdan JB, Zreik TG (2007): Lateral distribution of endometriomas as a function of age. *Fertil Steril* 87: 419–421.

62. Beach FA (1976): Sexual attractivity, proceptivity, and receptivity in female mammals. *Hormones & Behavior* 7:105–138.

63. Beljic T, Babic T, Babic D, Knezevic N, Drezgic M (2004): Effect of hormone replacement therapy on lipids and left ventricular function in postmenopausal smokers. *Climacteric* 7:366–374.

64. Bell DR, Gochenaur KE, Hecht J (2002): O2(-)-mediated impairment of coronary arterial relaxation is prevented by overnight treatment with 1 nM beta-estradiol. *J Appl Physiol* 93(6):1952–1958.

65. Bell RJ, Donath S, Davison SL, Davis SR (2006): Endogenous androgen levels and well-being: Differences between premenopausal and postmenopausal women. *Menopause* 13:65–71.

66. Benard VB, Eheman CR, Lawson HW, Blackman DK, Anderson C, Helsel W, Thames SF, Lee NC (2004): Cervical screening in the National Breast and Cervical Cancer Early Detection Program, 1995–2001. *Obstet & Gyn* 103:564–570.
67. Beral V (2003): Breast cancer and hormone-replacement therapy in the Million Women Study. *Lancet* 362(9382):419–427.
68. Beral V, Bull D, Doll R, Key T, Peto R, Reeves G (1997): Breast cancer and hormone replacement therapy: Collaborative reanalysis of data from 51 epidemiological studies of 52,705 women with breast cancer and 108,411 women without breast cancer. *Lancet* 350:1047–1059.
69. Berg GA, Siseles N, Gonzalez AI, Ortiz OC, Tempone A, Wikinski RW (2001): Higher values of hepatic lipase activity in postmenopause: Relationship with atherogenic intermediate density and low density lipoproteins. *Menopause* 8:51–57.
70. Berman JR, Berman L, Goldstein I (1999): Female sexual dysfunction: Incidence, pathophysiology, evaluation, and treatment options. *Urology* 54:385–391.
71. Berman L, Berman J, Felder S, Pollets D, Chhabra S, Miles M, Powell JA (2003): Seeking help for sexual function complaints: What gynecologists need to know about the female patient's experience. *Fertil Steril* 79(3):572–576.
72. Bernini GP, Moretti A, Sgro M, Argenio GF, Barlascini CO, Cristofani R, Salvetti A (2001): Influence of endogenous androgens on carotid wall in postmenopausal women. *Menopause* 8:43–50.
73. Bethea CL, Mirkes SJ, Su A, Michelson D (2002): Effects of oral estrogen, raloxifene and arzoxifene on gene expression in serotonin neurons in macaques. *Psychneuroendocrinology* 27:431–445.
74. Bilezikian JP(2005): PTH in clinical practice. *Suppl to Menopause Management* 7:22–24.
75. Birkhaeuser M (2005): Invited editorial: The Women's Health Initiative conundrum. *Arch Women* 8:7–14.
76. Birnbaum GE (2003): The meaning of heterosexual intercourse among women with female orgasmic disorder. *Arch Sexual Behavior* 32(1):61–71.
77. Bischoff HA, Stahelin HB, Dick W, Akos R, Knecht M, Salis C, Nebiker M, Theiler R, Pfeifer M, Begerow B, Lew RA, Conzelmann M (2003): Effects of vitamin D and calcium supplementation on falls: A randomized controlled trial. *J Bone Min* 18:2:343–351.
78. Bischoff-Ferrari HA, Dietrich T, Orav EJ, Hu FB, Zhang Y, Karlson EW, Dawson-Hughes B (2004): Higher 25-hydroxyvitamin D concentrations are associated with better lower-extremity function in both active and inactive persons aged ≥ 60 y. *Am J Clin Nutr* 80:3:752–758.
79. Bjarnason NH, Jorgensen C, Kremmer H, Alexanderson P, Christiansen C (2004): Smoking reduces breast tenderness during oral estrogen-progestogen therapy. *Climacteric* 7:390–396.
80. Bladbjerg EM, Skouby SO, Andersen LF, Jespersen J (2002): Effects of different progestin regimens in hormone replacement therapy on blood coagulation factor VII and tissue factor pathway inhibitor. *Human Reproduction* 17(12):3235–3241.
81. Blandau RJ, Moghissi K (1973): *The Biology of the Cervix*. Chicago: University of Chicago Press, 1–450.
82. Blumel JE, Castelo-Branco C, Binfa L, Gramegna G, Tacla X, Aracena B, Cumsille MA, Sanjuan A (2000): Quality of life after menopause: A population study. *Maturitas* 34:17–23.

83. Blumel JE, Castelo-Branco C, Cancelo MJ, Romero H, Aprikian D, Sarra S (2004): Impairment of sexual activity in middle-aged women in Chile. *Menopause* 11:78–81.
84. Blumenfeld Z (2004): Hormonal suppressive therapy for endometriosis may not improve patient health. *Fertil Steril* 81(3):487–504.
85. Boccardi M, Ghidoni R, Govoni S, Testa C, Benussi L, Bonetti M, Binetti G, Frisoni GB (2006): Effects of hormone therapy on brain morphology of healthy postmenopausal women: A Voxel-based morphometry study. *Menopause* 13:584–592.
86. Boothby LA, Doering PL, Kipersztok S (2004): Bioidentical hormone therapy: A review. *Menopause* 11(3):356–367.
87. Boudreaux-Nippert DJ, Norton PA, Sharp HT, Peltier MA (2006): Tension-free vaginal tape: Complications reported in the manufacturers and users' device experience database. *Obstet Gynecol* 107:(4):10S.
88. Bourdrez P, Bongers MY, Mol BWJ (2004): Treatment of dysfunctional uterine bleeding: Patient preferences for endometrial ablation, a levonorgestrel-releasing intrauterine device, or hysterectomy. *Fertil Steril* 82(1):160–166.
89. Bouxsein ML, Kaufman J, Tosi L, Cummings S, Lane J, Johnell O (2004): Recommendations for optimal care of the fragility fracture patient to reduce the risk of future fracture. *J Am Acad Orthop Surg* 12:6:385–395.
90. Boyd NF, Byng JW, Jong RA, Fishell EK, Little LE, Miller AB, Lockwood GA, Tritchler DL, Yaffe MJ (1995): Quantitative classification of mammographic densities and breast cancer risk: Results from the Canadian National Breast Screening Study. *J Natl Cancer Inst* 87(9):670–675.
91. Boyle WJ, Simonet S, Lacey DL (2003): Osteoclast differentiation and activation. *Nature* 423:337–342.
92. Bradley CS, Zimmerman MB, Qi Y, Nygaard IE (2007): Natural history of pelvic organ prolapse in postmenopausal women. *Obstetrics & Gynecology* 109: 848–854.
93. Braendle, W (2003): The Million Women Study, an additional observational study with the implications and limits of an observational study. *Maturitas* 46:101–102.
94. Breen KJ (2003): Ethical issues in the use of complementary medicines. *Climacteric* 6:268–272.
95. Brincat M, Galea R, Baron YM, Xuereb A (1997): Changes in bone collagen markers and in bone density in hormone treated and untreated postmenopausal women. *Maturitas* 27:171–177.
96. Brincat MP, Baron YM, Galea R (2005): Estrogens and the skin. *Climacteric* 8:110–123.
97. Broder MS, Goodwin S, Chen G, Tang LJ, Constantino MM, Nguyen MH, Yegul TN, Erberich H (2002): Comparison of long-term outcomes of myomectomy and uterine artery embolization. *Obstet Gynecol* 100(5):864–868.
98. Brown L, Rosner B, Willett WW, Sacks FM (1999): Cholesterol-lowering effects of dietary fiber: A meta-analysis. *Am J Clin* 69:30–42.
99. Bruyere O, Pavelka K, Rovati LC, Deroisy R, Olejarova M, Gatterova J, Giacovelli G, Reginster JY (2004): Glucosamine sulfate reduces osteoarthritis progression in postmenopausal women with knee osteoarthritis: Evidence from two 3-year studies. *Menopause* 11:138–143.

100. Brzezinski A, Danenberg HA (2005): Editorial: Estrogen, progesterone, and cardiovascular health: When shall we complete the puzzle? *Menopause* 12:488–491.
101. Buchsbaum GM, Duecy EE, Kerr LA, Huang LS, Guzick DS (2005): Urinary incontinence in nulliparous women and their parous sisters. *Obstet Gynecol* 106:1235–1258.
102. Buist DSM, Newton KM, Miglioretti DL, Beverly K, Connelly MT, Andrade S, Hartsfield CL, Wei F, Chan A, Kessler L (2004): Hormone therapy prescribing patterns in the United States. *Obstet Gyn* 104(5):1042–1050.
103. Burger HG (2007): Should testosterone be added to estrogen-progestin therapy for breast protection? *Menopause* 14:159–162.
104. Burger HG, Robertson DM, Baksheev L, Collins A, Csemiczky G, Landgren B (2005): The relationship between the endocrine characteristics and the regularity of menstrual cycles in the approach to menopause. *Menopause* 12:267–274.
105. Burgio KL, Goode PS, Locher JL, Richter HE, Roth DL, Wright KC, Varner RE (2003): Predictors of outcome in the behavioral treatment of urinary incontinence in women. *Obstet Gynecol* 102:940–947.
106. Burrows LJ, Meyn LA, Walters MD, Weber AM (2004): Pelvic symptoms in women with pelvic organ prolapse. *Obstet Gynecol* 104(5):982–87.
107. Bush TL, Whiteman M, Flaws JA (2001): Hormone replacement therapy and breast cancer: A qualitative review. *Obstet Gynecol* 98(3):498–508.
108. Buster JE, Kingsberg SA, Aguirre O, Brown C, Breaux J, Buch A, Rodenberg CA, Wekselman K, Casson P (2005): Testosterone patch for low sexual desire in surgically menopausal women: A randomized trial. *Obstet Gyn* 105:944–952.
109. Cagnacci A, Tonie AD, Caretto S, Menozzi R, Bondi M, Corradini B, Alessandrini C, Volpe A (2006): Cyclic progestin administration increases energy expenditure and decreases body fat mass in perimenopausal women. *Menopause* 13:197–201.
110. Cagnacci A, Zanni AL, Alessandrini C, Caretti S, Volpe A (2004): Comparison of the effect of oral and transdermal hormone therapy on fasting and postmethionine homocysteine levels. *Fertil Steril* 81:99–103.
111. Cameron DR, Braunstein GD (2004): Androgen replacement therapy in women. *Fertil Steril* 82(2):273–289.
112. Canonico M, Oger E, Plu-Bureau G, Conard J, Meyer G, Levesque H, Trillot N, Barrellier M, Wahl D, Emmerich J, Scarabin P (2007): Hormone therapy and venous thromboembolism among postmenopausal women. Impact of the route of estrogen administration and progestogens: The ESTHER study. *Circulation* 115:840–845.
113. Carlson KJ, Miller BA, Fowler FJ (1994): The Maine women's health study: 1. Outcomes of hysterectomy. *Obstet Gynecol* 83:556–565.
114. Carlson LE, Speca M, Patel KD, Goodey E (2003): Mindfulness-based stress reduction in relation to quality of life, mood, symptoms of stress and levels of cortisol, dehydroepiandrosterone sulfate (DHEAS), and melatonin in breast and prostate cancer outpatients. *Psychoneur* 29:448–474.
115. Carmody J, Crawford S, Churchill L (2006): A pilot study of mindfulness-based stress reduction for hot flashes. *Menopause* 13:760–769.
116. Carpenter JS, Gilchrist JM, Chen K, Gautam S, Freedman RR (2004): Hot flashes, core body temperature, and metabolic parameters in breast cancer survivors. *Menopause* 11:375–381.

117. Caruso S, Maiolino L, Agnello C, Garozzo A, Di Mari L, Serra A (2003): Effects of patch or gel estrogen therapies on auditory brainstem response in surgically postmenopausal women: A prospective, randomized study. *Fertil Steril* 79(3):556–561.

118. Caruso S, Roccasalva L, Di Fazio E, Sapienza G, Agnello C, Ficarra S, Di Mari L, Serra A (2003): Cytologic aspects of the nasal respiratory epithelium in postmenopausal women treated with hormone therapy. *Fertil Steril* 79:543–549.

119. Caruso S, Roccasalva L, Sapienza G, Zappala M, Nuciforo G, Biondi S (2000): Laryngeal cytological aspects in women with surgically induced menopause who were treated with transdermal estrogen replacement therapy. *Fertil Steril* 74 (6):1073–1079.

120. Casini ML, Marelli G, Papaleo E, Ferrari A, D'Ambrosio F, Unfer V (2006): Psychological assessment of the effects of treatment with phytoestrogens on postmenopausal women: A randomized, double-blind, crossover, placebo-controlled study. *Fertil Steril* 85:972–978.

121. Castelo-Branco C, Peralta S, Ferrer J, Palacios S, Cornago S, Quereda F (2006): The dilemma of menopause and hormone replacement—a challenge for women and health-care providers: Knowledge of menopause and hormone therapy in Spanish menopausal women. *Climacteric* 9:380–387.

122. Castelo-Branco C, Pons F, Gonzalez-Merlo J (1993): Bone mineral density in surgically postmenopausal women receiving hormone replacement therapy as assessed by dual photon absorptiometry. *Maturitas* 16:133–137.

123. Catherino WH, Segars JH (2003): Microarray analysis in fibroids: Which gene list is the correct list? *Fertil Steril* 80(2):293–294.

124. Cermik D, Arici A, Taylor HS (2002): Coordinated regulation of HOX gene expression in myometrium and uterine leiomyoma. *Fertil Steril* 78(5):979–984.

125. Chalas E, Costantino JP, Wickerham DL, Wolmark N, Lewis GC, Bergman C, et al. (2005): Tamoxifen and benign gynecologic conditions. *Am J Obst* 192: 1230–1237.

126. Chalmers C, Lindsay M, Usher D, Warner P, Evans D, Ferguson M (2002): Hysterectomy and ovarian function: Levels of follicle stimulating hormone and incidence of menopausal symptoms are not affected by hysterectomy in women under 45 years. *Climacteric* 5:366–373.

127. Chan JK, Cheung MK, Husain A, Teng NN, West D, Whittemore AS, Berek JS, Osann K (2006): Patterns and progress in ovarian cancer over 14 years. *Obstet Gynecol* 108:521–528.

128. Chan LY, Yuen PM (2004): Influence of the Women's Health Initiative trial on the practice of prophylactic oophorectomy and the prescription of estrogen therapy. *Fertil Steril* 81(6): 1699–1700.

129. Chang CJ, Chiu JH, Tseng LM, Chang CH, Chien TM, Chen CC, Wu CW, Lui WY (2006): Si-Wu-Tang and its constituents promote mammary duct cell proliferation by up-regulation of HER-2 signaling. *Menopause* 13:967–976.

130. Chang WC, Huang SC, Sheu BC, Chen CL, Torng PL, Hsu WC, Chang DY (2005): Transvaginal hysterectomy or laparoscopically assisted vaginal hysterectomy for nonprolapsed uteri. *Obstet Gyn* 106:321–326.

131. Chao HT, Kuo CD, Su YJ, Chuang SS, Fang YJ, Ho LT (2005): Short-term effect of transdermal estrogen on autonomic nervous modulation in postmenopausal women. *Fertil Steril* 84:1477–1483.

132. Chapuy MC, Arlot ME, Duboeufs F, Burn J, Crouzet B, Arnaud S, Delmas PD, Meunier PJ (1992): Vitamin D3 and calcium to prevent hip fractures in elderly women. *NEJM* 327:1637–1642.

133. Chataigneau T, Zerr M, Chataigneau M, Hudlett F, Hirn C, Pernot F, Schini-Kerth VB (2004): Chronic treatment with progesterone but not medroxyprogesterone acetate restores the endothelial control of vascular tone in the mesenteric artery of ovariectomized rats. *Menopause* 11(3):255–263.

134. Chen CL, Weiss NS, Newcomb P, Barlow W, White E (2002): Hormone replacement therapy in relation to breast cancer. *JAMA* 287:734–741.

135. This reference was removed at author's request.

136. Chen WY, Manson JE, Hankinson SE, Rosner B, Holmes MD, Willett WC, Colditz GA (2006): Unopposed estrogen therapy and the risk of invasive breast cancer. *Arch Intern Med* 166:1027–1032.

137. Chen Y, Ho SC, Lam SSH, Ho SSS, Woo JLF (2004): Beneficial effect of soy isoflavones on bone mineral content was modified by years since menopause, body weight, and calcium intake: A double-blind, randomized, controlled trial. *Menopause* 11(3):246–254.

138. Cherrier MM, Plymate S, Mohan S, Asthana S, Matsumoto AM, Bremner W, Peskind E, Raskind M, Latendresse S, Haley AP, Craft S (2004): Relationship between testosterone supplementation and insulin-like growth factor-I levels and cognition in healthy older men. *Psychneuroendocrinology* 29:65–82.

139. Chiantera V, Sarti CD, Fornaro F, Farzati A, De Franciscis P, Sepe E, Borrelli AL, Colacurci N (2003): Long-term effects of oral and transdermal hormone replacement therapy on plasma homocysteine levels. *Menopause* 10(4): 286–291.

140. Chlebowski RT, Col N (2004): Menopausal hormone therapy after breast cancer. *Lancet* 363:9407:410–411.

141. Cho E, Seddon JM, Rosner B, Willett WC, Hankinson SE (2004): Prospective study of intake of fruits, vegetables, vitamins, and carotenoids and risk of age-related maculopathy. *Arch Ophth* 122:883–892.

142. Cho E, Spiegelman D, Hunter DJ, Chen WY, Stampfer MJ, Colditz GA, Willett WC (2003): Premenopausal fat intake and risk of breast cancer. *J Natl Cancer Inst* 95(14):1079–1085.

143. Clarke RB (2004): Human breast cell proliferation and its relationship to steroid receptor expression. *Climacteric* 7:129–137.

144. Clarke SC, Kelleher J, Lloyd-Jones H, Slack M, Schofield PM (2002): A study of hormone replacement therapy in postmenopausal women with ischaemic heart disease: The Papworth HRT Atherosclerosis Study. *Climacteric* 109:1056–1062.

145. Clarkson T (2006): Estrogen effects on arteries vary with stage of reproductive life and extent of subclinical atherosclerosis progression. (Abstract of keynote address NAMS 2006). *Menopause* 13:981.

146. Clarkson TB (2002): Stage of atherogenesis and effectiveness of ERT/HRT. *Menopause* 9:466.

147. Clarkson TB (2007): Estrogen effects on arteries vary with stage of reproductive life and extent of subclinical atherosclerosis progression. *Menopause* 14: 373–384.

148. Clement U (2002): Sex in long-term relationships: A systemic approach to sexual desire problems. *Arch Sexual Behavior* 31(3):241–246.

149. Cohen SM, O'Connor AM, Hart J, Merel NH, Te HS (2004): Autoimmune hepatitis associated with the use of black cohosh: A case study. *Menopause* 11: 575–577.

150. Colacurci N, Chiantera A, Fornaro F, de Novellis V, Manzella D, Arciello A, Chiantera V, Improta L, Paolisso G (2005): Effects of soy isoflavones on endothelial function in healthy postmenopausal women. *Menopause* 12:299–307.

151. Colditz GA, Hankinson SE, Hunter DJ, Willett WC, Manson JE, Stampfer MJ, Hennekens C, Rosner B, Speizer FE (1995): The use of estrogens and progestins and the risk of breast cancer in postmenopausal women. *NEJM* 332:1589–1593.

152. Compton J, Murphy D (2003): Editorial: Imaging the brain in healthy postmenopausal users and non-users of hormone replacement therapy. *Climacteric* 6:180–183.

153. Conner P, Svane G, Azavedo E, Soderqvist G, Carlstrom K, Graser T, Walter F, von Schoultz B (2004): Mammographic breast density, hormones, and growth factors during continuous combined hormone therapy. *Fertil Steril* 81(6): 1617–1623.

154. Coombs NJ, Taylor R, Wilcken N, Boyages J (2005): Hormone replacement therapy and breast cancer: Estimate of risk. *BMJ* 331:347–349.

155. Corbo RM, Scacchi R, Cresta M (2004): Differential reproductive efficiency associated with common apolipoprotein E alleles in postreproductive-aged subjects. *Fertil Steril* 81(1):104–107.

156. Cortes E, Reid WMN, Singh K, Berger L (2004): Clinical examination and dynamic magnetic resonance imaging in vaginal vault prolapse. *Obstet Gynecol* 103 (1):41–46.

157. Cottier C, Shapiro K, Julius S (1984): Treatment of mild hypertension with progressive muscle relaxation. *Arch Inter* 177:1954–1958.

158. Coyne JC, Stefanek M, Palmer SC (2007): Psychotherapy and survival in cancer: The conflict between hope and evidence. *Psychological Bulletin* 133:367–394.

159. Craig MC, Cutter WJ, Wickham H, van Amelsvoort TAMJ, Rymer J, Whitehead M, Murphy DGM (2004): Effect of long-term estrogen therapy on dopaminergic responsivity in post-menopausal women—a preliminary study. *Psychoneur* 29:1309–1316.

160. Crandall C, Palla S, Reboussin B, Hu P, Barrett-Connor E, Reuben D, Greendale G (2006): Cross-sectional association between markers of inflammation and serum sex steroid levels in the postmenopausal estrogen/progestin interventions trial. *Journal of Women's Health* 15:14–23.

161. Crisafulli A, Altavilla D, Marini H, Bitto A, Cucinotta D, Frisina N, Corrado F, D'Anna R, Squadrito G, Adamo E, Marini R, Romeo A, Cancellieri F, Buemi M, Squadrito F (2005): Effects of the phytoestrogen genistein on cardiovascular risk factors in postmenopausal women. *Menopause* 12:186–192.

162. Crisafulli A, Marini H, Bitto A, Altavilla D, Squadrito G, Romeo A, Adamo EB, Marini R, D'Anna R, Corrado F, Bartolone S, Frisina N, Squadrito F (2004): Effects of genistein on hot flashes in early postmenopausal women: A randomized, double-blind EPT- and placebo-controlled study. *Menopause* 11: 400–404.

163. Cucinelli F, Soranna L, Perri C, Romualdi D, Barini A, Mancuso S, Lanzone A (2002): Naloxone decreases insulin secretion in hyperinsulinemic postmenopausal women and may positively affect hormone replacement therapy. *Fertil Steril* 78:1017–1024.

164. Cummings SR, Black DM, Nevitt MC, Genant HK, Mascioli SR, Scott JC, See-ley DG, Steiger P, et al. (1990): Appendicular bone density and age predict hip fracture in women. The Study of Osteoporotic Fractures Research Group. *JAMA* 263:665–668.

165. Cundiff GW, Fenner D (2004): Evaluation and treatment of women with rec-tocele: Focus on associated defecatory and sexual dysfunction. *Obstet Gynecol* 104:1403–1421.

166. Curb JD, Prentice RL, Bray PF, Langer RD, Van Horn L, Barnabei VM, Bloch MJ, Cyr MG, Gass M, Lepine L, Rodabough RJ, Sidney S, Uwaifo GI, Rosendaal FR (2006): Venous thrombosis and conjugated equine estrogen in women without a uterus. *Arch Inter* 166:772–780.

167. Curcio JJ, Smolinski D, Dye J (2005): Letters to the Editor. *Menopause* 12:12: 774–775.

168. Cutler WB (1990): *Hysterectomy: Before and After*. New York: HarperPerennial.

169. Cutler WB (1991): *Love Cycles: The Science of Intimacy*. Random House/Villard: New York: Athena Institute Press.

170. Cutler WB (1996): Oophorectomy at hysterectomy after age 40? A practice that does not withstand scrutiny. *Menopause* 5:10–14.

171. Cutler WB, Garcia CR (1992): *Menopause: A Guide for Women and the Men Who Love Them—Revised and Expanded*. W W Norton: August 1993.

172. Cutler WB, Friedmann E, Felmet K (1993): Kyphosis in a healthy sample of pre and post menopausal women. *Am J Phys Med Rehab* 72:219–225.

173. Cutler WB, Genovese-Stone E (1998): Wellness in women after 40 years of age: The role of sex hormones and pheromones. *Disease-a-Month* 44:421–548.

174. Cutler WB, Genovese-Stone E (2000): Wellness in women after 40 years of age: The role of sex hormones and pheromones: Part I. The sex hormones, adre-nal sex hormones and pheromonal modulation of brain and behavior. *Current Problems in Obstetrics, Gynecology and Fertility* 23:1–32.

175. Cutler WB, Genovese-Stone E (2000): Wellness in women after 40 years of age: The role of sex hormones and pheromones: Part II. Hormone replacement therapy; Part III. Hysterectomy. *Current Problems in Obstetrics, Gynecology and Fertility* 23:33–88.

176. Cutler WB, Karp J, Stine R (1988): Single photon absorptiometry imaging as a screen for diminished dual photon density measures. *Maturitas* 10:143–155.

177. Cutler WB, McCoy NL, Friedmann E, Genovese-Stone E, Zacher MJ (2000): Sexual response in women. *Obstet Gynecol* 95:2000, 19S.

178. Cutler WB, McCoy NL, Friedmann E, Genovese-Stone E, Zacher MJ (2001): The impact of hysterectomy on the sexual life of women. *Obstet Gynec* 97:April 2001:23S.

179. Dalais FS, Rice GE, Wahlqvist ML, Grehan M, Murkies AL, Medley G, Ayton R, Strauss BJG (1998): Effects of dietary phytoestrogens in postmenopausal women. *Climacteric* 1:124–129.

180. Daley A, MacArthur C, McManus R, Stokes-Lampard H, Wilson S, Roalfe A, Mutrie N (2006): Factors associated with the use of complementary medicine and non-pharmacological interventions in symptomatic menopausal women. *Climacteric* 9:336–346.

181. Daling JR, Malone KE, Doody DR, Voigt LF, Bernstein L, Coates RJ, Marchbanks PA, Norman SA, Weiss LK, Ursin G, Berlin JA, Burkman RT, Deapen D, Folger SG, McDonald JA, Simon MS, Strom BL, Wingo PA, Spirtas R (2002):

Relation of regimens of combined hormone replacement therapy to lobular, ductal, and other histologic types of breast carcinoma. *Cancer* 92:2455–2464.

182. Daling JR, Malone KE, Doody DR, Voigt LF, Bernstein L, Marchbanks PA, Coates RJ, Norman SA, Weiss LK, Ursin G, Burkman RT, Deapen D, Folger SG, McDonald JA, Simon MS, Strom BL, Spirtas R (2003): Association of regimens of hormone replacement therapy to prognostic factors among women diagnosed with breast cancer aged 50–64 years. *Cancer Epidemiology, Biomarkers and Prevention* 12:1175–1181.

183. Danesh MB, Wheeler JG, Hirschfield GM, Eda S, Eiriksdottir G, Rumley A, Lowe GDO, Pepys MB, Gudnason V (2004): C-reactive protein and other circulating markers of inflammation in the prediction of coronary heart disease. *NEJM* 350:1387–1397.

184. Danforth KN, Shah AD, Townsend MK, Lifford KL, Curhan GC, Resnick NM, Grodstein F (2007): Physical activity and urinary incontinence among healthy, older women. *Obstet Gynecol* 109:721–727.

185. Davis SR (2005): Editorial: Determining the effects of androgen therapy on sexual well-being: A complex challenge. *Menopause* 12(4):359–360.

186. Davis SR, Goldstat R, Newman A, Berry K, Burger HG, Meredith I, Koch K (2002): Differing effects of low-dose estrogen-progestin therapy and pravastatin in postmenopausal hypercholesterolemic women. *Climacteric* 5:341–350.

187. Davis SR, McCloud P, Strauss BJG, Burger H (1995): Testosterone enhances estradiol's effects on postmenopausal bone density and sexuality. *Maturitas* 21:227–236.

188. Davis SR, van der Mooren MJ, van Lunsen RHW, Lopes P, Ribot J, Rees M, Moufarege A, Rodenberg C, Buch A, Purdie DW (2006): Efficacy and safety of a testosterone patch for the treatment of hypoactive sexual desire disorder in surgically menopausal women: A randomized, placebo-controlled trial. *Menopause* 13(3):387–396.

189. Davison S, Davis SR (2003): New markers for cardiovascular disease risk in women: Impact of endogenous estrogen status and exogenous postmenopausal hormone therapy. *J Clin End* 88:2470–2478.

190. Davy M, Oehler MK (2006): Controversial issues: Invited commentary. Does retention of the ovaries improve long-term survival after hysterectomy? A gynecological oncological perspective. *Climacteric* 9:167–169.

191. Dawson-Hughes B, Harris SS, Krall EA, Dallal GE (1997): Effect of calcium and vitamin D supplementation on bone density in men and women 65 years of age or older. *NEJM* 337:10:670–676.

192. De Lignieres B (2002): Editorial: Effects of progesterone on the postmenopausal breast. *Climacteric* 5:229–235.

193. De Lignieres B, de Vathaire F, Fournier S, Urbinelli R, Allaert F, Le MG, Kuttenn F (2002): Combined hormone replacement therapy and risk of breast cancer in a French cohort study of 3175 women. *Climacteric* 5:332–340.

194. De Wit H, Schmitt L, Purdy R, Hauger R (2001): Effects of acute progesterone administration in healthy postmenopausal women and normally-cycling women. *Psychneuroendocrinology* 26:697–710.

195. DeCherney AH, Bachmann G, Isaacson K, Gall S (2002): Postoperative fatigue negatively impacts the daily lives of patients recovering from hysterectomy. *Obstet Gynecol* 99(1):51–57.

196. Decker DA, Pettinga JE, Cox TC, Burdakin JH, Jaiyesimi IA (1997): Hormone replacement therapy in breast cancer survivors. *Breast* 3(2):63–68.
197. Decker DA, Pettinga JE, Vander Velde N, Huang RR, Kestin L, Burdakin JH (2003): Estrogen replacement therapy in breast cancer survivors: A matched-controlled series. *Menopause* 10(4):277–285.
198. DeLancey JOL, Kearney R, Chou Q, Speights S, Binno S (2003): The appearance of levator ani muscle abnormalities in magnetic resonance images after vaginal delivery. *Obstet Gynecol* 101(1):46–53.
199. Delmas PD (2005): Bone mineral density versus bone quality. *Menopause Management* 14:15–17.
200. Dennerstein L, Dudley E, Burger H (2001): Are changes in sexual functioning during midlife due to aging or menopause? *Fertil Steril* 76(3):456–460.
201. Dennerstein L, Guthrie JR, Clark M, Lehert P, Henderson VW (2004): A population-based study of depressed mood in middle-aged, Australian-born women. *Menopause* 11(5):563–568.
202. Dennerstein L, Lehert P (2004): Women's sexual functioning, lifestyle, mid-age, and menopause in 12 European countries. *Menopause* 11(6):778–785.
203. Dennerstein L, Lehert P, Burger H (2005): The relative effects of hormones and relationship factors on sexual function of women through the natural menopausal transition. *Fertil Steril* 84:174–180.
204. Dennerstein L, Lehert P, Burger H, Dudley E (1999): Factors affecting sexual functioning of women in the mid-life years. *Climacteric* 2:254–262.
205. Dessole S, Rubattu G, Ambrosini G, Gallo O, Capobianco G, Cherchi PL, Marci R, Cosmi E (2004): Efficacy of low-dose intravaginal estriol on urogenital aging in postmenopausal women. *Menopause* 11(1):49–56.
206. Detillion CE, Craft TKS, Glasper ER, Prendergast BJ, DeVries AC (2004): Social facilitation of wound healing. *Psychoneur* 29:1004–1011.
207. Dew JE, Wren BG, Eden JA (2003): A cohort study of topical vaginal estrogen therapy in women previously treated for breast cancer. *Climacteric* 6:45–52.
208. DeWaay DJ, Syrop CH, Nygaard IE, Davis WA, Van Voorhis BJ (2002): Natural history of uterine polyps and leiomyomata. *Obstet Gynecol* 100(1):3–17.
209. Dewell A, Hollenbeck CB (2003): Soy and isoflavones: A review of the potential role of phytoestrogens in the management of hypercholesterolemia. *Menopause* 12:10–14.
210. Deyhim F, Stoecker BJ, Brusewitz GH, Devareddy L, Arjmandi BH (2005): Dried plum reverses bone loss in an osteopenic rat model of osteoporosis. *Menopause* 12:755–762.
211. Di Carlo C, Sammartino A, Di Spiezio Sardo A, Tommaselli GA, Guida M, Mandato VD, D'Elia A, Nappi C (2005): Bleeding patterns during continuous estradiol with different sequential progestogens therapy. *Menopause* 12:520–525.
212. Dietz DM, Stahlfeld KR, Bansal SK, Christopherson WA (2004): Buttock necrosis after uterine artery embolization. *Obstet Gynecol* 104(5).
213. Dimitrakakis C, Jones RA, Liu A, Bondy CA (2004): Breast cancer incidence in postmenopausal women using testosterone in addition to usual hormone therapy. *Menopause* 11(5):531–535.
214. Dimitrakakis C, Zhou J, Wang J, Belanger A, LaBrie F, Cheng C, Powell D, Bondy C (2003): A physiologic role for testosterone in limiting estrogenic stimulation of the breast. *Menopause* 10(4):292–298.

215. Dog TL, Powell KL, Weisman SM (2003): Critical evaluation of the safety of Cimicifuga racemosa in menopause symptom relief. *Menopause* 10:299–313.
216. Domoney C, Studd WW, Mocroft A (2003): Continuation of hormone replacement therapy after hysterectomy. *Climacteric* 6:58–66.
217. Dorgan JF, Stanczyk FZ, Longcope C, Stephenson Jr HE, Chang L, Miller R, Franz C, Falk RT, Kahle L (1997): Relationship of serum dehydroepiandrosterone (DHEA), DHEA sulfate, and 5-androstene-3 b 17 beta-diol to risk of breast cancer in postmenopausal women. *Cancer Epidemiology, Biomarkers and Prevention* 6:177–181.
218. Draelos ZD (2005): Topical and oral estrogens revisited for antiaging purposes. *Fertil Steril* 84:291–292.
219. Druckmann R (2003): Progestins and their effects on the breast. *Maturitas* 46:59–69.
220. Dunkin J, Rasgon N, Wagner-Steh K, David S, Altshuler L, Rapkin A (2005): Reproductive events modify the effects of estrogen replacement therapy on cognition in healthy postmenopausal women. *Psychneuroendocrinology* 30:284–296.
221. Durant LE, Carey MP (2000): Self-administered questionnaires versus face-to-face interviews in assessing sexual behavior in young women. *Arch Sexual Behavior* 29:309–322.
222. Durna EM, Heller GZ, Leader LR, Sjoblom P, Eden JA, Wren BG (2004): Breast cancer in premenopausal women: Recurrence and survival rates and relationship to hormone replacement therapy. *Climacteric* 7:284–291.
223. Durna EM, Wren BG, Heller GZ, Leader LR, Sjoblom P, Eden JA (2002): Hormone replacement therapy after a diagnosis of breast cancer: Cancer recurrence and mortality. *Med J Aust* 177:403–409.
224. Duvernoy CS, Kulkarni PM, Dowsett SA, Keech CA (2005): Vascular events in the Multiple Outcomes of Raloxifene Evaluation (MORE) Trial: Incidence, patient characteristics, and effect of raloxifene. *Menopause* 12:444–452.
225. Ebrecht M, Hextall J, Kirtely LG, Taylor A, Dyson M, Weinman J (2004): Perceived stress and cortisol levels predict speed of wound healing in healthy male adults. *Psychoneur* 29:798–809.
226. Edwards RD, Moss JG, Lumsden MA, Wu O, Murray LS, Twaddle S, Murray GD (2007): Uterine-artery embolization versus surgery for symptomatic uterine fibroids. *NEJM* 356:360–370.
227. Elavsky S, McAuley E (2007): Physical activity and mental health outcomes during menopause: A randomized controlled trial. *Ann Behav Med* 33:132–142.
228. Espeland MA, Rapp SR, Shumaker SA, Brunner R, Manson JE, Sherwin BB, Hsia J, Margolis KL, Hogan PE, Wallace R, Dailey M, Freeman R, Hays J (2004): Conjugated equine estrogens and global cognitive function in postmenopausal women. *JAMA* 291(24):2959–2968.
229. Ettinger B, Black DM, Mitlak BH, Knickerbocker RK, Nickelsen T, Genant HK, Christiansen C, Delmas PD, Zanchetta JR, Stakkestad J, Gluer CC, Krueger K, Cohen FJ, Eckert S, Ensrud KE, Avioli LV, Lips P, Cummings SR (1999): Reduction of vertebral fracture risk in postmenopausal women with osteoporosis treated with raloxifene: Results from a 3-year randomized clinical trial. *JAMA* 282(7):216–220.
230. Ettinger B, Ensrud KE, Wallace R, Johnson KC, Cummings SR, Yankov V, Wittinghoff E, Grady D (2004): Effects of ultralow-dose transdermal estradiol on bone mineral density: A randomized clinical trial. *Obstet Gynecol* 104:443–451.

231. Executive Committee of the International Menopause Society (2004): Position Statement; Guidelines for the hormone treatment of women in the menopausal transition and beyond. *Climacteric* 7:8–11.

232. Exton MS, Kruger THC, Koch M, Paulson E, Knapp W, Hartmann U, Schedlowski M (2001): Coitus-induced orgasm stimulates prolactin secretion in healthy subjects. *Psychneuroendocrinology* 26:287–294.

233. Falcone T (2004): Laparoscopic hysterectomy: Why is it not more popular? *Gyne Trends* 8:1:1–6.

234. Falkeborn M, Lithell H, Persson I, Vessby B, Naessen T (2002): Lipids and anti-oxidative effects of estradiol and sequential norethisterone acetate treatment in a 3-month randomized controlled trial. *Climacteric* 5:240–248.

235. Farmer R (2005): Invited editorial: The Million Women Study—is it believable? *Climacteric* 8:210–213.

236. Farquhar CM, Sadler L, Harvey SA, Stewart AW (2005): The association of hysterectomy and menopause: A prospective cohort study. *BJOG* 112:956–962.

237. Ferrero S, Abbamonte LH, Parisi M, Ragni N, Remorgida V (2007): Dyspareunia and quality of sex life after laparoscopic excision of endometriosis and postoperative administration of triptorelin. *Fertil Steril* 87:227–229.

238. Ferrero S, Abbamonte LH, Parisi M, Ragni N, Remorgida V (2007): Response to commentaries on retention of the ovaries and long-term survival. *Fertil Steril* 87:227–229.

239. Ferrero S, Abbamonte LH, Giordano M, Parisi M, Ragni N, Remorgida V (2006): Uterine myomas, dyspareunia, and sexual function. *Fertil Steril* 86:1504–1510.

240. Filer RB, Wu CH (1989): Coitus during menses: Its effect on endometriosis and pelvic inflammatory disease. *J Reprod M* 34:887–890.

241. Finset A, Overlie I, Holte A (2004): Musculo-skeletal pain, psychological distress, and hormones during the menopausal transition. *Psychneuroendocrinology* 29:49–64.

242. Fitzpatrick LA, Good A (1999): Micronized progesterone: Clinical indications and comparison with current treatments. *Fertil Steril* 72(3):389–397.

243. Floter A, Nathorst-Boos J, Carlstrom K, von Schoultz B (2002): Addition of testosterone to estrogen replacement therapy in oophorectomized women: Effects on sexuality and well-being. *Climacteric* 5:357–365.

244. Foidart JM, Colin C, Denoo X, Desreux J, Beliard A, Fournier S, de Lignieres B (1998): Estradiol and progesterone regulate the proliferation of human breast epithelial cells. *Fertil Steril* 69(5):963–969.

245. Fournier A, Clavel-Chapelon F, et al. (2003): "Menopause hormonal treatment and risk of breast cancer: Comments on the results of the Million Women Study." *Bull Cancer* 90(10):924–926.

246. Francois K, Ortiz J, Harris C, Foley M, Elliott J (2005): Is peripartum hysterectomy more common in multiple gestations? *Obstet Gynecol* 105:1369–1372.

247. Franklin, Benjamin (1909): *Benjamin Franklin, His Autobiography: 1706–1757*, by Benjamin Franklin. The Harvard classics, edited by Charles W. Eliot. 1: New York: Collier & Son.

248. Fraser IS, Bonnar J, Peyvandi F (2005): Requirements for research investigations to clarify the relationships and management of menstrual abnormalities in women with hemostatic disorders. *Fertil Steril* 84:1360–1365.

249. Freeman EW, Sammel MD, Rinaudo PJ, Sheng L (2004): Premenstrual syndrome as a predictor of menopausal symptoms. *Obstet Gynecol* 103(5):960–966.

250. Freeman ML, Saed GM, Elhammady EF, Diamond MP (2003): Expression of transforming growth factor beta isoform mRNA in injured peritoneum that healed with adhesions and without adhesions and in uninjured peritoneum. *Fertil Steril* 80:708–713.

251. Freije WA (2003): Genome biology and gynecology: The application of oligonucleotide microarrays to leiomyomata. *Fertil Steril* 80(2):277–278.

252. Friedmann E, Thomas SA, Stein PK, Kleiger RE (2003): Relation between pet ownership and heart rate variability in patients with healed myocardial infarcts. *The Americ* 91:718–721.

253. Fultz NH, Fisher GG, Jenkins KR (2004): Does urinary incontinence affect middle-aged and older women's time use and activity patterns? *Am Col Obs* 104:1327–1334.

254. Gallagher JC, Satpathy R, Rafferty K, Haynatzka V (2004): The effect of soy protein isolate on bone metabolism. *Menopause* 11:290–298.

255. Gallicchio L, Schilling C, Miller SR, Zacur H, Flaws JA (2007): Correlates of sexual functioning among mid-life women. *Climacteric* 10:132–142.

256. Gambacciani M, Genazzani AR (2003): "The study with a million women (and hopefully fewer mistakes)." *Gynecol Endocrinol* 17(5):359–362.

257. Gambrell DR (2003): Editorial: Progesterone skin cream and measurements of absorption. *Menopause* 10:1–3.

258. Gambrell RD, Natrajan PK (2006): Moderate dosage estrogen-androgen therapy improves continuation rates in postmenopausal women: Impact of the WHI reports. *Climacteric* 9:224–233.

259. Gao Z, Matsuo H, Wang Y, Nakago S, Maruo T (2001): Up-regulation by IGF-I of proliferating cell nuclear antigen and Bcl-2 protein expression in human uterine leiomyoma cells. *JCEM* 86:5593–5599.

260. Garcia PM, Gimenez J, Bonacasa B, Carbonell LF, Miguel SG, Quesada T, Hernandez I (2005): 17b-Estradiol exerts a beneficial effect on coronary vascular remodeling in the early stages of hypertension in spontaneously hypertensive rats. *Menopause* 12:453–459.

261. Garry R (2006): Diagnosis of endometriosis and pelvic pain. *Fertil Steril* 86:1307–1309.

262. Geerlings MI, Ruitenberg A, Witteman JCM, van Swieten JC, Hofman A, van Duijn CM, Breteler MMB, Launer LJ (2001): Reproductive period and risk of dementia in postmenopausal women. *JAMA* 285:1475–1481.

263. Geller S, Studee L (2006): Soy and red clover for mid-life and aging. *Climacteric* 9:245–263.

264. Geller SE, Studee L, Chandra G (2005): Knowledge, attitudes, and behaviors of healthcare providers for botanical and dietary supplement use for postmenopausal health. *Menopause* 12:49–55.

265. Genazzani AR, Gambacciani M, Schneider HPG, Christiansen C (2005): Controversial issues in climacteric medicine IV: Postmenopausal osteoporosis: Therapeutic options. *Climacteric* 8:99–109.

266. Genazzani AR, Gambacciani M, Simoncini T, Schneider HPG (eds.): (2003): Position Paper: Controversial issues in climacteric medicine III: Hormone replacement therapy in climacteric and aging brain. *Climacteric* 6:188–203.

267. Gerber JR, Johnson JV, Bunn JY, O'Brien SL (2005): A longitudinal study of the effects of free testosterone and other psychosocial variables on sexual function during the natural traverse of menopause. *Fertil Steril* 83(3):643–648.

268. Gertig DM, Fletcher AS, English DR, MacInnis RJ, Hopper JL, Giles GG (2006): Hormone therapy and breast cancer: What factors modify the association? *Menopause* 13:178–184.

269. Gierhart BS (2006): When does a "less than perfect" sex life become female sexual dysfunction? *Obstet Gynecol* 107:750–751.

270. Gilmour DT, Das S, Flowerdew G (2006): Rates of urinary tract injury from gynecologic surgery and the role of intraoperative cystoscopy. *Obstet Gynecol* 107:1366–1372.

271. Going S, Lohman T, Houtkooper L, Metcalfe L, Flint-Wager H, Blew R, Cussler E, Martin J, Teixeira P, Harris M, Milliken L, Figueroa-Galvez A, Weber J (2003): Effects of exercise on bone mineral density in calcium-replete postmenopausal women with and without hormone replacement therapy. *Osteoporosis Int* 14:8:637–643.

272. Goldstat R, Briganti E, Tran J, Wolfe R, Davis SR (2003): Transdermal testosterone therapy improves well-being, mood, and sexual function in premenopausal women. *Menopause* 10(5):390–398.

273. Goldstein J (2006): Hospital infections' costs tallied. *Phila Inquirer* 11/15/06: page 1.

274. Goldstein J, Sites CK, Toth MJ (2004): Progesterone stimulates cardiac muscle protein synthesis via receptor-dependent pathway. *Fertil Steril* 82(2):430–436.

275. Goldstein S, Johnson S, Watts N, Ciaccia A, Elmerick D, Muram D (2005): Incidence of urinary incontinence in postmenopausal women treated with raloxifene or estrogen. *Menopause* 12:160–164.

276. Gomes MKO, Ferriani RA, de Silva JCR, de Sa' Rosa e Silva ACJ, Vieira CS, dos Reis FJC (2007): The levonorgestrel-releasing intrauterine system and endometriosis staging. *Fertil Ster* 87:1231–1234.

277. Goode PS, Burgio KL, Locher JL, et al. (2003): Effect of behavioral training with or without pelvic floor electrical stimulation on stress incontinence in women: A randomized controlled trial. *JAMA* 290:345–352.

278. Goodwin, SC (2003): Uterine artery embolization for the treatment of uterine fibroids. *Fertil Steril* 79(1):136–137.

279. Goodwin SC (2006): Uterine artery embolization: A legitimate option for the treatment of uterine fibroids. *Fertil Steril* 85:48.

280. Gorodeski GI (2004): Is progesterone a vasodilator? *Menopause* 11(3):242–243.

281. Gorodeski GI (2005): Effects of estrogen on proton secretion via the apical membrane in vaginal-ectocervical epithelial cells of postmenopausal women. *Menopause* 12:679–684.

282. Goss AN (2007): Bisphosphonate-associated osteonecrosis of the jaws. *Climacteric* 10:5–8.

283. Gracia CR, Freeman EW, Sammel MD, Lin H, Mogul M (2007): Hormones and sexuality during transition to menopause. *Obstet Gynecol* 109:831–840.

284. Gracia CR, Sammel MD, Freeman EW, Liu L, Hollander L, Nelson DB (2004): Predictors of decreased libido in women during the late reproductive years. *Menopause* 11(2):144–150.

285. Grady D, Ettinger B, Moscarelli E, Plouffe Jr L, Sarkar S, Ciaccia A, Cummings S (2004): Safety and adverse effects associated with raloxifene: Multiple outcomes of raloxifene evaluation. *Obstet Gynecol* 104(4):837–844.

286. Grady D, Herrington D, Bittner V, Blumenthal R, Davidson M, Hlatky M, Hsia J, Hulley S, Herd A, Khan S, Newby LK, Waters D, Vittinghoff E, Wenger N (2002):

Cardiovascular disease outcomes during 6.8 years of hormone therapy: Heart and estrogen/progestin replacement study follow-up (HERS II). *JAMA* 288: 49–57.

287. Graham CA, Sanders SA, Milhausen RR, McBride KR (2004): Turning on and turning off: A focus group study of the factors that affect women's sexual arousal. *Arch Sexual Behavior* 33:527–538.

288. Grambsch P, Young EA, Meller WH (2003): Pulsatile luteinizing hormone disruption in depression. *Psychoneur* 29:825–829.

289. Granger DA, Shirtcliff EA, Booth A, Kivlighan KT, Schwartz EB (2004): The "trouble" with salivary testosterone. *Psychneuroendocrinology* 29:1229–1240.

290. Grant WB (2002): An ecologic study of dietary and solar ultraviolet-B links to breast carcinoma mortality rates. *Cancer* 94:1:272–81.

291. Grant WB (2002): An estimate of premature cancer mortality in the U.S. due to inadequate doses of solar ultraviolet-B radiation. *Cancer* 94:6:1867–1875.

292. Gray A, Cundy T, Evans M, Reid I (1996): Medroxyprogesterone acetate enhances the spinal bone mineral density response to oestrogen in late post-menopausal women. *Clin Endoc* 44:293–296.

293. Graziotti A, Basson R (2004): Sexual dysfunction in women with premature menopause. *Menopause* 11(6):766–777.

294. Greenwald MA, Gluck OS, Lang E, Rakov V (2005): Oral hormone therapy with 17 beta-estradiol and 17 beta-estradiol in combination with norethindrone acetate in the prevention of bone loss in early postmenopausal women: Dose-dependent effects. *Menopause* 12:741–748.

295. Grigorieva V, Chen-Mok M, Tarasova M, Mikhailov A (2003): Use of a levonorgestrel-releasing intrauterine system to treat bleeding related to uterine leiomyomas. *Fertil Steril* 79(5):1194–1198.

296. Grigorova M, Sherwin BB (2006): No differences in performance on test of working memory and executive functioning between healthy elderly postmenopausal women using or not using hormone therapy. *Climacteric* 9:181–194.

297. Grodstein F, Lifford K, Resnick NM, Curhan GC (2004): Postmenopausal hormone therapy and risk of developing urinary incontinence. *Obstet Gyn* 103(2):254–260.

298. Grodstein F, Stampfer MJ, Colditz GA, Willett WC, Manson JE, Joffe M, Rosner B, Fuchs C, Hankinson SE, Hunter DJ, Hennekens CH, Speizer FE (1997): Postmenopausal hormone therapy and mortality. *NEJM* 336(25):1769–1775.

299. Guaschino S, Grimaldi E, Sartore A, Mugittu R, Mangino F, Bortoli P, Pensiero S, Vinciguerra A, Perissutti P (2003): Visual function in menopause: The role of hormone replacement therapy. *Menopause* 10(1):53–64.

300. Guidozzi, F (1999): Award article: Estrogen replacement therapy in breast cancer survivors. *Int J Gynecol Obstet* 64:59–63.

301. Guthrie JR, Clark MS, Dennerstein L (2007): A prospective study of outcomes after hysterectomy in mid-aged Australian-born women. *Climacteric* 10:171–177.

302. Guthrie JR, Clark MS, Dennerstein L, Burger HG (2005): Serum C-reactive protein and plasma homocysteine levels are associated with hormone therapy use and other factors: A population-based study of middle-aged Australian-born women. *Climacteric* 8:263–270.

303. Guthrie JR, Dennerstein L, Taffe JR, Ebeling PR, Randolph JF, Burger HG, Wark JD (2003): Central abdominal fat and endogenous hormones during the menopausal transition. *Fertil Steril* 79(6):1335–1340.

304. Guthrie JR, Taffe JR, Lehert P, Burger HG, Dennerstein L (2004): Association between hormonal changes at menopause and the risk of a coronary event: A longitudinal study. *Menopause* 11(3):315–322.
305. Guzick DS (2005): Can postmenopausal women patch up their sex lives with testosterone? *Obstet Gynecol* 105(5):938–940.
306. Halbreich U (2004): The fountain of mental youth: Search for homeostatic and adaptational hormonal processes. *Psycho* 29:697–704.
307. Hale RW (2004): Editorial: Cardiovascular disease prevention in women. *ACOG Clini* 9:1–15.
308. Hall G, Blomback M, Landgren B, Bremme K (2002): Effects of vaginally administered high estradiol doses on hormonal pharmacokinetics and hemostasis in postmenopausal women. *Fertil Steril* 78(6):1172–1177.
309. Halpern CT, Udry JR, Suchindran C (1998): Monthly measures of salivary testosterone predict sexual activity in adolescent males. *Arch Sexual Behavior* 27(5):445–465.
310. Hammerfald K, Eberle C, Grau M, Kinsperger A, Zimmermann A, Ehlert U, Gaab J (2006): Persistent effects of cognitive-behavioral stress management on cortisol responses to acute stress in healthy subjects—a randomized controlled trial. *Psychoneur* 31:333–339.
311. Hammoud A, Gago A, Diamond MP (2004): Adhesions in patients with chronic pelvic pain: A role for adhesiolysis? *Fertil Steril* 82:1483–1491.
312. Hanafi M (2005): Predictors of leiomyoma recurrence after myomectomy. *Obstet Gynecol* 105:877–881.
313. Hanggi W, Bersinger N, Altermatt HJ, Birkhauser MH (1997): Comparison of transvaginal ultrasonography and endometrial biopsy in endometrial surveillance in postmenopausal HRT users. *Maturitas* 27:133–143.
314. Hao J, Janssen WGM, Tang Y, Roberts JA, McKay H, Lasley B, Allen PB, Greengard P, Rapp PR, Kordower JH, Hof PR, Morrison JH (2003): Estrogen increases the number of spinophilin-immunoreactive spines in the hippocampus of young and aged female rhesus monkeys. *JCN* 465:540–550.
315. Harman SM, Tsitouras PD (1980): Reproductive hormones in aging men. Measurement of sex steroids, basal luteinizing hormone, and leydig cell response to human chorionic gonadotropin. *J Clin End* 35–40.
316. Hartmann KE, Birnbaum H, Ben-Hamadi R, Wu EQ, Farrell MH, Spalding J, Stang P (2006): Annual costs associated with diagnosis of uterine leiomyomata. *Obstet Gynecol* 108:930–937.
317. Hartmann U, Philippsohn S, Heiser K, Ruffer-Hesse C (2004): Low sexual desire in midlife and older women: Personality factors, psychosocial development, present sexuality. *Menopause* 11(6):726–740.
318. Harvey JA, Bovbjerg VE (2004): Quantitative assessment of mammographic breast density: Relationship with breast cancer risk. *Radiology* 230:29–41.
319. Harvey JA, Scheurer C, Kawakami FT, Quebe-Fehling E, Ibarra de Palacios P, Ragavan VV (2005): Hormone replacement therapy and breast density changes. *Climacteric* 8:185–192.
320. Hashimoto K, Nozaki M, Nakano H (2004): Positive effects of conjugated equine estrogen on triglyceride metabolism in oophorectomized women based on a stratification analysis of pretreatment values. *Fertil Steril* 81(4):1041–1046.
321. Hawton K, Gath D, Day A (1994): Sexual function in a community sample of middle-aged women with partners: Effects of age, marital, socioeconomic,

psychiatric, gynecological and menopausal factors. *Arch Sexual Behavior* 23: 375–395.

322. Hayes RD, Dennerstein, L, Bennett CM, Koochaki PE, Leiblum SR, Graziottin A (2007): Relationship between hypoactive sexual desire disorder and aging. *Fertil Steril* 87:107–112.

323. He FJ, MacGregor GA (2003): Potassium: More beneficial effects. *Climacteric* 6(Suppl 3):36–48.

324. He H, Yang F, Liu X, Zeng X, Hu Q, Zhu Q, Tu B (2007): Sex hormone ratio changes in men and postmenopausal women with coronary artery disease. *Menopause* 14:385–390.

325. Reference was removed at author's request.

326. Heaney RP (2003): Long-latency deficiency disease: Insights from calcium and vitamin D. *Am J Clin Nutr* 78:912–919.

327. Heaney RP (2003): Normalizing calcium intake: Projected population effects for body weight. *J Nutr* 133:268S–270S.

328. Heaney RP (2004): Functional indices of vitamin D status and ramifications of vitamin D deficiency. *Am J Clin Nutr* 80:6:1706S–1709S.

329. Heaney RP (2004): The vitamin D requirement in health and disease. *J Steroid Biochem Mol Biol* 97:13–19.

330. Heaney RP, Davies KM, Barger MJ (2002): Calcium and weight: Clinical studies. *Journal of the American College of Nutrition* 21:152S–155S.

331. Heaney RP, Davies KM, Chen TC, Holick MF, Barger-Lux MJ (2003): Human serum 25-hydroxycholecalciferol response to extended oral dosing with cholecalciferol. *Am J Clin Nutr* 77:204–210.

332. Heaney RP, Dowell S, Bierman J, Hale CA, Bendich A (2001): Absorbability and cost effectiveness in calcium supplementation. *J Am Coll Nutr* 20:3:239–246.

333. Heaney RP, Dowell S, Hale CA, Bendich A (2003): Calcium absorption varies within the reference range for serum 25-Hydroxyvitamin D. *J Am Coll Nutr* 22:2:142–146.

334. Heiman JR, Meston CM (1997): Evaluating sexual dysfunction in women. *Obstet Gynecol* 40(3):616–629.

335. Heit M, Rosenquist C, Culligan P, Graham C, Murphy M, Shott S (2003): Predicting treatment choice for patients with pelvic organ prolapse. *Obstet Gyn* 101:1279–1284.

336. Heitmann C, Greiser E, Doren M (2005): The impact of the Women's Health Initiative Randomized Controlled Trial 2002 on perceived risk communication and use of postmenopausal hormone therapy in Germany. *Menopause* 12:405–411.

337. Hellebrekers BWJ, Emeis JJ, Kooistra T, Trimbos JB, Moore NR, Zwinderman KH, Trimbos-Kemper TCM (2005): A role for the fibrinolytic system in postsurgical adhesion formation. *Fertil Steril* 83:122–129.

338. Heller HJ, Greer LG, Haynes SD, Poindexter JR, Pak CYC (2000): Pharmacokinetic and pharmacodynamic comparison of two calcium supplements in postmenopausal women. *J Clin Pharm* 40:1237–1244.

339. Heller HJ, Stewart A, Haynes S, Pak CYC (1999): Pharmacokinetics of calcium absorption from two commercial calcium supplements. *J Clin Pharm* 39:1151–1154.

340. Hemelaar M, Kenemans P, de Bie L, van de Weijer PHM, van der Mooren MJ (2006): Intranasal continuous combined 17b-estradiol/norethisterone therapy improves the lipid profile in healthy postmenopausal women. *Fertil Steril* 85:979–988.

341. Hemelaar M, van der Mooren MJ, Mijatovic V, Bouman AA, Schijf CPT, Kroeks MVAM, Franke HR, Kenemans P (2003): Oral, more than transdermal, estrogen therapy improves lipids and lipoprotein(a) in postmenopausal women: A randomized, placebo-controlled study. *Menopause* 10(6):550–558.

342. Henderson JA, Shively CA (2004): Triphasic oral contraceptive treatment alters the behavior and neurobiology of female cynomolgus monkeys. *Psychneuroendocrinology* 29:21–34.

343. Henderson VW, Sherwin BB (2007): Surgical versus natural menopause: Cognitive issues. *Menopause* 14:572–579.

344. Henmi H, Endo T, Kitajima Y, Manase K, Hata H, Kudo R (2003): Effects of ascorbic acid supplementation on serum progesterone levels in patients with a luteal phase defect. *Fertil Steril* 80:459–461.

345. Herlitz A, Thilers P, Habib R (2007): Endogenous estrogen is not associated with cognitive performance before, during, or after menopause. *Menopause* 14: 425–431.

346. Herrington DM, Howard TD, Hawkins GA, Reboussin DM, Xu J, Zheng SL, Brosnihan KB, Meyers DA, Bleecker ER (2002): Estrogen-receptor polymorphisms and effects of estrogen replacement on high-density lipoprotein cholesterol in women with coronary disease. *NEJM* 346(13):967–974.

347. Herrington DM, Reboussin DM, Brosnihan KB, Sharp PC, Shumaker SA, Snyder TE, Furberg CD, Kowalchuk GJ, Stuckey TD, Rogers WJ, Givens DH, Waters D (2000): Effects of estrogen replacement on the progression of coronary-artery atherosclerosis. *NEJM* 343:522–529.

348. Hickok LR, Toomey C, Speroff L (1993): A comparison of esterified estrogens with and without methyltestosterone: Effects on endometrial histology and serum lipoproteins in postmenopausal women. *Acta Theriologica* 82: 919–924.

349. Hodis HN, Mack WJ, Azen SP, Lobo RA, Shoupe D, Mahrer PR, Faxon DP, Cashin-Hemphill L, Sanmarco ME, French WJ, Shook TL, Gaarder TD, Mehra AO, Rabbani R, Sevanian A, Shil AB, Torres M, Vogelbach KH, Selzer RH (2003): Hormone therapy and the progression of coronary-artery atherosclerosis in postmenopausal women. *NEJM* 35–545.

350. Hofbauer LC, Schoppet M (2004): Clinical implications of the osteoprotegerin/RANKL/RANK system for bone and vascular disease. *JAMA* 292:4:490–495.

351. Hoffman PJ, Milliken DB, Gregg LC, Davis RR, Gregg JP (2004): Molecular characterization of uterine fibroids and its implication for underlying mechanisms of pathogenesis. *Fertil Steril* 83(3):639–649.

352. Hofling M, Hirschberg AL, Skoog L, Tani E, Hagerstrom T, von Schoultz B (2007): Testosterone inhibits estrogen/progestogen-induced breast cell proliferation in postmenopausal women. *Menopause* 14:183–190.

353. Hofseth LJ, Raafat AM, Osuch JR, Pathak DR, Slomski CA, Haslam SZ (1999): Hormone replacement therapy with estrogen or estrogen plus medroxyprogesterone acetate is associated with increased epithelial proliferation in the normal postmenopausal breast. *JCEM* 84(12):4559–4565.

354. Hogervorst E, Williams J, Budge M, Riedel W, Jolles J (2000): The nature of the effect of female gonadal hormone replacement therapy on cognitive function in post-menopausal women: A meta-analysis. *Neuroscience* 101(3):485–512.

355. Holick MF (2004): Vitamin D: Importance in the prevention of cancers, type 1 diabetes, heart disease, and osteoporosis. *Am J Clin Nutr* 79:362–371.

356. Holick MF, Siris ES, Binkley N, Beard MK, Khan A, Katzer JT, Petruschke RA, Chen E, de Papp AE (2005): Prevalence of vitamin D inadequacy among postmenopausal North American women receiving osteoporosis therapy. *JCEM* 90:3215–3224.

357. Holmberg L, Anderson H (2004): HABITS (hormonal replacement therapy after breast cancer—is it safe?), a randomized comparison: Trial stopped. *Lancet* 363:453–455.

358. Hoskins D, Chilvers CED, Christiansen C, et al. (1998): Prevention of bone loss with alendronate in postmenopausal women under 60 years of age. *NEJM* 338:485–491.

359. Howes JB, Bray K, Lorenz L, Smerdely P, Howes LG (2004): The effects of dietary supplementation with isoflavones from red clover on cognitive function in postmenopausal women. *Climacteric* 7:70–77.

360. Hsu K, Huang S, Hsiao J, Cheng Y, Wang SPH, Chou C (2003): Clinical significance of serum human papilloma virus DNA in cervical carcinoma. *Obstet Gyn* 102:1344–1351.

361. Hsu Y, Fenner DE, Weadock WJ, DeLancey JOL (2005): Magnetic resonance imaging and 3-dimensional analysis of external anal sphincter anatomy. *Obstet Gynecol* 6:1259–1265.

362. Huang JYJ, Kafy S, Dugas A, Valenti D, Tulandi T (2006): Failure of uterine fibroid embolization. *Fertil Steril* 85:30–35.

363. Huang JYJ, Valenti D, Tulandi T (2006): Treatment of uterine fibroids for the interest of patients and not specialists. *Fertil Steril* 85:50.

364. Huang MI, Nir Y, Chen B, Schnyer R, Manber R (2006): A randomized controlled pilot study of acupuncture for postmenopausal hot flashes: Effect on nocturnal hot flashes and sleep quality. *Fertil Steril* 86:701–710.

365. Hucklebridge F, Hussain T, Evans P, Clow A (2005): The diurnal patterns of the adrenal steroids cortisol and dehydroepiandrosterone (DHEA) in relation to awakening. *Psychoneuro* 30:51–57.

366. Hulley S, Furberg C, Barrett-Connor E, Cauley J, Grady D, Haskell W, Knopp K, Lowery M, Satterfield S, Schrott H, Vittinghoff E, Hunninghake D (2002): Noncardiovascular disease outcomes during 6.8 years of hormone therapy: Heart and estrogen/progestin replacement study follow-up (HERS II). *JAMA* 288:58–65.

367. Hulley S, Grady D, Bush T, Furberg C, Herrington D, Riggs B, Vittinghoff E (1998): Randomized trial of estrogen plus progestin for secondary prevention of coronary heart disease in postmenopausal women. *JAMA*:605–613.

368. Humphrey LL, Helfand M, Chan BKS, Woolf SH (2002): Breast cancer screening: A summary of the evidence for the U.S. preventative services task force. *Ann Intern* 137(5):347–367.

369. Huntley AL, Ernst E (2003): A systematic review of herbal medicinal products for the treatment of menopausal symptoms. *Menopause* 10(5):465–476.

370. Hurst BS, Matthews ML, Marshburn PB (2005): Laparoscopic myomectomy for symptomatic uterine myomas. *Fertil Steril* 83:1–23.

371. Irvin W, Andersen W, Taylor P, Rice L (2004): Minimizing the risk of neurologic injury in gynecologic surgery. *Obstet & Gyn* 103:374–382.

372. Isik-Akbay EF, Harmanli OH, Panganamamula UR, Akbay M, Gaughan J, Chatwani AJ (2004): Hysterectomy in obese women: A comparison of abdominal and vaginal routes. *Obstet Gynecol* 104:710–714.

373. Iverson RE, Chelmow D, Strohbehn D, Waldman L, Evantash E (2004): Relative morbidity of abdominal hysterectomy and myomectomy for management of uterine leiomyomas. *Obstet Gynecol* 88(3):415–419.

374. Jackson SL, Scholes D, Boyko EJ, Abraham L, Fihn S (2006): Predictors of urinary incontinence in a prospective cohort of postmenopausal women. *Obstet Gynecol* 108:855–862.

375. Jacobs DM, Tang MX, Stern Y, Sano M, Marder K, Bell KL, Schofield P, Dooneief G, Gurland B, Mayeux R (1998): Cognitive function in nondemented older women who took estrogen after menopause. *Neurology* 50(2):368–373.

376. Jacobs DR, Pereira MA, Meyer KA, Kushi LH (2000): Fiber from whole grains, but not refined grains, is inversely associated with all-cause mortality in older women: The Iowa Women's Health Study. *Am J Clin Nutr* 19(3):326S–330S.

377. Jadoul P, Donnez J (2003): Conservative treatment may be beneficial for young women with atypical endometrial hyperplasia or endometrial adenocarcinoma. *Fertil Steril* 80:1315–1324.

378. Jeanes HL, Wanikiat P, Sharif I, Gray G (2006): Medroxyprogesterone acetate inhibits the cardioprotective effect of estrogen in experimental ischemia-reperfusion injury. *Menopause* 13:80–86.

379. Jirecek S, Lee A, Pavo I, Crans G, Eppel W, Wenzl R (2004): Raloxifene prevents the growth of uterine leiomyomas in premenopausal women. *Fertil Steril* 81:132–136.

380. Joffe H, Hall JE, Gruber S, Sarmiento IA, Cohen LS, Yurgelun-Todd D, Martin KA (2006): Estrogen therapy selectively enhances prefrontal cognitive processes: A randomized, double-blind, placebo-controlled study with functional magnetic resonance imaging in perimenopausal and recently postmenopausal women. *Menopause* 13(3):411–422.

381. Johnson SR, Ettinger B, Macer JL, Ensrud KE, Quan J, Grady D (2005): Uterine and vaginal effects of unopposed ultralow-dose transdermal estradiol. *Obstet Gynecol* 105:779–787.

382. Kabat-Zinn J (2005): *Coming to Our Senses: Healing Ourselves and the World through Mindfulness.* New York: Hyperion Books.

383. Kadir RA, Lukes AS, Kouides PA, Fernandez H, Goudemand J (2005): Management of excessive menstrual bleeding in women with hemostatic disorders. *Fertil Steril* 84:1352–1359.

384. Kanaya AM, Herrington D, Vittinghoff E, Lin F, Grady D, Bittner V, Cauley JA, Barrett-Connor E (2003): Glycemic effects of postmenopausal hormone therapy: The heart and estrogen/progestin replacement study. A randomized, double-blind, placebo-controlled trial. *Ann Intern* 138:1–9.

385. Kanis JA, Johnell O, Black DM, Downs RW, Sarkar S, Fuerst T, Secrest RJ, Pavo I (2003): Effect of raloxifene on the risk of new vertebral fracture in postmenopausal women with osteopenia or osteoporosis: A reanalysis of the Multiple Outcomes of Raloxifene Evaluation trial. *Bone* 33:293–300.

386. Kanis JA, Johnell O, Oden A, De Laet C, Jonsson B, Dawson A (2002): Ten-year risk of osteoporotic fracture and the effect of risk factors on screening strategies. *Bone* 30:2:251–258.

387. Kaptchuk TJ (2002): The placebo effect in alternative medicine: Can the performance of a healing ritual have clinical significance? *Ann Intern* 136:817–825.

388. Karim R, Mack WJ, Lobo RA, Hwang J, Liu C, Liu C, Sevanian A, Hodis HN (2005): Determinants of the effect of estrogen on the progression of subclinical

atherosclerosis: Estrogen in the Prevention of Atherosclerosis Trial. *Menopause* 12:366–373.

389. Karlamangla AS, Singer BH, Greendale GA, Seeman TE (2005): Increase in epinephrine excretion is associated with cognitive decline in elderly men: MacArthur studies of successful aging. *Psychoneur* 30:453–460.

390. Kaspers-Kreijkamp S, Kok L, Grobbee DE, de Haan EHF, Aleman A, Lampe JW, van der Schouw YT (2004): Effect of soy protein containing isoflavones on cognitive function, bone mineral density, and plasma lipids in postmenopausal women. *JAMA* 292:1 292:65–74.

391. Kaunitz AM (2006): Editorial: Hormone therapy and breast cancer risk: Trumping fear with facts. *Menopause* 13:160–163.

392. Kawas C, Resnick S, Morrison A, Brookmeyer R, Corrada M, Zonderman A, Bacal C, Lingle DD, Metter E (1997): A prospective study of estrogen replacement therapy and the risk of developing Alzheimer's disease: The Baltimore Longitudinal Study of Aging. *Neurology* 48:1517–1521.

393. Ke RW, Pace DT, Ahokas RA (2003): Effect of short-term hormone replacement therapy on oxidative stress and endothelial function in African American and Caucasian postmenopausal women. *Fertil Steril* 79:1118–1122.

394. Keenan NL, Mark S, Fugh-Berman A, Browne D, Kaczmarczyk J, Hunter C (2003): Severity of menopausal symptoms and use of both conventional and complementary/alternative therapies. *Menopause* 10:507–515.

395. Keenan PA, Ezzat WH, Ginsburg K, Moore GJ (2001): Prefrontal cortex as the site of the estrogen's effect on cognition. *Psychneuroendocrinology* 26:577–590.

396. Kennedy ADM, Sculpher MJ, Coulter A, Dwyer N, Rees M, Abrams KR, Horsley S, Cowley D, Kidson C, Kirwin C, Naish C, Stirrat G (2002): Effects of decision aids for menorrhagia on treatment choices, health outcomes, and cost. *JAMA* 288(21):2701–2709.

397. Kennedy S (2006): Should a diagnosis of endometriosis be sought in all symptomatic women? *Fertil Steril* 86:1312–1313.

398. Kenny AM, Prestwood KM, Biskup B, Robbins B, Zayas E, Kleppinger A, Burleson JA, Raisz LG (2004): Comparison of the effects of calcium loading with calcium citrate or calcium carbonate on bone turnover in postmenopausal women. *Osteoporosis Int* 15:4:290–294.

399. Kerlikowske K, Smith-Bindman R, Ljung BM, Grady D (2003): Evaluation of abnormal mammography results and palpable breast abnormalities. *Ann Intern* 139(4):274–285.

400. Keshavarz H, Hillis SD, Kieke BA, Marchbanks PA (2002): Hysterectomy Surveillance—United States, 1994–1999. *Morbidity and Mortality Weekly Report* 51:1–8.

401. Keshavarzi A, Vaezy S, Noble ML, Paun MK, Fujimoto VY (2003): Treatment of uterine fibroid tumors in an in situ rat model using high-intensity focused ultrasound. *Fertil Steril* 80(2):761–767.

402. Klaiber EL, Vogel W, Rako S (2005): A critique of the Women's Health Initiative hormone therapy study. *Fertil Steril* 84:1589–1601.

403. Klein BE, Klein R, Ritter LL (1994): Is there evidence of an estrogen effect on age-related lens opacities? The Beaver Dam Eye Study. *Arch Ophth* 112:85–91.

404. Kluger R (1996): *Ashes to Ashes: America's Hundred-Year Cigarette War, the Public Health, and the Unabashed Triumph of Philip Morris*. New York: A. Knopf.

405. Klusmann D (2002): Sexual motivation and the duration of partnership. *Arch Sexual Behavior* 31(3):275–287.
406. Knekt P, Kumpulainen J, Jarvinen R, Rissanen H, Heliovaara M, Reunanen A, Hakulinen T, Aromaa A (2002): Flavonoid intake and risk of chronic diseases. *Am J Clin* 76:560–568.
407. Knoops KT, de Groot LC, Kromhout D, Perrin AE, Moreiras-Varela O, Menoti A, van Staveren WA (2004): Mediterranean diet, lifestyle factors, and 10-year mortality in elderly European men and women: The HALE project. *JAMA* 292:1 292:1433–1439.
408. Knopman D (2005): Memory and the older woman: Diagnosis and treatment. *Menopause* 14:21–24.
409. Koertge J, Al-Khalili F, Ahnve S, Janszky I, Svane B, Schenck-Gustafsson K (2002): Cortisol and vital exhaustion in relation to significant coronary artery stenosis in middle-aged women with acute coronary syndrome. *Psychneuroendocrinology* 27:893–906.
410. Kok HS, Kuh D, Cooper R, van der Schouw YT, Grobbee DE, Wadsworth ME, Richards M (2006): Cognitive function across the life course and the menopausal transition in a British birth cohort. *Menopause* 13:19–27.
411. Kok L, Kreijkamp-Kaspers S, Grobbee DE, Lampe JW, van der Schouw YT (2005): A randomized, placebo-controlled trial on the effects of soy protein containing isoflavones on quality of life in postmenopausal women. *Menopause* 12:56–62.
412. Komisaruk BR, Whipple B (1995): The suppression of pain by genital stimulation in females. *Annual Review of Sex Research* 56:151–186.
413. Komisaruk BR, Gerdes CA, Whipple B (1997): "Complete" spinal cord injury does not block perceptual responses to genital self-stimulation in women. *Arch Neuro* 54:1513–1520.
414. Komisaruk BR, Whipple B (2000): How does vaginal stimulation produce pleasure, pain, and analgesia? *Sex, Gender, and Pain: Progress in Pain Research Management*. Seattle: IASP Press, 109–134.
415. Kon Koh K (2003): Can a healthy endothelium influence the cardiovascular effects of hormone replacement therapy? *Int J Cardiol* 87:1–8.
416. Kouides PA, Conard J, Peyvandi F, Lukes A, Kadir R (2005): Hemostasis and menstruation: Appropriate investigation for underlying disorders of hemostasis in women with excessive menstrual bleeding. *Fertil Steril* 84:1345–1351.
417. Kraemer EA, Seeger H, Deuringer FU, Mueck AO (2004): Possible influence of stromal derived growth factors on progestogen-induced breast cancer cell proliferation. *Abstracts of the Annual Meeting of the North American Menopause Society*: Menopause Society.
418. Kraemer EA, Seeger H, Kramer B, Wallwiener D, Mueck AO (2005): The effects of progesterone, medroxyprogesterone acetate, and norethisterone on growth factor- and estradiol-treated human cancerous and noncancerous breast cells. *Menopause* 12:468–474.
419. Kraemer GR, Kraemer RR, Ogden BW, Kilpatrick RE, Gimpel TL, Castracane VD (2003): Variability of serum estrogens among postmenopausal women treated with the same transdermal estrogen therapy and the effect on androgens and sex hormone binding globulin. *Fertil Steril* 79:534–542.
420. Kreijkamp-Kaspers S, Kok L, Grobbee DE, de Haan EHF, Aleman A, Lampe JW, van der Schouw YT (2004): Effect of soy protein containing isoflavones on

cognitive function, bone mineral density, and plasma lipids in postmenopausal women. *JAMA* 292:65–74.

421. Kritz-Silverstein D, Von Muhlen D, Barrett-Connor E, Bressel MAB (2003): Isoflavones and cognitive function in older women: The Soy and Postmenopausal Health in Aging (SOPHIA) study. *Menopause* 10:196–202.

422. Kubzansky LD, Wright RJ, Cohen S, Weiss S, Rosner B, Sparrow D (2002): Breathing easy: A prospective study of optimism and pulmonary function in the Normative Aging Study. *Ann Behav* 24:345–353.

423. Kudielka BM, Kirschbaum C (2003): Awakening cortisol responses are influenced by health status and awakening time but not by menstrual cycle phase. *Psychneuroendocrinology* 28:35–47.

424. Kuh D, Butterworth S, Kok H, Richards M, Hardy R, Wadsworth MEJ, Leon DA (2005): Childhood cognitive ability and age at menopause: Evidence from two cohort studies. *Menopause* 12:475–482.

425. Kuhl H (2005): Pharmacology of estrogens and progestogens: Influence of different routes of administration. *Cancer Causes and Control* 8:3–63.

426. Kukuvitis A, Kourtis A, Papaiconomou N, Zournatzi V, Makedos G, Panidis D (2003): Differential effects of unopposed versus opposed hormone therapy, tibolone, ad raloxifene on substance p levels. *Fertil Steril* 80:96–98.

427. Kuppermann M, Summitt R, Varner R, McNeeley S, Goodman-Gruen D, Learman L, Ireland C, Vittinghoff E, Lin F, Richter H, Showstack J, Hulley S, Washington A (2005): Sexual functioning after total compared with supracervical hysterectomy: A randomized trial. *Obstet Gynecol* 105:1309–1318.

428. Kuppermann M, Varner RE, Summitt RL, Learman LA, Ireland C, Vittinghoff E, Stewart AL, Lin F, Richter HE, Showstack J, Hulley SB, Washington AE (2004): Effect of hysterectomy vs medical treatment on health-related quality of life and sexual functioning: The Medicine or Surgery (MS) Randomized Trial. *JAMA* 291:1447–1455.

429. Kurachi O, Matsuo H, Samoto T, Maruo T (2001): Tumor necrosis factor-expression in human uterine leiomyoma and its down-regulation by progesterone. *JCEM* 86:2275–2280.

430. Laan E, Everaerd W, van Bellen G, Hanewald G (1994): Women's arousal and emotional responses to male and female-produced erotica. *Arch Sexual Behavior* 21:153–169.

431. Lacey JV, Mink PJ, Lubin JH, Sherman ME, Troisi R, Hartge P, Schatzkin A, Schairer C (2002): Menopausal hormone replacement therapy and risk of ovarian cancer. *JAMA* 288:334–341.

432. Lacut K, Oger E, Le Gal G, Blouch MT, Abgrall JF, Kerlan V, et al. (2003): Differential effects on oral and transdermal postmenopausal estrogen replacement therapies on C-reactive protein. *Thromb Haemost* 98:124–131.

433. Lakoski SG, Herrington DM (2005): Effects of hormone therapy on C-reactive protein and IL-6 in postmenopausal women: A review article. *Climacteric* 8: 317–326.

434. Lambert PA, Conway BR (2003): Pharmaceutical quality of ceftriaxone generic drug products compared with Rocephin. *J Chemother* 4:357–368.

435. Laoag-Fernandez JB, Maruo T, Pakarinen P, Spitz IM, Johansson E (2003): Effects of levonorgestrel-releasing intra-uterine system on the expression of vascular endothelial growth factor and andrenomedullin in the endometrium in adenomyosis. *Hum Reprod* 18:694–699.

436. Laumann EO, Paik A, Glasser DB, Kang J, Wang T, Levinson B, Moreira ED, Nicolosi A, Gingell C (2006): A cross-national study of subjective sexual well-being among older women and men: Findings from the global study of sexual attitudes and behaviors. *Arch Sexual Behavior* 35:145–161.

437. Lauritzen C (2005): Letter to the editors: Importance of the progestogen added to the estrogen in hormone therapy. *Climacteric* 8:398–400.

438. Le Gal G, Gourlet V, Hogrel P, Plu-Bureau G, Touboul PJ, Scarabin PY (2003): Hormone replacement therapy use is associated with a lower occurrence of carotid atherosclerotic plaques but not with intima-media thickness progression among postmenopausal women. The vascular aging (EVA) study. *Atherosclerosis* 166:163–170.

439. Learman LA, Summitt Jr RL, Varner E, Richter HE, Lin F, Ireland CC, Kuppermann M, Vittinghoff E, Showstack J, Washington AE, Hulley SB (2004): Hysterectomy versus expanded medical treatment for abnormal uterine bleeding: Clinical outcomes in the medicine or surgery trial. *Obstet Gynecol* 103(5):824–833.

440. Ledger WJ, Monif GRG (2004): A growing concern: Inability to diagnose vulvovaginal infections correctly. *Obstet Gynecol* 103:782–784.

441. Legorreta AP, Chernicoff HO, Trinh JB, Parker RG (2004): Diagnosis, clinical staging, and treatment of breast cancer. A retrospective multiyear study of a large controlled population. *Am J Clin Oncol* 27(2):185–190.

442. Legros J (2001): Inhibitory effect of oxytocin on corticotrope function in humans: Are vasopressin and oxytocin yin-yang neurohormones? *Psychneuroendocrinology* 26:649–655.

443. Leiblum SR, Koochaki PA, Rodenberg CA, Barton IP, Rosen R (2006): Hypoactive sexual desire disorder in postmenopausal women: US results from the Women's International Study of Health and Sexuality (WISHeS). *Menopause* 13:46–56.

444. Lemaitre RN, Weiss NS, Smith NL, Psaty BM, Lumley T, Larson EB, Heckbert SR (2006): Esterified estrogen and conjugated equine estrogen and the risk of incident myocardial infarction and stroke. *Arch Inter* 166:399–404.

445. Leonetti HB, Wilson KJ, Anasti JN (2003): Topical progesterone cream has an antiproliferative effect on estrogen-stimulated endometrium. *Fertil Steril* 79:221–222.

446. Lepine LA, Hillis SD, Marchbanks PA, Koonin LM, Morrow B, Kieke BA, Wilcox LS (1997): Hysterectomy surveillance—United States, 1980–1993. *Morbidity* 46:1–15.

447. Leung PL, Tam Wh, Yuen PM (2003): Hysteroscopic appearance of the endometrial cavity following thermal balloon endometrial ablation. *Fertil Steril* 79(5):1226–1228.

448. Levine SB (2003): The nature of sexual desire: A clinician's perspective. *Arch Sexual Behavior* 32(3):279–285.

449. Li CI, Malone KE, Porter PL, Weiss NS, Tang MC, Cushing-Haugen KL, Daling JR (2003): Relationship between long durations and different regimens of hormone therapy and risk of breast cancer. *JAMA* 289:3254–3263.

450. Li F, Harmer P, McAuley E, Duncan TE, Duncan SC, Chaumeton N, Fisher KJ (2001): An evaluation of the effects of tai chi exercise on physical function among older persons: A randomized controlled trial. *Ann Behav* 23:139–146.

451. Lin PC, Thyer A, Soules MR (2004): Intrapretative ultrasound during a laparoscopic myomectomy. *Fertil Steril* 81(6):1671–1674.

452. Lindenfeld EA, Langer RD (2002): Bleeding patterns of the hormone replacement therapies in the postmenopausal estrogen and progestin interventions trial. *Obstet Gynecol* 100:853–863.

453. Lindsay R (2005): Bone strength: Therapeutic implications. *Menopause Management* 14:18–19.

454. Ling S, Little PJ, Williams MRI, Dai A, Hashimura K, Liu JP, Komesaroff PA, Sudhir K (2002): High glucose abolishes the antiproliferative effect of 17B-estradiol in human vascular smooth muscle cells. *Am J Physiol Endocrinal Metab* 282(2):746–751.

455. Linsey C, Brownbill RA, Bohannon RA, Illich JZ (2005): Physical performance affects bone density: Association of physical performance measures with bone mineral density in postmenopausal women. *Archives of Physical Medicine and Rehabilitation* 86:1102–1107.

456. Lippman SA, Warner M, Samuels S, Olive D, Vercellini P, Eskenazi B (2003): Uterine fibroids and gynecologic pain symptoms in a population-based study. *Fertil Steril* 80(6):1488–1494.

457. Lithgow DM, Politzer WM (1977): Vitamin A in the treatment of menorrhagia. *SA Medical* 51:191–193.

458. Liu C (2003): Does quality of marital sex decline with duration? *Arch Sexual Behavior* 32(1):55–60.

459. Liu CC, Kuo TBJ, Yang CCH (2003): Effects of estrogen on gender-related autonomic differences in humans. *Am J Physiol Heart* 285:2188–2193.

460. Liu S, Willett WC, Manson JE, Hu FB, Rosner B, Colditz G (2003): Relation between changes in intakes of dietary fiber and grain products and changes in weight and development of obesity among middle aged women. *Am J Clin* 78:920–927.

461. Liu W-M, Tzeng C-R, Yi-Jen C, Wang P-H (2004): Combining the uterine depletion procedure and myomectomy may be useful for treating symptomatic fibroids. *Fertil Steril* 82(1):205–210.

462. Liu W-M, Wang P-H, Chou C-S, Tang W-L, Wang I-T, Tzeng C-R (2007): Efficacy of combined laparoscopic uterine artery occlusion and myomectomy via mini laparotomy in the treatment of recurrent uterine myomas. *Fertil Steril* 87:356–366.

463. Lloyd Davies H (2003): Potential risks of phytoestrogens: Experience from animal models. *Climacteric* 6:6:81.

464. Lobo RA (2003): Editorial: Homocysteine in women's health. *Menopause* 10(4):271–273.

465. Lobo RA, Rosen RC, Yang H, Block B, Van Der Hoop RG (2003): Comparative effects of oral esterified estrogens with and without methyltestosterone on endocrine profiles and dimensions of sexual function in postmenopausal women with hypoactive sexual desire. *Fertil Steril* 79(6):1341–1342.

466. Lochner D, Brubaker KL (2006): Incidence of malignancy in hormone therapy users with indeterminate calcifications on mammogram. *Obstet Gynecol* 194:82–85.

467. Reference removed at author's request.

468. Long C, Liu C, Hsu S, Chen Y, Wu C, Tsai E (2006): A randomized comparative study of the effects of oral and topical estrogen therapy on the lower urinary tract of hysterectomized postmenopausal women. *Fertil Steril* 85:155–160.

469. Longcope C (2003): Editorial: Androgens, estrogens, and mammary epithelial proliferation. *Menopause* 10(4):274–276.

470. Lopez-Jaramillo P, Diaz LA, Pardo A, Parra G, Jaimes H, Chaudhuri G (2004): Estrogen therapy increases plasma concentrations of nitric oxide metabolites in postmenopausal women but increases flow-mediated vasodilation only in younger women. *Fertil Steril* 82(6):1550–1555.

471. Low LF, Anstey KJ, Jorm AF, Rodgers B, Christensen H (2005): Reproductive period and cognitive function in a representative sample of naturally postmenopausal women aged 60–64 years. *Climacteric* 8:380–389.

472. Luckey M, Kagan R, Greenspan S, Bone H, Kiel RDP, Simon J, Sackarowitz J, Palmisano J, Chen E, Petruschke RA, de Papp AE (2004): Once-weekly alendronate 70 mg and raloxifene 60 mg daily in the treatment of postmenopausal osteoporosis. *Menopause* 11:405–415.

473. Lukes AS, Kadir RA, Peyvandi F, Kouides PA (2005): Disorders of hemostasis and excessive menstrual bleeding: Prevalence and clinical impact. *Fertil Steril* 84:1338–1343.

474. Lundstrom E, Soderqvist G, Svane G, Azavedo E, Olovsson M, Skoog L, von Schoultz E, von Schoultz B (2006): Digitized assessment of mammographic breast density in patients who received low-dose intrauterine levonorgestrel in continuous combination with oral estradiol valerate: A pilot study. *Fertil Steril* 85:989–995.

475. Lupien SJ, Fiocco A, Wan N, Maheu F, Lord C, Schramek T, Thanh Tu M (2005): Stress hormones and human memory function across the lifespan. *Psychneuroendocrinology* 30:225–242.

476. Luyer MDP, Khosla S, Owen WG, Miller VM (2001): Prospective randomized study of effects of unopposed estrogen replacement therapy on markers of coagulation and inflammation in postmenopausal women. *JCEM* 86(8):3629–3634.

477. Lynch NA, Ryan AS, Berman DM, Sorkin JD, Nicklas BJ (2002): Comparison of VO2 max and disease risk factors between perimenopausal and postmenopausal women. *Menopause* 9:456–462.

478. Lyytinen, H, Pukkala E, Ylikorkala O (2006): Breast cancer risk in postmenopausal women using estrogen-only therapy. *Obstet & Gyn* 108:1345–1360.

479. Maas AHEM, van der Schouw YT, Grobbee DE, van der Graaf Y (2004): "Rise and fall" of hormone therapy in postmenopausal women with cardiovascular disease. *Menopause* 11:228–235.

480. Mack WJ, Hameed AB, Xiang M, Roy S, Slater CC, Stanczyk FZ, Lobo RA, Liu CR, Liu CH, Hodis HN (2003): Does elevated body mass modify the influence of postmenopausal estrogen replacement on atherosclerosis progression: Results from the Estrogen in the Prevention of Atherosclerosis Trial. *Atherosclerosis* 168(1):91–98.

481. Mack WJ, Slater CC, Xiang M, Shoupe D, Lobo RA, Hodis HN (2004): Elevated subclinical atherosclerosis associated with oophorectomy is related to time since menopause rather than type of menopause. *Fertil Steril* 82(2):391–397.

482. MacLennan AH, Henderson VW, Paine BJ, Mathias J, Ramsey EN, Ryan P, Stocks NP, Taylor AW (2006): Hormone therapy, timing of initiation, and cognition in women aged older than 60 years: The REMEMBER pilot study. *Menopause* 13:28–36.

483. MacLennan AH, Sturdee DW (2006): Editorial: The "bioidentical/bioequivalent" hormone scan. *Climacteric* 9:1–3.

484. Maddalozzo GF, Cardinal BJ, Li F, Snow CM (2004): The association between hormone therapy use and changes in strength and body composition in early postmenopausal women. *Menopause* 11:438–446.

485. Magnusson C, Baron JA, Correia N, Bergstrom R, Adami H-O, Persson I (1999): Breast-cancer risk following long-term oestrogen- and oestrogen-progestin-replacement therapy. *Int J Cancer* 81:339–344.

486. Maki, PM (2006): Editorial: Potential importance of early initiation of hormone therapy for cognitive benefit. *Menopause* 13:6–7.

487. Maklan CW, Else B (1995): Treatment of common non-cancerous uterine conditions: Issues for research [conference summary]. Rockville, MD: U.S. Dept. of Health and Human Services, Public Health Service, Agency for Health Care Policy and Research; 1995. AHCPR publication 95-0067.

488. Malamitsi-Puchner A, Sarandakou A, Tziotis J, Stavreus-Evers A, Tzonou A, Landgren B (2004): Circulating angiogenic factors during periovulation and the luteal phase of normal menstrual cycles. *Fertil Steril* 81(5):1322–1327.

489. Mallinckrodt CH, Clark SW, Carroll RJ, Molenbergh G (2003): Assessing response profiles from incomplete longitudinal clinical trial data under regulatory considerations. *J Biopharm Stat* 13:179–190.

490. Manderson L (2005): Editorial: The social and cultural context of sexual function among middle-aged women. *Menopause* 12(4):361–362.

491. Mansfield PK, Koch PB, Voda AM (1998): Qualities midlife women desire in their sexual relationships and their changing sexual response. *Psychology of Women Quarterly* 22:285–303.

492. Mansfield PK, Koch PB, Voda AM (2000): Midlife women's attributions for their sexual response changes. *Health Care for Women International* 21:543–559.

493. Manson JE, Bassuk SS, Harman SM, Brinton EA, Cedars MI, Lobo R, Merriam GR, Miller VM, Naftolin F, Santoro N (2006): Personal perspective: Postmenopausal hormone therapy: New questions and the case for new clinical trials. *Menopause* 13:139–147.

494. Manson JE, Hsia J, Johnson KC, Rossouw JE, Assaf AR, Lasser NL, Trevisan M, Black HR, Heckbert SR, Detrano R, Strickland OL, Wong ND, Crouse JR, Stein E, Cushman M (2003): Estrogen plus progestin and the risk of coronary heart disease. *NEJM* 349(6):523–534.

495. Marazziti D, Canale D (2004): Hormonal changes when falling in love. *Psychoneur* 29:931–936.

496. Marchbanks PA, McDonald JA, Wilson HG, Folger SG, Mandel MG, Daling JR, Bernstein L, Malone KE, Ursin G, Strom BL, Norman SA, Weiss LK (2002): Oral contraceptives and the risk of breast cancer. *NEJM* 346(26):2025–2032.

497. Margolis KL, Manson JE, Greenland P, Rodabough R, Bray P, Safford M, Grimm R, Howard B, Assaf A, Prentice R (2005): Leukocyte count as a predictor of cardiovascular events and mortality in postmenopausal women. *Arch Intern Med* 106:500–508.

498. Maruo T, Laoag-Fernandez JB, Pakarinen P, Murakshi H, Spitz IM, Johansson E (2001): Effects of the levonorgestrel-releasing intrauterine system on proliferation and apoptosis in the endometrium. *Hum Reprod* 16(10):2103–2108.

499. Maruo T, Matsuo H, Samoto T, Shimomura Y, Kurachi O, Gao Z, Wang Y, Spitz I, Johansson E (2000): Effects of progesterone on uterine leiomyoma growth and apoptosis. *Steroids* 65:585–592.

500. Masera RG, Prolo P, Sartori ML, Staurenghi A, Griot G, Ravizza L, Dovio A, Chiappelli F, Angeli A (2002): Mental deterioration correlates with response of natural killer (NK): Cell activity to physiological modifiers in patients with short history of Alzheimer's disease. *Psychneuroendocrinology* 27:447–461.

501. Maslow KD, Lyons EA (2003): Effect of oral contraceptives and intrauterine devices on midcycle myometrial contractions. *Fertil Steril* 80(5):1224–1227.
502. Masters KS, Hill RD, Kircher JC, Lensegrav Benson TL, Fallon JA (2004): Religious orientation, aging and blood pressure reactivity to interpersonal and cognitive stressors. *Ann Behav Med* 28(3):171–174.
503. Matsuo H, Maruo T, Samoto T (1997): Increased expression of Bcl-2 protein in human uterine leiomyoma and its up-regulation by progesterone. *JCEM* 82:293–299.
504. Matsuzaki S, Canis M, Pouly JL, Rabischong B, Botchorishvili R, Mage G (2006): Relationship between delay of surgical diagnosis and severity of disease in patients with symptomatic deep infiltrating endometriosis. *Fertil Steril* 86: 1314–1316.
505. Mazer NA, Leiblum SR, Rosen RC (2000): The Brief Index of Sexual Functioning for Women (BISF-W): A new scoring algorithm and comparison of normative and surgically menopausal populations. *Menopause* 7(5):350–363.
506. McAuley E, Konopack JF, Motl RW, Morris KS, Doerksen SE, Rosengren KR (2006): Physical activity and quality of life in older adults: Influence of health status and self-efficacy. *Annals Behav Med* 31:99–103.
507. McCoy NL (2001): Female sexuality during aging. In *Functional Neurobiology of Aging*. Academic Press:769–779.
508. McCoy NL, Matyas JR (1996): Oral contraceptives and sexuality in university women. *Arch Sexual Behavior* 25:73–90.
509. McHorney CA, Koochaki PE (2002): Oophorectomized women experience a diminished quality of life. *Menopause* 9:473.
510. McHorney CA, Rust J, Golombok S, Davis S, Bouchard C, Brown C, Basson R, Sarti CD, Kuznicki J, Rodenberg C, Derogatis L (2004): Profile of Female Sexual Function: A patient-based, international, psychometric instrument for the assessment of hypoactive sexual desire in oophorectomized women. *Menopause* 11:474–483.
511. McKane WR, Khosla S, Egan KS, Robins SP, Burritt MF, Riggs BL (1996): Role of calcium intake in modulating age-related increases in parathyroid function and bone resorption. *JCEM* 81:5:1699–1703.
512. McSorley PT, Young IS, Bell PM, Fee JPH, McCance DR (2003): Vitamin C improves endothelial function in healthy estrogen-deficient postmenopausal women. *Climacteric* 6:238–247.
513. Mendelsohn ME, Karas RH (1999): The protective effects of estrogen on the cardiovascular system. *NEJM* 340(23):1801–1811.
514. Merck Research Laboratories (2003): *Bones change. Merck Manual of Medical Information*, 2nd Home Edition:343.
515. Meschia M, Buonaguidi A, Pifarotti P, Somigliana E, Spennacchio M, Amicarelli F (2002): Prevalence of anal incontinence in women with symptoms of urinary incontinence and genital prolapse. *Obstet Gynecol* 100(4):719–723.
516. Meston C (2004): The effects of hysterectomy on the subjective and physiological sexual function of women with benign uterine fibroids. *Arch Sexual Behavior* 33:31–42.
517. Meston CM, Gorzalka BB (1995): The effects of sympathetic activation on physiological and subjective sexual arousal in women. *Behav Res Ther* 33:651–664.
518. Meston CM, Heiman JR, Trapnell PD, Paulhus DL (1998): Socially desirable responding and sexuality self-reports. *J Sex Research* 35(2):148–157.

519. Miller AB, To T, Baines CJ, Wall C (2002): The Canadian national breast screening study-1: Breast cancer mortality after 11 to 16 years of follow-up. A randomized screening trial of mammography in women age 40 to 49 years. *Ann Intern Med* 137:101:194.

520. Miller AP, Chen YF, Xing D, Feng W, Oparil S (2003): Hormone replacement therapy and inflammation: Interactions in cardiovascular disease. *Hypertension* 42:657–663.

521. Miller MM, Monjan AA, Buckholtz NS (2001): Estrogen replacement therapy for the potential treatment or prevention of Alzheimer's disease. *Annals of NYAS* 949:223–234.

522. Million Women Study Collaborators (2002): Patterns of use of hormone replacement therapy in one million women in Britain, 1996–2000. *BJOG* 109: 1319–1330.

523. Mirkin S, Archer DF (2004): Effects of levonorgestrel, medroxyprogesterone acetate, norethindrone, progesterone, and 17-estradiol on thrombospondin-1 mRNA in Ishikawa cells. *Fertil Steril* 82(1):220–222.

524. Missmer SA, Eliassen AH, Barbieri RL, Hankinson SE (2004): Endogenous estrogen, androgen, and progesterone concentrations and breast cancer risk among postmenopausal women. *J Natl Cancer Inst* 96:1856–1865.

525. Misso M, Jang C, Adams J, Tran J, Murata Y, Bell R, Boon W, Simpson E, Davis S (2005): Adipose aromatase gene expression is greater in older women and is unaffected by postmenopausal estrogen therapy. *Menopause* 12(2):210–215.

526. Moalli PA, Shand SH, Zyczynski HM, Gordy SC, Meyn LA (2005): Remodeling of vaginal connective tissue in patients with prolapse. *Obstet Gynecol* 106: 953–963.

527. Montplaisir J, Lorrain J, Denesle R, Petit D (2001): Sleep in menopause: Differential effects of two forms of hormone replacement therapy. *Menopause* 8: 10–16.

528. Mook D, Felger J, Graves F, Wallen K, Wilson ME (2005): Tamoxifen fails to affect central serotonergic tone but increases indices of anxiety in female rhesus macaques. *PNEC* 30:273–283.

529. Morabia A, Costanza MC (2006): Recent reversal of trends in hormone therapy use in a European population. *Menopause* 13:111–115.

530. Moreau K, Gavin K, Plum A, Seals D (2006): Oxidative stress explains differences in large elastic artery compliance between sedentary and habitually exercising postmenopausal women. *Menopause* 13:951–958.

531. Moreau KL, Donato AJ, Seals DR, Dinenno FA, Blackett SD, Hoetzer GL, Desouza CA, Tanaka H (2002): Arterial intima-media thickness: Site-specific associations with HRT and habitual exercise. *Am J Physiol Heart* 283(4):H1409–1417.

532. Moreau KL, Donato AJ, Tanaka H, Jones PP, Gates PE, Seals DR (2003): Basal leg blood flow in healthy women is related to age and hormone replacement therapy status. *J Physiol* 547(1):306–316.

533. Morgan III CA, Southwick S, Hazlett G, Rasmusson A, Hoyt G, Zimolo Z, Charney D (2004): Relationships among plasma dehydroepiandrosterone sulfate and cortisol levels, symptoms of dissociation, and objective performance in humans exposed to acute stress. *Arch Gen Psych* 61:819–825.

534. Morin S (2004): Editorial: Isoflavones and bone health. *Menopause* 11(3): 239–241.

535. Morkved S, Bo K, Fjortoft T (2002): Effect of adding biofeedback to pelvic floor muscle training to treat urodynamic stress incontinence. *Obstet Gynecol* 100(4): 730–739.

536. Morrison JE Jr, Jacobs VR (2002): 437 classic intrafascial supracervical hysterectomies in 8 years. *J Am Assoc of Gynecol Laparoscopists* 9(3):401.

537. Morse AN, Labin LC, Young SB, Aronson MP, Gurwitz JH (2004): Exclusion of elderly women from published randomized trials of stress incontinence surgery. *Obstet Gynecol* 104(3):498–503.

538. Morse CA, Rice K (2005): Memory after menopause: Preliminary considerations of hormone influence on cognitive functioning. *Arch Women's Ment Health* 8:155–162.

539. Mueck AO, Seeger H, Wallwiener D (2002): Medroxyprogesterone acetate versus norethisterone: Effect on estradiol-induced changes of markers for endothelial function and atherosclerotic plaque characteristics in human female coronary endothelial cell cultures. *Menopause* 9(4):273–281.

540. Mueck AO, Seeger H, Wallwiener D (2003): Comparison of the proliferative effects of estradiol and conjugated equine estrogens on human breast cancer cells and impact of continuous combined progestogen addition. *Climacteric* 6:221–227.

541. Mulnard RA, Cotman CW, Kawas C, van Dyck CH, Sano M, Doody R, Koss E, Pfeiffer E, Jin S, Gamst A, Grundman M, Thomas R, Thal LJ (2000): Estrogen replacement therapy for treatment of mild to moderate Alzheimer disease. *JAMA* 283:1007–1015.

542. Munk-Jensen N, Pors-Nielsen S, Obel EB, Bonne-Riksen P (1988): Reversal of post-menopausal vertebral bone loss by oestrogen and progestogen: A double-blind placebo controlled study. *BMJ* 296:1150–1152.

543. Munro MG (2006): Management of leiomyomas: Is there a panacea in Pandora's box? *Fertil Steril* 85:40–43.

544. Munro MG, Lukes AS (2005): Abnormal uterine bleeding and underlying hemostatic disorders: Report of a consensus process. *Fertil Steril* 84:1335–1337.

545. Munro, MG, Mainor N, Basu R, Brisinger M, Barreda L (2006): Oral medroxyprogesterone acetate and combination oral contraceptives for acute uterine bleeding. A randomized controlled trial. *Obstet Gynecol* 108:924–929.

546. Musgrove EA, Lee CS, Sutherland RL (1991): Progestins both stimulate and inhibit breast cancer cell cycle progression while increasing expression of transforming growth factor a, epidermal growth factor receptor, c-fos, and c-myc genes. *Molecular* 11(10):5032–5043.

547. Myers ER, Barber MD, Gustilo-Ashby T, Couchman G, Matchar DB, McCrory DC (2002): Management of uterine leiomyomata: What do we really know? *Obstet Gynecol* 100:8–17.

548. Naftolin F (2005): Prevention during the menopause is critical for good health: Skin studies support protracted hormone therapy. *Fertil Steril* 84:293–294.

549. Naftolin F, Schneider HPG, Sturdee DW, Birkhauser M, Brincat MP, Gambacciani M, Genazzani AR, Limpaphayom KK, O'Neill S, Palacios S, Pines A, Siseles N, Tan D, Burger HG (2004): Guidelines for hormone treatment of women in the menopausal transition and beyond. *Climacteric* 7:333–337.

550. Naftolin F, Taylor HS, Karas R, Brinton E, Newman I, Clarkson TB, Mendelsohn M, Lobo RA, Judelson DR, Nachtigall LE, Heward CB, Hecht H,

Jaff MR, Harman SM (2004): The Women's Health Initiative could not have detected cardioprotective effects of starting hormone therapy during the menopausal transition. *Fertil Steril* 81:1498–1501.

551. Nappi C, Di Spiezio Sardo A, Guerra G, Bifulco G, Testa D, Di Carlo C (2003): Functional and morphologic evaluation of the nasal mucosa before and after hormone therapy in postmenopausal women with nasal symptoms. *Fertil Steril* 80(3):669–671.

552. Nappi C, Di Spiezio Sardo A, Guerra G, Di Carlo C, Bifulco G, Acunzo G, Sammartino A, Galli V (2004): Comparison of intranasal and transdermal estradiol on nasal mucosa in postmenopausal women. *Menopause* 11:447–455.

553. Natale V, Albertazzi P, Zini M, Di Micco R (2001): Exploration of cyclical changes in memory and mood in postmenopausal women taking sequential combined oestrogen and progestogen preparations. *BJOG* 108(3):286–290.

554. National Center for Health Statistics (2005): Table 29 (page 1 of 4). Age-related death rates for selected causes of death, according to sex, race, and Hispanic origin: United States, selected years 1950–2003. Health.

555. Naunton M, Hadithy AFYA, Brouwers JRBJ, Archer DF (2006): Estradiol gel: Review of the pharmacology, pharmacokinetics, efficacy, and safety in menopausal women. *Menopause* 13:517–527.

556. Nelson ME, Wernick S (2000): *Strong Women Stay Young*. Rev. ed. New York: Bantam Books.

557. Neves-e-Castro M (2003): Some comments on the Million Women Study. *Climacteric* 6:357.

558. Nichols CM, Gill EJ (2002): Thermal balloon endometrial ablation for management of acute uterine hemorrhage. *Obstet Gynecol* 100(5):1092–1094.

559. Nikander E, Kilkkinen A, Metsa-Heikkila M, Adlercreutz H, Pietinen P, Tiitinen A, Ylikorkala O (2003): A randomized placebo-controlled crossover trial with phytoestrogens in treatment of menopause in breast cancer patients. *Obstet Gynecol* 101:1213–1220.

560. Nikander E, Rutanen EM, Nieminen P, Wahlstrom T, Ylikorkala O, Tiitinen A (2005): Lack of effect of isoflavonoids on the vagina and endometrium in postmenopausal women. *Fertil Steril* 83:137–142.

561. Norman SA, Berlin JA, Weber AL, Strom BL, Daling JR, Weiss LK, Marchbanks PA, Bernstein L, Voigt LF, McDonald JA, Ursin G, Liff JM, Burkman RT, Malone KE, Simon MS, Folger SG, Deapen D, Wingo PA, Spirtas R (2003): Combined effect of oral contraceptive use and hormone replacement therapy on breast cancer risk in postmenopausal women. *Cancer Causes and Control* 14:933–943.

562. Norton P (2006): New technology in gynecologic surgery. Is new necessarily better? *Obstet Gynecol* 108:707–708.

563. Notelovitz M, John VA, Good WR (2002): Effectiveness of Alora estradiol matrix transdermal delivery system in improving lumbar bone mineral density in healthy, postmenopausal women. *Menopause* 9:343–353.

564. Nozaki M, Hashimoto K, Nakano H (2004): Relationship between bone resorption and adrenal sex steroids and their derivatives in oophorectomized women. *Fertil Steril* 82:1556–1560.

565. Nygaard I (2006): Editorial: Urogynecology—The importance of long-term follow up. *Obstet Gynecol* 108:244–245.

566. Nygaard I, Bradley C, Brandt D (2004): Pelvic organ prolapse in older women: Prevalence and risk factors. *Obstet Gynecol* 100(3):489–497.

567. Nygaard I, Girts T, Fultz NH, Kinchen K, Pohl G, Sternfeld B (2005): Is urinary incontinence a barrier to exercise in women? *Obstet Gynecol* 106:307–314.

568. Nygaard IE, Heit M (2004): Stress urinary incontinence. *Obstet Gynecol* 104: 607–620.

569. Nystrom L, Andersson I, Frisell J, Nordenskjold B, Rutqvist LE (2002): Long-term effects of mammography screening: Updated overview of the Swedish randomized trials. *Lancet* 359:15–16.

570. O'Hanlan KA, Lopez L, Dibble SL, Garnier A, Huang GS, Leuchtenberger M (2003): Total laparoscopic hysterectomy: Body mass index and outcomes. *Obstet Gynecol* 102:1384–1392.

571. O'Meara ES, Rossing MA, Daling JR, Elmore JG, Barlow WE, Weiss NS (2001): Hormone replacement therapy after a diagnosis of breast cancer in relation to recurrence and mortality. *JNCI* 93(10):754–762.

572. Obermeyer CM, Reynolds RF, Price K, Abraham A (2004): Therapeutic decisions for menopause: Results of the DAMES project in central Massachusetts. *Menopause* 11:456–465.

573. Olive DL (2005): Editorial: Dogma, skepsis, and the analytic method: The role of prophylactic oophorectomy at the time of hysterectomy. *Obstet Gynecol* 106:1–2.

574. Omodei U, Ferrazzi E, Ramazzotto F, Becorpi A, Grimaldi E, Scarselli G, Spagnolo D, Spagnolo L, Torri W (2004): Endometrial evaluation with transvaginal ultrasound during hormone therapy: A prospective multicenter study. *Fertil Steril* 81(6):1632–1637.

575. Ondrizek RR, Chan PJ, Patton WC, King A (1999): An alternative medicine study of herbal effects on the penetration of zona-free hamster oocytes and the integrity of sperm deoxyribonucleic acid. *Fertil Steril* 71:517–518.

576. Oparil S (1999): Hormones and vasoprotection. *Hypertension* 33:170–176.

577. Ornan D, White R, Pollak J, Tal M (2003): Pelvic embolization for intractable postpartum hemorrhage: Long-term follow-up and implications for fertility. *Obstet Gynecol* 102.

578. Os I, Os A, Abdelnoor M, Larsen A, Birkeland K, Westheim A (2003): Plasma leptin in postmenopausal women with coronary artery disease: Effect of transdermal 17b-estradiol and intermittent medroxyprogesterone acetate. *Climacteric* 6:204–210.

579. Ossewaarde ME, Bots ML, Verbeek AL, Peeters PH, van der Graaf Y, van der Schouw YT (2005): Age at menopause, cause-specific mortality and total life expectancy. *Epidem* 16:556–662.

580. Owen L (1993): *Her Blood Is Gold*. New York: HarperCollins.

581. Paffenberger R, Hyde R, Wiag L, Steinmetz C (1984): A natural history of athleticism and cardiovascular health. *JAMA* 252:491–495.

582. Paganini-Hill A, Corrada MM, Kawas CH (2006): Increased longevity in older users of postmenopausal estrogen therapy: The Leisure World Cohort Study. *Menopause* 13:12–18.

583. Page JH, Colditz GA, Rifai N, Barbieri RL, Willett WC, Hankinson SE (2004): Plasma adrenal androgens and risk of breast cancer in premenopausal women. *Cancer Epidemiology, Biomarkers and Prevention* 13(6):1032–1036.

584. Pal L (2006): Editorial: Progesterone: A "weight watcher's pill" for reproductively aging women. *Menopause* 13(2):166–167.

585. Palacios S (2003): The "Million Women" Study should not change HRT prescription. *Maturitas* 46(2):97–98.

586. Palacios S, Castelo-Branco C, Cifuentes I, von Helde S, Baro L, Tapia-Ruano C, Menendez C, Rueda C (2005): Changes in bone turnover markers after calcium-enriched milk supplementation in healthy postmenopausal women: A randomized, double-blind, prospective clinical trial. *Menopause* 12:63–68.

587. Pan H, Li C, Cheng Y, Wu M, Chang F (2003): Quantification of ovarian stromal Doppler signals in postmenopausal women receiving hormone replacement therapy. *Menopause* 10:366–372.

588. Parasrampuria J, Schwartz K, Petesch R (1998): Letter to the editor: Quality control of dehydroepiandrosterone dietary supplement products. *JAMA* 280:1565.

589. Parekh M, Minassian VA, Poplawsky D (2006): Bilateral bladder erosion of a transobturator tape mesh. *Obstet Gynecol* 108:713–715.

590. Parisky YR, Sardi A, Hamm R, Hughes K, Esserman L, Rust S, Callahan K (2003): Efficacy of computerized infrared imaging analysis to evaluate mammographically suspicious lesions. *AJR* 180:263–269.

591. Park M, Ross GW, Petrovitch H, White LR, Masaki KH, Nelson JS, Tanner CM, Curb JD, Blanchette PL, Abbott RD (2005): Consumption of milk and calcium in midlife and the future risk of Parkinson's disease. *Neurology* 64:1047–1051.

592. Parker WH, Broder MS, Liu Z, Shoupe D, Farquhar C, Berek JS (2006): Letters to the editors: Response to commentaries on retention of the ovaries and long-term survival after hysterectomy. *Climacteric* 9:396–400.

593. Parker WH, Broder MS, Lui Z, Shoupe D, Farquhar C, Berek J (2005): Ovarian conservation at the time of hysterectomy for benign disease. *Obstet Gynecol* 106: April 2006.

594. Payne JF, Haney AF (2003): Serious complications of uterine artery embolization for conservative treatment of fibroids. *Fertil Steril* 79(1):128–131.

595. Peale NV (1956): *The Power of Positive Thinking.* New York: Random House.

596. Pearson Murphy BE, Abbott FV, Allison CM, Watts C, Ghadirian AM (2004): Elevated levels of some neuroactive progesterone metabolites, particularly isopregnanolone, in women with chronic fatigue syndrome. *Psychneuroendocrinology* 29:245–268.

597. Peeyananjarassri K, Baber R (2005): Effects of low-dose hormone therapy on menopausal symptoms, bone mineral density, endometrium, and the cardiovascular system: A review of randomized clinical trials. *Climacteric* 8:13–23.

598. Pelage JP, Le Dref O, Soyer P, Kardache M, Dahan H, Abitbol M, Merland MM, Ravina JH, Rymer R (2000): Fibroid-related menorrhagia: Treatment with superselective embolization of the uterine arteries and midterm follow-up. *Radiology* 215:428–431.

599. Penteado SRL, Fonseca AM, Bagnoli VR, Assis JS, Pinotti JA (2003): Sexuality in healthy postmenopausal women. *Climacteric* 6:321–329.

600. Perry HM III, Horowitz M, Morley JH, et al. (1996): Aging and bone metabolism in African American and Caucasian women. *J Clin End* 81:1108–1117.

601. Peyote M, Fabio E, Mokena AB, Renaldo M, Moodier U, Viand P (2003): Effect of soy-derived isoflavones on hot flushes, endometrial thickness, and the pulsatility index of the uterine and cerebral arteries. *Fertil Steril* 79:1112–1117.

602. Phillips LS, Langer RD (2005): Postmenopausal hormone therapy: Critical reappraisal and a unified hypothesis. *Fertil Steril* 83(3):558–566.

603. Pines A (2005): Editorial: Compliance with hormone therapy after Women's Health Initiative: Who is to blame? *Menopause* 12:363–365.

604. Pines A, Sturdee DW, Birkhauser M (2006): WHI and breast cancer: A response to a recent publication from the WHI. *Climacteric* 6:242–243.
605. Polan ML, Warrington JA, Chen B, Mahadevappa M, Wang H, Wen Y (2003): Bench to bedside: Clinical opportunities for microarray analysis. *Fertil Steril* 80(2):291–292.
606. Poli A, Bruschi F, Cesana B, Rossi M, Paoletti R, Crosignani PG (2003): Plasma low-density lipoprotein cholesterol and bone mass densitometry in postmenopausal women. *Obstet Gynecol* 102(5):922–926.
607. Polo-Kantola P, Rauhala E, Helenius H, Erkkola R, Irjala K (2003): Breathing during sleep in menopause: A randomized, controlled, crossover trial with estrogen therapy. *Obstet Gynecol* 102:68–75.
608. Pors-Nielsen S, Barenholdt O, Hermansen F, Munk-Jensen N (1994): Magnitude and pattern of skeletal response to long-term continuous and cyclic sequential oestrogen/progestin treatment. *Br J Obste* 101:319–324.
609. Porthouse J, Cockayne S, King C, Saxon L, Steele E, Aspray T, Baverstock M, Birks Y, Dumville J, Francis R, Iglesias C, Puffer S, Sutcliffe A, Watt I, Torgerson D (2005): Randomised controlled trial of calcium and supplementation with cholecalciferol (Vitamin D3) for prevention of fractures in primary care. *BMJ* 330:1003–1010.
610. Post HS, van der Mooren MJ, Stehouwer CD, van Baal WM, Mijatovic V, Schalkwijk CG, Kenemans P. (2002): Effects of transdermal and oral oestrogen replacement therapy on C-reactive protein levels in postmenopausal women: A randomised, placebo-controlled trial. *Throm Haemost* 88:605–610.
611. Pradhan AD, Manson JE, Rossouw JE, Siscovick DS, Mouton CP, Rifai N, Wallace RB, Jackson RD, Pettinger MB, Ridker PM (2002): Inflammatory biomarkers, hormone replacement therapy, and incident coronary heart disease: Prospective analysis from the Women's Health Initiative Observational Study. *JAMA* 288(8):980–987.
612. Primatesta P, Falaschetti E, Poulter NR (2003): Influence of hormone replacement therapy on C-reactive protein: Population-based data. *J Cardiovasc Risk* 10:57–60.
613. Prior JC (1990): Progesterone as a bone trophic hormone. *Endocr Rev* 11:386–398.
614. Prior JC (1993): Progesterone and its role in bone remodelling. In Ziegler R et al., eds. *Sex, Steroids, and Bone.* Springer Verlag:29–56.
615. Prior JC (1998): Perimenopause: The complex endocrinology of the menopausal transition. *Endocr Rev* 19:397–428.
616. Prior JC, Nielsen JD, Hitchcock CL, Williams LA, Vigna YM, Dean CB (2007): Medroxyprogesterone and conjugated estrogen are equivalent for hot flushes—a one-year randomized double blind trial following premenopausal ovariectomy. *Clinical Science* 1–21.
617. Prior JC, Vigna YM, Barr SI, Rexworthy C, Lentle, BC (1994): Cyclic medroxyprogesterone treatment increases bone density: A controlled trial in active women with menstrual cycle disturbances. *Am J Med* 96:521–530.
618. Prior JC, Vigna YM, Schecter MT, Burgess AE (1990): Spinal bone loss and ovulatory disturbances. *NEJM* 323:1221–1227.
619. Prior JC, Vigna YM, Wark JD, et al. (1997): Premenopausal ovariectomy-related bone loss: A randomized, double-blind, one-year trial of conjugated estrogen or medroxyprogesterone acetate. *J Bone Min* 12:1851–1863.

620. Proctor DN, Koch DW, Newcomer SC, Le KU, Leuenberger UA (2003): Impaired leg vasodilation during dynamic exercise in healthy older women. *J Appl Physiol* 95:1963–1970.

621. Pron, G (2006): New uterine-preserving therapies raise questions about interdisciplinary management and the role of surgery for symptomatic fibroids. *Fertil Steril* 85:44–45.

622. Pron G, Cohen M, Soucie J, Garvin G, Vanderburgh L, Bell S (2003): The Ontario Uterine Fibroid Embolization Trial. Part 1. Baseline patient characteristics, fibroid burden, and impact on life. *Fertil Steril* 79(1):112–119.

623. Province MA, Hadley EC, Hornbrook MC, et al. (1995): The effects of exercise on falls in elderly patients: A preplanned meta-analysis of the FICSIT trials. *JAMA* 273:1341–1347.

624. Punnonen R, et al. (1997): Impaired ovarian function and risk factors for atherosclerosis in pre-menopausal women. *Maturitas* 27:238. Reprinted.

625. Queenan JT (2003): Smoking: The cloudy, smelly plague. *Obstet Gynecol* 102:893–894.

626. Rafii A, Jacob D, Deval B (2006): Obturator abscess after transobturator tape for stress urinary incontinence. *Obstet Gynecol* 108:720–723.

627. Rako S (1996): *The Hormone of Desire: The Truth about Testosterone, Sexuality, and Menopause.* New York: Rivers Press.

628. Rapp PR, Morrison JH, Roberts JA (2003): Cyclic estrogen replacement improves cognitive function in aged ovariectomized rhesus monkeys. *Neuroscience* 23(13):5708–5714.

629. Rapp SR, Espeland MA, Shumaker SA, Henderson VW, Brunner RL, Manson JE, Gass MLS, Stefanick ML, Lane DS, Hays J, Johnson KC, Coker LH, Dailey M, Bowen D (2003): Effect of estrogen plus progestin on global cognitive function in postmenopausal women. The Women's Health Initiative Memory Study: A randomized controlled trial. *JAMA* 289(20):2663–2672.

630. Rasgon N, Magnusson C, Johansson A, Pedersen N, Elman S, Gatz M (2005): Endogenous and exogenous hormone exposure and risk of cognitive impairment in Swedish twins: A preliminary study. *Psychoneur* 30:558–567.

631. Ravina JH, Bouret JM, Ciraru-Vigneron N, Repiquet D, Herbreteau D, Aymard A, le Dref O, Merland JJ, Ferrand J (1997): Recourse to particular arterial embolization in the treatment of some uterine leiomyoma. *Bull Acad* 181:233–243.

632. Ravina JH, Bouret JM, Fried D, Benifla JL, Darai E, Pennehouat G, Madelenat P, Herbreteau D, Houdard E, Merland JJ (1995): Value of preoperative embolization of uterine fibroma: Report of a multicenter series of 31 cases. *Contracept Fertile Sex* 23(1):45–49.

633. Ravina JH, Ciraru-Vigneron N, Aymard A, Ferrand J, Merland JJ (1999): Uterine artery embolization for fibroid disease: Results of a 6 year study. *Min Invas Ther & Allied Technol* 8:441–447.

634. Ravina JH, Herbreteau D, Ciraru-Vigneron N, Bouret JM, Houdart E, Aymard A, Merland JJ (1995): Arterial embolisation to treat uterine myomata. *Lancet* 346:671–672.

635. Ravina JH, Vigneron NC, Aymard A, le Dref O, Merland JJ (2000): Pregnancy after embolization of uterine myoma: Report of 12 cases. *Fertil Steril* 73:1241–1243.

636. Raymundo N, Yu-cheng B, Zi-yan H, Lai C, Leung K, Subramaniam R, Bin-rong C, Ling YS, Nasri N, Calimon N (2004): Treatment of atrophic vaginitis

with topical conjugated equine estrogens in postmenopausal Asian women. *Climacteric* 7:312–318.

637. RECORD Trial Group (2005): Oral vitamin D3 and calcium for secondary prevention of low-trauma fractures in elderly people (Randomized Evaluation of Calcium Or vitamin D, RECORD): A randomized placebo-controlled trial. *Lancet* 365: www.thelancet.com.

638. Reed SD, Cushing-Haugen KL, Daling JR, Scholes D, Schwartz SM (2004): Postmenopausal estrogen and progestogen therapy and the risk of uterine leiomyomas. *Menopause* 11(2):214–226.

639. Regitz-Zagrosek V (2003): Cardiovascular disease in postmenopausal women. *Climacteric* 6:13–20.

640. Reid IR, Mason B, Horne A, Ames R, Clearwater J, Bava U, Orr-Walker B, Wu F, Evans MC, Gamble GD (2002): Effects of calcium supplementation on serum lipid concentrations in normal older women: A randomized controlled trial. *Am J Med* 112(5):343–347.

641. Rhodes JC, Kjerulff KH, Langenberg PW, Guzinski GM (1999): Hysterectomy and sexual functioning. *JAMA* 282:1934–1941.

642. Rice MM, Graves AB, McCurry SM, et al. (1997): Estrogen replacement therapy and cognitive function in postmenopausal women without dementia. *Am J Med* 103:26S–35S.

643. Rice MM, Graves AB, McCurry SM, Gibbons LE, Bowen JD, McCormick WC, Larson EB (2000): Postmenopausal estrogen and estrogen-progestin use and 2-year rate of cognitive change in a cohort of older Japanese American women. *Arch Intern Med*:1641–1649.

644. Richman S, Edusa V, Fadiel A, Naftolin F (2006): Personal perspective: Low-dose estrogen therapy for prevention of osteoporosis: Working our way back to monotherapy. *Menopause* 13:148–155.

645. Richter HE, Burgio KL, Clements RH, Goode PS, Redden DT, Varner RE (2005): Urinary and anal incontinence in morbidly obese women considering weight loss surgery. *Obstet Gynecol* 106:1272–1278.

646. Richy F, Bruyere O, Ethgen O, et al. (2003): Structural and symptomatic efficacy of glucosamine and chondroitin in knee osteoarthritis: A comprehensive meta-analysis. *Arch Inter* 163:1514–1522.

647. Ringa V, Legare F, Dodin S, Norton J, Godin D, Breart G (2004): Hormone therapy prescription among physicians in France and Quebec. *Menopause* 11(1):89–97.

648. Robinson D, Friedman L, Marcus R, Tinklenberg J, Yesavage J (1994): Estrogen replacement therapy and memory in older women. *J Am Ger Soc* 42(9):919–922.

649. Robinson G (1996): Cross cultural perspectives on menopause. *JNMD* 184(8):453–458.

650. Rolnick SJ, Kopher RA, DeFor TA, Kelley ME (2005): Hormone use and patient concerns after the findings of the Women's Health Initiative. *Menopause* 12: 399–404.

651. Romero AA, Hardart A, Kobak W, Qualls C, Rogers R (2003): Validation of a Spanish version of the pelvic organ prolapse incontinence sexual questionnaire. *Obstet Gynecol* 102(5):1000–1005.

652. Rortveit G, Brown JS, Thom DH, Van Den Eeden SK, Creasman JM, Subak LL (2007): Symptomatic pelvic organ prolapse: Prevalence and risk factors in a population-based, racially diverse cohort. *Obstet Gynecol* 1396–1403.

653. Rosenberg L, Park S (2002): Verbal and spatial functions across the menstrual cycle in healthy young women. *Psychneuroendocrinology* 27:835–841.

654. Ross RK, Paganini-Hill A, Wan PC, Pike MC (2000): Effect of hormone replacement therapy on breast cancer risk: Estrogen versus estrogen plus progestin. *JNCI* 92(4):328–332.

655. Rossetti A, Sizzi O, Soranna L, Cucinelli F, Mancuso S, Lanzone A (2001): Long-term results of laparoscopic myomectomy: Recurrence rate in comparison with abdominal myomectomy. *Human Reproduction* 16(4):4–770.

656. Rossouw et al. (2002): Risks and benefits of estrogen plus progestin in healthy postmenopausal women: Principal results from the WHI randomised controlled trial. *JAMA* 288:321–333.

657. Roy KH, Mattox JH (2003): Endometrial ablation for perimenopausal menorrhagia. *Menopause* 12(5):13–17.

658. Rudolph I, Palombo-Kinne E, Kirsch B, Mellinger U, Breitbarth H, Graser T (2004): Influence of a continuous combined HRT (2 mg estradiol valerate and 2 mg dienogest) on postmenopausal depression. *Climacteric* 7(3):301–311.

659. Ruml LA, Sakhaee K, Peterson R, Adams-Huet B, Pak CY (1999): The effect of calcium citrate on bone density in the early and mid-postmenopausal period: A randomized placebo-controlled study. *Am J Ther* 6:6:325–326.

660. Rupprecht R (2003): Neuroactive steroids: Mechanisms of action and neuropsychopharmacological properties. *Psychneuroendocrinology* 28:139–168.

661. Saed GM, Diamond MP (2003): Effect of glucose on the expression of type I collagen and transforming growth factor b1 in cultured human peritoneal fibroblasts. *Fertil Steril* 79:158–163.

662. Saed GM, Diamond MP (2003): Modulation of the expression of tissue plasminogen activator and its inhibitor by hypoxia in human peritoneal and adhesion fibroblasts. *Fertil Steril* 79(1):164–157.

663. Sagiv R, Sadan O, Boaz M, Dishi M, Schechter E, Golan A (2006): A new approach to office hysteroscopy compared with traditional hysteroscopy. *Obstet Gynecol* 108:387–391.

664. Salpeter S (2005): Invited editorial: Hormone therapy for younger postmenopausal women: How can we make sense out of the evidence? *Climacteric* 8: 307–310.

665. Sambrook P (2005): Vitamin D and fractures: Quo vadis? *Lancet* 365: 1599–1600.

666. Samsioe G (2001): Editorial: Lipid oxidation and the road to arteriosclerosis. *Menopause* 8:395–397.

667. Samsioe G (2004): Transdermal hormone therapy: Gels and patches. *Climacteric* 7:347–356.

668. Sanada M, Tsuda M, Kodama I, Sakashita T, Nakagawa H, Ohama K (2004): Substitution of transdermal estradiol during oral estrogen-progestin therapy in postmenopausal women: Effects on hypertriglyceridemia. *Menopause* 11(3):331–336.

669. Sandmark H, Hogstedt C, Lewold S, Vingard E (1999): Osteoarthrosis of the knee in men and women in association with overweight, smoking, hormone therapy. *Ann Rheum Dis* 58:151–155.

670. Sarrel PM (2003): Care of the surgically menopausal woman. *Menopause Mgmt* 12(2):26–31.

671. Sarrel PM (2005): Sexual dysfunction: Treat or refer. *Obstet Gynecol* 106:834–839.
672. Sarrel PM (2006): Editorial: Testosterone therapy for postmenopausal decline in sexual desire: Implications of a new study. *Menopause* 13(3):328–330.
673. Sarti CD, Chiantera A, Graziottin A, Ognisanti F, Sidoli C, Mincigrucci M, Parazzini F (2005): Hormone therapy and sleep quality in women around menopause. *Menopause* 12(5):545–551.
674. Scambia G, Gallo D (2006): The role of phytochemicals in menopause: A new actor on the scene of alternative treatment options. *Menopause* 13:724–726.
675. Schaumberg DA, Buring JE, Sullivan DA, Dana MR (2001): Hormone replacement therapy and dry eye syndrome. *JAMA* 286:2114–2119.
676. Schiff R, Bulpitt CJ, Wesnes KA, Rajkumar C (2005): Short-term transdermal estradiol therapy, cognition and depressive symptoms in healthy older women. A randomized placebo controlled pilot cross-over study. *Psychneuroendocrinology* 30:309–315.
677. Schmidt JB, Binder M, Demschik G, Bieglmayer C, Reiner A (1996): Treatment of skin aging with topical estrogens. *Int J Derm* 35(9):669–674.
678. Schmidt PJ, Daly CR, Bloch M, Smith MJ, Danaceau MA, St. Clair LS, Murphy JH, Haq N, Rubinow DR (2005): Dehydroepiandrosterone monotherapy in midlife-onset major and minor depression. *Arch Gen Psych* 62:154–162.
679. Schmidt PJ, Murphy JH, Haq N, Danaceau MA, Simpson St. Clair L (2002): Basal plasma hormone levels in depressed perimenopausal women. *Psychneuroendocrinology* 27:907–920.
680. Schneeman BO (1999): Editorial: Building scientific consensus: The importance of dietary fiber. *Am J Clin* 69:1.
681. Schneider DL, Barrett-Connor EL, Morton DJ (1997): Timing of postmenopausal estrogen for optimal bone mineral density. The Rancho Bernardo study. *JAMA* 277:543–547.
682. Schneider HPG, Mueck AO, Kuhl H (2005): Presidential comment: IARC monographs program on carcinogenicity of combined hormonal contraceptives and menopausal therapy. *Climacteric* 8:311–316.
683. Schousboe JT, DeBold CR, Bowles C, Glickstein S, Rubino RK (2002): Prevalence of vertebral compression fracture deformity by X-ray absorptiometry of lateral thoracic and lumbar spines in a population referred for bone densitometry. *Journal of Clinical Densitometry* 5:239–46.
684. Schwartz LM, Woloshin S, Fowler FJ, Welch HG (2004): Enthusiasm for cancer screening in the United States. *JAMA* 291(1):71–78.
685. Scialli AR (2004): Clues as to the molecular basis for uterine fibroids. *Fertil Steril* 81(5):1432.
686. Seeger H, Wallwiener D, Mueck AO (2001): Effect of medroxyprogesterone acetate and norethisterone on serum-stimulated and estradiol-inhibited proliferation of human coronary artery smooth muscle cells. *Menopause* 8:5–9.
687. Sendag F, Terek MC, Ozsener S, Oztekin K, Bilgin O, Bilgen I, Memis A (2001): Mammographic density changes during different postmenopausal hormone replacement therapies. *Fertil Steril* 76:445–450.
688. Shah NR, Borenstein J, Dubois RW (2005): Postmenopausal hormone therapy and breast cancer: A systematic review and meta-analysis. *Menopause* 12:668–678.
689. Shakir YA, Samsioe G, Nerbrand C, Lidfeldt J (2004): Combined hormone therapy in postmenopausal women with features of metabolic syndrome. Results

from a population-based study of Swedish women: Women's Health in the Lund Area study. *Menopause* 11(5):549–555.

690. Shakir YA, Samsioe G, Nyberg P, Lidfeldt J, Nerbrand C (2004): Cardiovascular risk factors in middle-aged women and the association with use of hormone therapy: Results from a population-based study of Swedish women. The Women's Health in the Lund Area (WHILA) Study. *Climacteric* 7(3):274–283.

691. Shapiro S (2004): The Million Women Study: Potential biases do not allow uncritical acceptance of the data. *Climacteric* 7:3–7.

692. Shapiro S (2006): Controversial issues: Invited commentary. Does retention of the ovaries improve long-term survival after hysterectomy? The validity of the epidemiological evidence. *Climacteric* 9:161–163.

693. Shaywitz SE, Naftolin F, Zelterman D, Marchione KE, Holahan JM, Palter SF, Shaywitz BA (2003): Better oral reading and short-term memory in midlife, postmenopausal women taking estrogen. *Menopause* 10(5):420–426.

694. Shifren JL (2003): Editorial: Is there a role for testosterone therapy in premenopausal women?. *Menopause* 10(5):383–384.

695. Shifren JL (2006): Editorial: Is testosterone or estradiol the hormone of desire? A novel study of the effects of testosterone treatment and aromatase inhibition in postmenopausal women. *Menopause* 13:8–9.

696. Shifren JL, Braunstein GD, Simon JA, Casson PA, Buster JE, Redmond GP, Burki RE, Ginsburg ES, Rosen RC, Leiblum SR, Caramelli KE, Mazer NA (2000): Transdermal testosterone treatment in women with impaired sexual function after oophorectomy. *NEJM* 343:682–688.

697. Shifren JL, Nahum R, Mazer NA (1998): Incidence of sexual dysfunction in surgically menopausal women. *Menopause* 5:189–190.

698. Shilling D (2005): *Medical Malpractice. Lawyers' Desk Book.* New York, Aspen Publishers.

699. Shimomura Y, Matsuo H, Samoto T, Maruo T (1998): Up-regulation by progesterone of proliferating cell nuclear antigen and epidermal growth factor expression in human uterine leiomyoma. *JCEM* 83:2192–2198.

700. Shin M, Holmes S, Hankinson K, Wu G, Colditz G, Willett C (2002): Intake of dairy products, calcium, and vitamin D and risk of breast cancer. *J Natl Cancer Inst* 94:1301–1311.

701. Shively CA (1998): Behavioral and neurobiological effects of estrogen replacement therapy and a history of triphasic oral contraceptive exposure. *Psychneuroendocrinology* 23:713–732.

702. Showstack J, Kuppermann M, Lin F, Vittinghoff E, Varner RE, Summitt Jr RL, McNeeley SG, Learman LA, Richter H, Hulley S, Washington AE (2004): Resource use for total and supracervical hysterectomies: Results of a randomized trial. *Obstet Gynecol* 103(5):834–841.

703. Shulman LP, Harari D (2004): Low-dose transdermal estradiol for symptomatic perimenopause. *Menopause* 11:34–39.

704. Shumaker SA, Legault C, Rapp SR, Thal L, Wallace RB, Ockene JK, Hendrix SL, Jones III BN, Assaf AR, Jackson RD, Kotchen JM, Wassertheil-Smoller S, Wactawski-Wende J (2003): Estrogen plus progestin and the incidence of dementia and mild cognitive impairment in postmenopausal women. *JAMA* 289(20):2651–2662.

705. Siddle N, Sarrel P, Whitehead M (1987): The effect of hysterectomy on the age of ovarian failure: Identification of a subgroup of women with premature loss of ovarian function and literature review. *Fertil Steril* 47:94–100.

706. Reference removed at author's request.
707. Sidelmann JJ, Jespersen J, Anderson LF, Skouby SO (2003): Hormone replacement therapy and hypercoagulability. Results from the Prospective Collaborative Danish Climacteric Study. *BJOG* 110:541–547.
708. Silva I, Mello LEAM, Freymuller E, Haidar MA, Baracat EC (2003): Onset of estrogen replacement as a critical effect on synaptic density of CA1 hippocampus in ovariectomized adult rats. *Menopause* 10(5):406–411.
709. Silva WA, Pauls RN, Segal JL, Rooney CM, Kleeman SD, Karram MM (2006): Uterosacral ligament vault suspension: Five-year outcomes. *Obstet Gynecol* 108:255–263.
710. Simkin-Silverman LR, Wing RR, Boraz MA, Kuller LH (2003): Lifestyle intervention can prevent weight gain during menopause: Results from a 5-year randomized clinical trial. *Ann Behav* 26:212–220.
711. Simko V (1978): Physical exercise and the prevention of atherosclerosis and cholesterol gallstone. *Postgrad M* 54:270–277.
712. Simoncini T, Fornari L, Mannella P, Caruso A, Garibaldi S, Baldacci C, Genazzani AR (2005): Activation of nitric oxide synthesis in human endothelial cells by red clover extracts. *Menopause* 12:69–77.
713. Sinaii N, Cleary SD, Younes N, Ballweg ML, Stratton P (2007): Treatment utilization for endometriosis symptoms: A cross-sectional survey study of lifetime experience. *Fertil Steril*, 87:1277–1286.
714. Sitruk-Ware R (2005): Editorial: Estrogen and progestogens—different routes of administration. *Climacteric* 8(Suppl 1):1–2.
715. Sitruk-Ware R, Husmann F, Thijssen JHH, Skouby SO, Fruzzetti F, Hanker J, Huber J, Druckmann R (2004): Role of progestins with partial antiandrogenic effects. *Climacteric* 7(3):238–254.
716. Sitruk-Ware RL (2003): Hormone therapy and the cardiovascular system: The critical role of progestins. *Climacteric* 6:21–28.
717. Slater CC, Souter I, Zhang C, Guan C, Stanczyk FZ, Mishell DR (2001): Pharmacokinetics of testosterone after percutaneous gel or buccal administration. *Fertil Steril* 76:32–37.
718. Smith G (2005): Letter to the editor: Ovarian conservation at the time of hysterectomy for the benign disease. *Obstet Gynecol* 106:1413.
719. Smith JC, Tarocco G, Merazzi F, Salzmann U (2006): Are generic formulations of carvedilol of inferior pharmaceutical quality compared with the branded formulation? *Curr Med Res Opin* 4:709–720.
720. Smith NL, Heckbert SR, Lemaitre RN, Reiner AP, Lumley T, Weiss NS, Larson EB, Rosendaal FR, Psaty BM (2004): Esterified estrogens and conjugated equine estrogens and the risk of venous thrombosis. *JAMA* 292(13):1581–1587.
721. Smith YR, Minoshima S, Kuhl DE, Zubieta JK (2001): Effects of long-term hormone therapy on cholinergic synaptic concentrations in healthy postmenopausal women. *JCEM* 86(2):679–684.
722. Smith-Bindman R, Chu PW, Miglioretti DL, Sickles EA, Blanks R, Ballard-Barbash R, Bobo JK, Lee NC, Wallis MG, Patnick J, Kerlikowske K (2003): Comparison of screening mammography in the United States and the United Kingdom. *JAMA* 290(16):2129–2137.
723. Smolders RGV, Sipkema P, Kenemans P, Stehouwer CDA, van der Mooren MJ (2004): Homocysteine impairs estrogen-induced vasodilation in isolated rat arterioles. *Menopause* 11(1):98–103.

724. Soliman NF, Hillard TC (2006): Hormone replacement therapy in women with past history of endometriosis. *Climacteric* 9:325–335.
725. Solis-Ortiz S, Guevara MA, Corsi-Cabrera M (2004): Performance in a test demanding prefrontal functions is favored by early luteal phase progesterone: An electroencephalographic study. *Psychneuroendocrinology* 29:1047–1057.
726. Solomon SD (2005): A new wave of behavior change intervention research. *Ann Behav* 29:1–3.
727. Sozen I, Arici A (2002): Interactions of cytokines, growth factors, and the extracellular matrix in the cellular biology of uterine leiomyomata. *Fertil Steril* 78(1):1–12.
728. Speroff L (2003): Efficacy and tolerability of a novel estradiol vaginal ring for relief of menopausal symptoms. *Obstet Gynecol* 102(4):823–834.
729. Speroff L (2005): Editorial: Postmenopausal hormone therapy and cardiovascular disease: One view of the elephant. *Menopause* 12(4):357–358.
730. Speroff L (2007): Gonads are the heart of the matter. *Menopause* 14:342–344.
731. Speroff L, Haney AF, Gilbert RD, Ellman H (2006): Efficacy of a new, oral estradiol acetate formulation for relief of menopause symptoms. *Menopause* 13: 442–450.
732. Spies JB, Bruno J, Czeyda-Pommersheim F, Magee ST, Ascher SA, Jha RC (2005): Long-term outcome of uterine artery embolization of leiomyomata. *Obstet Gynecol* 106:933–939.
733. Spies JB, Spector A, Roth AR, Baker CM, Mauro L, Murphy-Skrynarz K (2002): Complications after uterine artery embolization for leiomyomas. *Obstet Gynecol* 100(5):873–880.
734. St. Germain A, Peterson CT, Robinson JG, Alekel DL (2001): Isoflavone-rich or isoflavone-poor soy protein does not reduce menopausal symptoms during 24 weeks of treatment. *Menopause* 8:17–26.
735. Stahlberg C, Lynge E, Andersen ZJ, Keiding N, Ottesen B, Rank F, Hundrup YA, Obel EB, Pedersen AT (2005): Breast cancer incidence, case-fatality and breast cancer mortality in Danish women using hormone replacement therapy—a prospective observational study. *International Journal of Epidemiology* 34:931–935.
736. Stahlberg C, Pedersen AT, Lynge E, Andersen ZJ, Keiding N, Hundrup YA, Obel EB, Ottesen B (2004): Increased risk of breast cancer following different regimens of hormone replacement therapy frequently used in Europe. *Int J Cancer* 109:721–727.
737. Stanczyk F, Paulson R, Roy S (2005): Percutaneous administration of progesterone: Blood levels and endometrial protection. *Menopause* 12:232–237.
738. Stanczyk FZ (2005): "Natural" versus "synthetic" estrogens for hormone therapy: Is there a difference? *Menopause Mgmt* 14:10–19.
739. Stanford JL, Weiss NS, Voigt LF, Daling JR, Habel LA, Rossing MA (1995): Combined estrogen and progestin hormone replacement therapy in relation to risk of breast cancer in middle-aged women. *JAMA* 274(2):137–142.
740. Steege JF (2006): Too soon, too late, too often, too seldom? *Fertil Steril* 86: 1310–1311.
741. Stefanick M, Anderson GL, Margolis K, Hendrix SL, Rodabough RJ, Paskett ED, Lane DS, Hubbell FA, Assaf AR, Sarto GE, Schenken RS, Yasmeen S, Lessin L, Chlebowski RT for the WHI Investigators (2006): Effects of conjugated equine estrogens on breast cancer and mammography screening in postmenopausal women with hysterectomy. *JAMA* 295:1647–1657.

742. Steffen LM, Jacobs DR, Stevens J, Shahar E, Carithers T, Folsom AR (2003): Associations of whole-grain, refined-grain, and fruit and vegetable consumption with risks of all-cause mortality and incident coronary artery disease and ischemic stroke: The Atherosclerosis Risk in Communities (ARIC) Study. *Am J Clin* 78:383–390.

743. Steffen PR, Masters KS (2005): Does compassion mediate the intrinsic religion-health relationship? *Ann Behav* 30:217–224.

744. Steinauer JE, Waetjen E, Vittinghoff E, Subak LL, Hulley SB, Grady D, Lin F, Brown JS (2005): Postmenopausal hormone therapy: Does it cause incontinence? *Obstet Gynecol* 106:940–945.

745. Steiner AS, Hodis HN, Lobo RA, Shoupe D, Xiang M, Mack WJ (2005): Postmenopausal oral estrogen therapy and blood pressure in normotensive and hypertensive subjects: The Estrogen in the Prevention of Atherosclerosis Trial. *Menopause* 12:728–733.

746. Stevenson JC, Rioux JE, Komer L, Gelfand M (2005): 1 and 2 mg 17b-estradiol combined with sequential dydrogesterone have similar effects on the serum lipid profile of postmenopausal women. *Climacteric* 8:352–359.

747. Stewart EA (2006): Magnetic resonance imaging-guided focused ultrasound: No panacea, but nevertheless a safe step forward. *Fertil Steril* 85:49.

748. Stewart EA, Gedroyc WMW, Tempany MC, Quade BJ, Inbar Y, Ehrenstein T, Shushan A, Hindley JT, Goldin RD, David M, Sklair M, Rabinovici J (2003): Focused ultrasound treatment of uterine fibroid tumors: Safety and feasibility of a noninvasive thermoablative technique. *Obstet Gynecol* 189:48–54.

749. Stewart EA, Rabinovici J, Tempany CMC, Inbar Y, Regan L, Gastout B, Hesley G, Kim HY, Hengst S, Gedroye WM (2006): Clinical outcomes of focused ultrasound surgery for the treatment of uterine fibroids. *Fertil Steril* 85:22–29.

750. Stoleru S, Gregoire MC, Gerard D, et al. (1999): Neuroanatomical correlates of visually evoked sexual arousal in human males. *Arch Sexual Behavior* 28:1–21.

751. Stratton P (2006): The tangled web of reasons for the delay in diagnosis of endometriosis in women with chronic pelvic pain: Will the suffering end? *Fertil Steril* 86:1302–1304.

752. Studd J (2006): Controversial issues: Invited commentary. Does retention of the ovaries improve long-term survival after hysterectomy? Prophylactic oophorectomy. *Climacteric* 9:164–166.

753. Studd J, Panay N (2004): Hormones and depression in women. *Climacteric* 7:338–346.

754. Sturdee DW, MacLennan AH (2005): Editorial: Prevention of osteoporosis is still a valid aim for hormone therapy. *Climacteric* 8:97–98.

755. Subak LL, Quesenberry CP, Posner SF, Cattolica E, Soghikian K (2002): The effect of behavioral therapy on urinary incontinence: A randomized controlled trial. *Obstet Gynecol* 100(1):72–78.

756. Sumic A, Michael YL, Carlson NE, Howieson DB, Kaye JA (2007): Physical activity and the risk of dementia in oldest old. *Journal of Aging and Health* 19:242–259.

757. Sun MJ, Chen GD, Lin KC (2006): Obturator hematoma after the transobturator suburethral tape procedure. *Obstet Gynecol* 108:716–718.

758. Suparto IH, Williams JK, Fox JL, Vinten-Johansen (2005): A comparison of two progestins on myocardial ischemia—reperfusion injury in ovariectomized monkeys receiving estrogen therapy. *Coron Artery Dis* 16:301–308.

759. Suvanto-Luukkonen E, Koivunen R, Sundstrom H, Bloigu R, Karjalainen E, Haiva-Mallinen L, Tapanainen JS (2005): Citalopram and fluoxetine in the treatment of postmenopausal symptoms: A prospective, randomized, 9-month, placebo-controlled, double-blind study. *Menopause* 12:18–26.

760. Sylvestre C, Child TJ, Tulandi T, Tan SL (2003): A prospective study to evaluate the efficacy of two- and three-dimensional sonohysterography in women with intrauterine lesions. *Fertil Steril* 79(5):1222–1225.

761. Szoeke C, Cicuttini F, Guthrie J, Dennerstein L (2005): Self-reported arthritis and the menopause. *Climacteric* 8:49–55.

762. Sztefko K, Rogatko I, Milewicz T, Krzysiek J, Tomasik PJ, Szafran Z (2005): Effect of hormone therapy on the enteroinsular axis. *Menopause* 12:630–638.

763. Taguchi A, Sanada M, Suei Y, Ohtsuka M, Nakamoto T, Lee K, Tsuda M, Ohama K, Tanimoto K, Bollen A (2004): Effect of estrogen use on tooth retention, oral bone height, and oral bone porosity in Japanese postmenopausal women. *Menopause* 11(5):556–562.

764. Tamimi RM, Hankinson SE, Chen WY, Rosner B, Colditz GA (2006): Combined estrogen and testosterone and risk of breast cancer in postmenopausal women. *Arch Inter Med* 166:1483–1489.

765. Tan TL, Rafla N (2004): Retained calcified fibroid fragments after uterine artery embolization for fibroids. *Fertil Steril* 81(4):1145–1148.

766. Tang M, Jacobs D, Stern Y, Marder K, Schofield P, Gurland B, Andrews H, Mayeux R (1996): Effect of oestrogen during menopause on risk and age at onset of Alzheimer's disease. *Lancet* 348:429–432.

767. Tang Y, Janssen WGM, Hao J, Roberts JA, McKay H, Lasley B, Allen PB, Greengard P, Rapp PR, Kordower JH, Hof PR, Morrison JH (2004): Estrogen replacement increases spinophilin-immunoreactive spine number in the prefrontal cortex of female rhesus monkeys. *Cerebral Cortex* 14(2):215–223.

768. Taniguchi F, Harada T, Iwabe I, Yoshida S, Mitsunari M, Terakawa N (2004): Use of LAP DISK (abdominal wall sealing device) in laparoscopically assisted myomectomy. *Fertil Steril* 81(4):1120–1124.

769. Tanko LB, Christiansen C (2004): An update on the antiestrogenic effect of smoking: A literature review with implications for researchers and practitioners. *Menopause* 11:104–109.

770. Tanko LB, Christiansen C (2006): Adipose tissue, insulin resistance and low-grade inflammation: Implications for atherogenesis and the cardiovascular harm of estrogen plus progestogen therapy. *Climacteric* 9:169–180.

771. Tanko LB, Karsdal MA, Christiansen C (2005): The clinical potential of estrogen for the prevention of osteoarthritis: What is known and what needs to be done? *Women's Health* 1:125–132.

772. Taylor HS (2005): Judging a book by its cover: Estrogen and skin aging. *Fertil Steril* 84(2):295.

773. Tempany CM, Stewart EA, McDannold E, Quade BJ, Jolesz FA, Hynynen K (2003): MR imaging-guided focused ultrasound surgery of uterine leiomyomas: A feasibility study. *Radiology* 226:897–905.

774. Thakar R, Ayers S, Clarkson P, Stanton S, Manyonda I (2002): Outcomes after total versus subtotal abdominal hysterectomy. *NEJM* 347:1318–1325.

775. The Million Women Study Collaborative Group (1999): The Million Women Study: Design and characteristics of the study population. *Breast Cancer Res* 1:73–80.

776. The Practice Committee of the American Society for Reproductive Medicine (2006): Treatment of pelvic pain associated with endometriosis. *Fertil Steril* 86:S18–S28.

777. Thilers PP, MacDonald SWS, Herlitz A (2006): The association between endogenous free testosterone and cognitive performance: A population-based study in 35 to 90 year-old men and women. *Psychoneur* 31:565–576.

778. Thomas T, Rhodin J, Clark L, Garces A (2003): Progestins initiate adverse events of menopausal estrogen therapy. *Climacteric* 6:293–301.

779. Tice JA, Ettinger B, Ensrud D, Wallace R, Blackwell T, Cummings SR (2003): Phytoestrogen supplements for the treatment of hot flashes: The Isoflavone Clover Extract (ICE) Study. *JAMA* 290:2 290:207–214.

780. Toobert D, Glasgow RE, Barrera M, Angell K (2005): Effects of the Mediterranean lifestyle program on multiple risk behaviors and psychosocial outcomes among women at risk for heart disease. *Ann Behav Med* 29:128–137.

781. Toprak A, Erenus M, Ilhan AH, Hakler G, Fak AS, Oktay A (2005): The effect of postmenopausal hormone therapy with or without folic acid supplementation on serum homocysteine level. *Climacteric* 8:279–286.

782. Tregon ML, Blumel JE, Tarin JJ, Cano A (2003): The early response of the postmenopausal endometrium to tamoxifen: expression of estrogen receptors, progesterone receptors, and Ki-67 antigen. *Menopause* 10(2):154–279.

783. Trichopoulou A, Costacou T, Bamia C, Trichopoulos D (2003): Adherence to a Mediterranean diet and survival in a Greek population. *NEJM* 348: 2599–2608.

784. Trimble CL, Genkinger JM, Burke AE, Hoffman SC, Helzlsouer KJ, Diener-West M, Comstock GW, Alberg AJ (2005): Active and passive cigarette smoking and the risk of cervical neoplasia. *Obstet Gynecol* 174–181.

785. Trivedi DP, Doll R, Khaw KT (2003): Effect of four monthly oral vitamin D3 (cholecalciferol) supplementation on fractures and mortality in men and women living in the community: Randomized double blind controlled trial. *BMJ* 326:469–474.

786. Tropeano G, Litwicka K, Di Stasi C, Romano D, Mancuso S (2003): Permanent amenorrhea associated with endometrial atrophy after uterine artery embolization for symptomatic uterine fibroids. *Fertil Steril* 79(1):132–135.

787. Tsibris JCM, Segars J, Coppola D, Mane S, Wilbanks GD, O'Brien WF, Spellacy WN (2002): Insights from gene arrays on the development and growth regulation of uterine leiomyomata. *Fertil Steril* 78(1):114–121.

788. Tsibris JCM, Segars J, Enkemann S, Coppola D, Wilbanks GD, O'Brien WF, Spellacy WN (2003): New and old regulators of uterine leiomyoma growth from screening with DNA arrays. *Fertil Steril* 80(2):279–281.

789. Tutuncu L, Ergur A, Mungen E, Gun I, Ertekin A, Yergok Y (2005): The effect of hormone therapy on plasma homocysteine levels: A randomized clinical trial. *Menopause* 12(2):216–222.

790. Unfer V, Casini ML, Costabile L, Mignosa M, Gerli S, Di Renzo GC (2004): Endometrial effects of long-term treatment with phytoestrogens: A randomized, double-blind, placebo-controlled study. *Fertil Steril* 82:145–148.

791. Utian WH, Lederman SA, Williams BM, Vega RY, Koltun WD, Leonard TW (2004): Relief of hot flushes with new plant-derived 10-component synthetic conjugated estrogens. *Obstet Gynecol* 103:245–253.

792. Utian WH, Speroff L, Ellman H, Dart C (2005): Comparative controlled trial of a novel oral estrogen therapy, estradiol acetate, for relief of menopause symptoms. *Menopause* 12:708–715.

793. Valdivia I, Campodonico I, Tapia A, Capetillo M, Espinoza A, Lavin P (2004): Effects of tibolone and continuous combined hormone therapy on mammographic breast density and breast histochemical markers in postmenopausal women. *Fertil Steril* 81:617–623.

794. Van Amelsvoort T, Murphy DGM, Robertson D, Daly E, Whitehead M, Abel K (2003): Effects of long-term estrogen replacement therapy on growth hormone response to pyridostigmine in healthy postmenopausal women. *Psychneuroendocrinology* 28:101–112.

795. Van Baal WM, Kenemans P, Peters-Muller ER, van Vugt JM, van der Mooren MJ (1999): Sequentially combined hormone replacement therapy reduces impedance to flow within the uterine and central retinal arteries in healthy postmenopausal women. *Obstet Gynecol* 181:1365–1373.

796. Van der Mooren MJ, Franke HR (2003): The Million Women Study: No new evidence to change current opinions. *Maturitas* 46(2):99–100.

797. Van der Mooren MJ, Kenemans P (2004): The Million Women Study: A license to kill other investigations? *Eur J Obstet Gynecol Reprod Biol* 113:3–5.

798. Van der Waal JM, Bot SDM, Terwee CB, van der Windt DAWM, Bouter LM, Dekker J (2006): The course and prognosis of hip complaints in general practice. *Ann Behav* 31:297–308.

799. Van Lunsen RHW, Laan E (2004): Genital vascular responsiveness and sexual feelings in midlife women: Psychophysiologic, brain, and genital imaging studies. *Menopause* 11(6):741–748.

800. Vandelanotte C, Bourdeaudhujj I, Stallis J, Spittaels H, Brug J (2005): Efficacy of sequential or simultaneous interactive computer-tailored interventions for increasing physical activity and decreasing fat intake. *Annals of Behav Med* 29(2):138–146.

801. Vercellini P, Trespidi L, Zaina B, Vicentini S, Stellato G, Crosignani PG (2003): Gonadotropin-releasing hormone agonist treatment before abdominal myomectomy: A controlled trial. *Fertil Steril* 79(6):1390–1395.

802. Verhoeven MO, van der Mooren MJ, van de Weijer PH, Verdegem PJ, van der Burgt LMJ, Kenemans P (2005): Effect of a combination of isoflavones and Actaea racemosa Linnaeus on climacteric symptoms in healthy symptomatic perimenopausal women: A 12-week randomized, placebo-controlled, double-blind study. *Menopause* 12:412–420.

803. Vieth R (2005): The role of vitamin D in the prevention of osteoporosis. *Annals of Internal Medicine* 37:278–285.

804. Villareal DT, Binder EF, Williams DB, Schechtman KB, Yarasheski KE, Kohrt WM (1997): Bone mineral density response to estrogen replacement in frail elderly women: A randomized controlled trial. *JAMA* 286:815–820.

805. Vincent A, Riggs BL, Atkinson EJ, Oberg AL, Khosla S (2003): Effect of estrogen replacement therapy on parathyroid hormone secretion in elderly postmenopausal women. *Menopause* 10:165–171.

806. Vingard E, Alfredsson L, Malchau H (1997): Lifestyle factors and hip arthrosis. A case referent study of body mass index, smoking and hormone therapy in 503 Swedish women. *Acta Orthop Scan* 68:216–220.

807. Viscoli CM, Brass LM, Kernan WN, Sarrel PM, Suissa S, Horwitz R (2001): A clinical trial of estrogen-replacement therapy after ischemic stroke. *NEJM* 345:1243–1249.
808. Vitale C, Cornoldi A, Gebara O, Silvestri A, Wajngarten M, Cerqutani E, Fini M, Ramires AF, Rosano MC (2005): Interleukin-6 and flow-mediated dilatation as markers of increased vascular inflammation in women receiving hormone therapy. *Menopause* 12:552–558.
809. Von Muhlen D, Morton D, Von Muhlen CA, Barrett-Connor E (2002): Postmenopausal estrogen and increased risk of clinical osteoarthritis at the hip, hand, and knee in older women. *J Women's Health* 11:511–518.
810. Waetjen LE, Brown JS, Vittinghoff E, Ensrud KE, Pinkerton J, Wallace R, Macer JL, Grady D (2005): The effect of ultralow-dose transdermal estradiol on urinary incontinence in postmenopausal women. *Obstet Gynecol* 106:946–952.
811. Wakatsuki A, Okatani Y, Ikenoue N, Fukaya T (2002): Different effects of oral conjugated equine estrogen and transdermal estrogen replacement therapy on size and oxidative susceptibility of low-density lipoprotein particles in postmenopausal women. *Circulation* 106:1771–1776.
812. Waldstein SR, Brown JRP, Maier KJ, Katzel LI (2005): Diagnosis of hypertension and high blood pressure levels negatively affect cognitive function in older adults. *Ann Behav* 29:174–180.
813. Wallach EE, Vlahos NF (2004): Uterine myomas: An overview of development, clinical features, and management. *Fertil Steril* 104(2):393–406.
814. Wang G, Pratt M, Macera CA, Zheng Z, Heath G (2004): Physical activity, cardiovascular disease, and medical expenditures in U.S. adults. *Ann Behav* 28: 88–94.
815. Wang H, Mahadevappa M, Yamamoto K, Wen Y, Chen B, Warrington JA, Polan ML (2003): Distinctive proliferative phase differences in gene expression in human myometrium and leiomyomata. *Fertil Steril* 80(2):266–276.
816. Wang Y, Matsuo H, Kurachi O, Maruo T (2002): Down-regulation of proliferation and up-regulation of apoptosis by gonadotropin-releasing hormone agonist in cultured uterine leiomyoma cells. *Euro J of Endocrin* 146:447–456.
817. Warnock JK, Swanson SG, Borel RW, Zipfel LM, Brennan JJ, ESTRATEST Clinical Study Group (2005): Combined esterified estrogens and methyltestosterone versus esterified estrogens alone in the treatment of loss of sexual interest in surgically menopausal women. *Menopause* 12(4):374–384.
818. Wasnich RD, Bagger YZ, Hosking DJ, McClung MR, Wu M, Mantz AM, Yates JJ, Ross PD, Alexandersen P, Ravn P, Christiansen C, Santora II AC (2004): Changes in bone density and turnover after alendronate or estrogen withdrawal. *Menopause* 11:622–630.
819. Wassertheil-Smoller S, Hendrix SL, Limacher M, Heiss G, Kooperberg C, Baird A, Kotchen T, Curb JD, Black H, Rossouw JE, Aragaki A, Safford M, Stein E, Laowattana S, Mysiw WJ (2003): Effect of estrogen plus progestin on stroke in postmenopausal women. The Women's Health Initiative: A randomized trial. *JAMA* 289(20):2673–2684.
820. Webber C, Blake J, Chambers L, Roberts J (1994): Effects of 2 yrs of hormone replacement upon bone mass, serum lipids and lipoproteins. *Maturitas* 19:13–23.
821. Weber AM, Lee J (1996): Use of alternative techniques of hysterectomy in Ohio, 1988–1994. *NEJM* 335:483–489.

822. Weber AM, Mitchinson A, Gidwani GP, Mascha E, Walters MD (1997): Uterine myomas and factors associated with hysterectomy in premenopausal women. *Obstet Gynecol* 176:1213–1219.

823. Weber AM, Richter HE (2005): Pelvic organ prolapse. *Obstet Gynecol* 106:615–634.

824. Weber AM, Walters MD (1997): Anterior vaginal prolapse: Review of anatomy and techniques of surgical repair. *Obstet Gynecol* 89(2):311–318.

825. Weber AM, Walters MD, Piedmonte MR (2000): Sexual function and vaginal anatomy in women before and after surgery for pelvic organ prolapse and urinary incontinence. *American J Obstet Gynecol* 182:1610–1615.

826. Weber AM, Walters MD, Schover LR, Church JM, Piedmonte MR (1999): Functional outcomes and satisfaction after abdominal hysterectomy. *Obstet Gynecol* 181:530–535.

827. Weber AM, Walters MD, Schover LR, Mitchinson A (1995): Sexual function in women with uterovaginal prolapse and urinary incontinence. *Obstet Gynecol* 85(4):483–487.

828. Weber AM, Walters MD, Schover LR, Mitchinson A (1995): Vaginal anatomy and sexual function. *Obstet Gynecol* 86:946–949.

829. Weber B, Lewicka S, Deuschle M, Colla M, Heuser I (2000): Testosterone, androstenedione and dihydrotestosterone concentrations are elevated in female patients with major depression. *Psychneuroendocrinology* 25:765–771.

830. Webster's (2005): *New World College Dictionary: Fourth Edition.* John Wiley: Books Worldwide. Hoboken, NJ.

831. Weisberg E, Ayton R, Darling G, Farrell E, Murkies A, O'Neill S, Kirkegard Y, Fraser I (2005): Endometrial and vaginal effects of low-dose estradiol delivered by vaginal ring or vaginal tablet. *Climacteric* 8:83–92.

832. Weiss LK, Burkman RT, Cushing-Haugen KL, Voigt LF, Simon MS, Daling JR, Norman SA, Bernstein L, Ursin G, Marchbanks PA, Strom BL, Berlin JA, Weber AL, Doody DR, Wingo PA, McDonald JA, Malone KE, Folger SG, Spirtas R (2002): Hormone replacement therapy regimens and breast cancer risk. *Obstet Gynecol* 100:1148–1158.

833. Weitz G, Elam M, Born J, Fehm HL, Dodt C (2001): Postmenopausal estrogen administration suppresses muscle sympathetic nerve activity. *JCEM* 86(1): 344–348.

834. Welty FK (2004): Preventing clinically evident coronary heart disease in the postmenopausal woman. *Menopause* 11:484–494.

835. West J, Otte C, Geher K, Johnson J, Mohr DC (2004): Effects of Hatha yoga and African dance on perceived stress, affect, and salivary cortisol. *Ann Behav* 28:114–118.

836. West S, Ruiz R, Parker WH (2006): Abdominal myomectomy in women with very large uterine size. *Fertil Steril* 85:36–39.

837. Whipple B, Gerdes CA, Komisaruk BR (1996): Sexual response to self-stimulation in women with complete spinal cord injury. *J Sex Research* 33:231–240.

838. Whipple B, Ogden G, Komisaruk BR (1992): Physiological correlates of imagery-induced orgasm in women. *Arch Sexual Behavior* 21:121–133.

839. White LR, Petrovitch H, Ross GW, Masaki K, Hardman J, Nelson J, Davis D, Markesbery W (2000): Brain aging and midlife tofu consumption. *J Am Coll Nutr* 19:242–255.

840. Whiteside J, Barber M, Paraiso M, Walters M (2005): Vaginal rugae: Measurement and significance. *Climacteric* 8:71–75.

841. Whiting SJ, Calvo MS (2005): Dietary recommendations for vitamin D: A critical need for functional end points to establish an estimated average requirement. *J Nutr* 135:2:304–309.
842. Wihlback A, Nyberg S, Backstrom T, Bixo M, Sundstrom-Poromaa I (2005): Estradiol and the addition of progesterone increase the sensitivity to a neurosteroid in postmenopausal women. *Psychon* 30:38–50.
843. Williams E, Magid K, Steptoe A (2005): The impact of time of waking and concurrent subjective stress on the cortisol response to awakening. *Psychneuroendocrinology* 30(2):139–148.
844. Williamson-Hughes P, Flickinger B, Messina M, Empie M (2006): Isoflavone supplements containing predominantly genistein reduce hot flash symptoms: A critical review of published studies. *Menopause* 13:831–839.
845. Wilson RS, Bennett DA, Mendes de Leon CF, Bienias JL, Morris MC, Evans DA (2005): Distress proneness and cognitive decline in a population of older persons. *Psychneuroendocrinology* 30:11–17.
846. Witek-Janusek L, Gabram S, Matthews HL (2007): Psychologic stress, reduced NK cell activity, and cytokine dysregulation in women experiencing diagnostic breast biopsy. *Psychoneur* 32:22–35.
847. Wolf OT, Kudielka BM, Hellhammer DH, Torber S, McEwen BS, Kirschbaum C (1999): Two weeks of transdermal estradiol treatment in postmenopausal elderly women and its effect on memory and mood: Verbal memory changes are associated with treatment induced estradiol levels. *Psychneuroendocrinology* 24:727–741.
848. Wolf OT, Schommer NC, Hellhammer DH, McEwen BS, Kirschbaum C (2001): The relationship between stress induced cortisol levels and memory differs between men and women. *Psychneuroendocrinology* 26:711–720.
849. Wolff EF, Narayan D, Taylor HS (2005): Long-term effects of hormone therapy on skin rigidity and wrinkles. *Fertil Steril* 84:285–288.
850. Worthington-Kirsch R, Spies J, Myers E, Mulgund J, Mauro M, Pron G, Peterson E, Goodwin S (2005): The Fibroid Registry for Outcomes Data (FIBROID) for uterine embolization: Short-term outcomes. *Obstet Gynecol* 106:52–59.
851. Worzala K, Hiller R, Sperduto RD, Mutalik K, Murabito JM, Moskowitz M, D'Agostino RB, Wilson PWF (2001): Postmenopausal estrogen use, type of menopause, and lens opacities. *Arch Intern Med* 161:1448–1454.
852. Wren BG (2003): Editorial: Progesterone creams: Do they work? *Climacteric* 6:184–187.
853. Wren BG (2004): Do female sex hormones initiate breast cancer? A review of the evidence. *Climacteric* 7(2):2–120.
854. Wren BG, Day RO, McLachlan AJ, Williams KM (2003): Pharmacokinetics of estradiol, progesterone, testosterone and dehydroepiandrosterone after transbuccal administration to postmenopausal women. *Climacteric* 6:104–111.
855. Wright CE, Kunz-Ebrecht SR, Iliffe S, Foese O, Steptoe A (2005): Physiological correlates of cognitive functioning in an elderly population. *Psychoneu* 30:826–838.
856. Writing Group for the Women's Health Initiative Investigators (2002): Risks and benefits of estrogen plus progestin in healthy postmenopausal women: Principal results from the Women's Health Initiative randomized controlled trial. *JAMA* 288:321–333.
857. Wu X, Wang H, Englund K, Blanck A, Lindblom B, Sahlin L (2002): Expression of progesterone receptors A and B and insulin-like growth factor-I in human

myometrium and fibroids after treatment with a gonadotropin-releasing hormone analogue. *Fertil Steril* 78(5):985–993.

858. Wust S, Federenko IS, van Rossum EFC, Koper JW, Hellhammer DH (2005): Habituation of cortisol responses to repeated psychosocial stress—further characterization and impact of genetic factors. *Psychneuroendocrinology* 30(2): 199–211.

859. Wyon Y, Wijma K, Nedstrand E, Hammar M (2004): A comparison of acupuncture and oral estradiol treatment of vasomotor symptoms in postmenopausal women. *Climacteric* 7:153–164.

860. Xiangying H, Lili H, Yifu S (2006): The effect of hysterectomy on ovarian blood supply and endocrine function. *Climacteric* 9:283–289.

861. Yaffe K, Haan M, Byers A, Tangen C, Kuller L (2000): Estrogen use, APOE, and cognitive decline. *Neurology* 54:1949–1954.

862. Yasmeen S, Romano PS, Pettinger M, Johnson SR, Hubbell A, Lane DS, Hendrix SL (2006): Incidence of cervical cytological abnormalities with aging in the Women's Health Initiative. A randomized controlled trial. *Obstet Gynecol* 108(2):410–419.

863. Yeagley TJ, Goldberg J, Klein TA, Bonn J (2002): Labial necrosis after uterine artery embolization for leiomyomata. *Obstet Gynecol* 100(5):881–882.

864. Yen, H (2007): Ex FDA chief sentenced to probation and fined. *Philadelphia Inquirer* daily:news section.

865. Yenen MC, Dede M, Goktolga U, Kucuk T, Pabuccu R (2003): Hormone replacement therapy in postmenopausal women with benign fibrocystic mastopathy. *Climacteric* 6:146–150.

866. Yildirim B, Abban G, Erdogan BS (2004): Immunohistochemical detection of 1,25-dihydroxyvitamin D receptor in rat vaginal epithelium. *Fertil Steril* 82:1602–1608.

867. Yilmazer M, Fenkci V, Fenkci S, Sonmezer M, Aktepe O, Altindis M, Kurtay G (2003): Hormone replacement therapy, C-reactive protein, and fibrinogen in healthy postmenopausal women. *Maturitas* 26:245–253.

868. Yoon B, Oh W, Kessel B, Roh C, Choi D, Lee J, Kim D (2001): 17b-estradiol inhibits proliferation of cultured vascular smooth muscle cells induced by lysophosphatidylcholine via a nongenomic antioxidant mechanism. *Menopause* 8:58–64.

869. Zahl P, Strand BH, Maehlen J (2004): Incidence of breast cancer in Norway and Sweden during introduction of nationwide screening: Prospective cohort study. *BMJ* 328:921–924.

870. Zahl P-H (2004): Overdiagnosis of breast cancer in Denmark. *Br J Cancer* 90:1686.

871. Zandi PP, Carlson MC, Plasssman BL, et al. (2002): Hormone replacement therapy and incidence of Alzheimer's disease in older women: The Cache County study. *JAMA* 288:2123–2129.

871b. Zahl P, Maehlen J, Welch G (2008): The natural history of invasive breast cancers detected by screening mammography. *Arch Intern Med* 168(21): 2311–2316.

872. Zang H, Carlstrom K, Arner P, Hirschberg AL (2006): Effects of treatment with testosterone alone or in combination with estrogen on insulin sensitivity in postmenopausal women. *Fertil Steril* 86:136–144.

873. Zekam N, Oyelese Y, Goodwin K, Colin C, Sinai I, Queenan JT (2003): Total versus subtotal hysterectomy: A survey of gynecologists. *Obstet Gynecol* 102(2):301–305.

874. Zemel MB (2002): Regulation of adiposity and obesity risk by dietary calcium: Mechanisms and implications. *JACN* 21(2):146S–151S.
875. Zemel MB (2004): Role of calcium and dairy products in energy partitioning and weight management. *Am J Clin* 79:907S–912S.
876. Zemel MB, Shi H, Greer B, Dirienzo D, Zemel PC (2000): Regulation of adiposity by dietary calcium. *FASEB* 14:1 14:1132–1138.
877. Zemel MB, Thompson W, Milstead A, Morris K, Campbell P (2004): Calcium and dairy acceleration of weight and fat loss during energy restriction in obese adults. *Obesity Res* 12:582–590.
878. Zullo MA, Plotti F, Calcagno M, Palaia I, Muzii L, Manci N, Angioli R, Panici PB (2005): Vaginal estrogen therapy and overactive bladder symptoms in postmenopausal patients after a tension-free vaginal tape procedure: A randomized clinical trial. *Menopause* 12:421–427.
879. Zumoff B, Strain GW, Miller LK, Rosner W (1995): Twenty-four-hour mean plasma testosterone concentration declines with age in normal premenopausal women. *J Clin End* 80:1429–1430.
880. Zupi E, Pocek M, Dauri M, Marconi D, Sbracia M, Piccione E, Simonetti G (2003): Selective uterine artery embolization in the management of uterine myomas. *Fertil Steril* 79 (1):107–111.

Index

Page numbers in *italics* refer to illustrations.

Printed in the USA
CPSIA information can be obtained
at www.ICGtesting.com
JSHW082227140824
68134JS00016B/764